SOPH'S PLANT KITCHEN

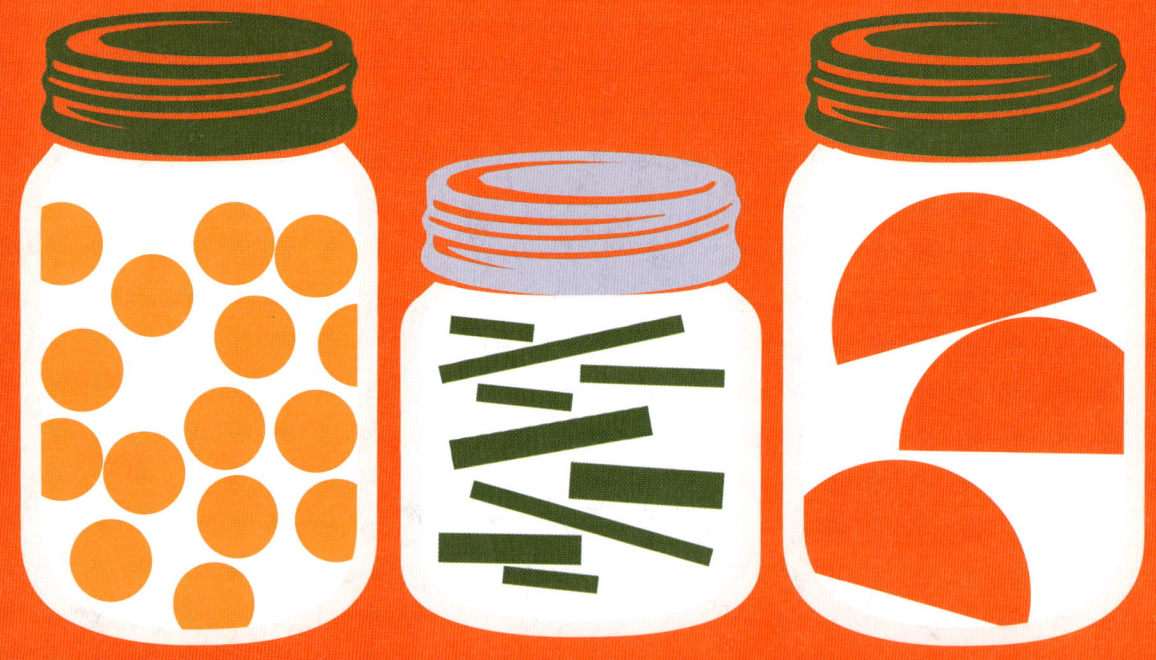

SOPH'S PLANT KITCHEN

**Delicious
high-protein
recipes to fuel
you for life**

Sophie Waplington

CONTENTS

Introduction

Welcome to your new bible on wholefood, plant-based, high-protein eating.

I'm Sophie, a plant-based cook, qualified personal trainer and recipe developer. You might know me from my social media accounts, where I post as @sophsplantkitchen.

My mission is to help as many people as I possibly can discover the benefits and joy of high-protein, wholefood, plant-based cooking, to fuel healthy, happy, active lifestyles.

Plant-based/vegan diets have gained a lot of media attention over the past decade or so and most people will have heard of the health, environmental and animal welfare benefits, as well as some of the less positive myths. I'll be exploring the benefits of adding plant-based protein into your diet, and while I personally follow a 100% plant-based diet, I know this isn't possible for everyone, and I very much respect this. This book intends to educate, enrich and delight, offering science-backed insight and my own professional knowledge as a personal trainer to help you make informed decisions to benefit your health.

Once we've uncovered some of the facts (and busted some of those myths!), it's time to give you all the tools you need to design a healthy, plant-forward diet to help fuel an active lifestyle. Every single one of these recipes is designed to slot into your weekly routine, to be made on repeat, make you feel incredible and give you the energy to put your best foot forward, every day. It's a collection of my best, most-used, most-loved recipes, many of which are brand-new and exclusive to this book.

There's something for everyone here: power bowls that can be prepped ahead for ease and convenience, portable salad jars, snacks, savoury and sweet breakfasts, quick dinners, delicious batch cooks with three ways to jazz them up and, of course, sweet treats, as life is all about balance!

After reading this book, and trying some of the delicious nutrient-dense recipes, you'll have the knowledge you need to live a happy, healthy and active life. It's the book I wish I had seven years ago, when I made the transition to plant-based eating, and I'm overjoyed I've been able to make it. Thank you all for your support.

Soph x

6

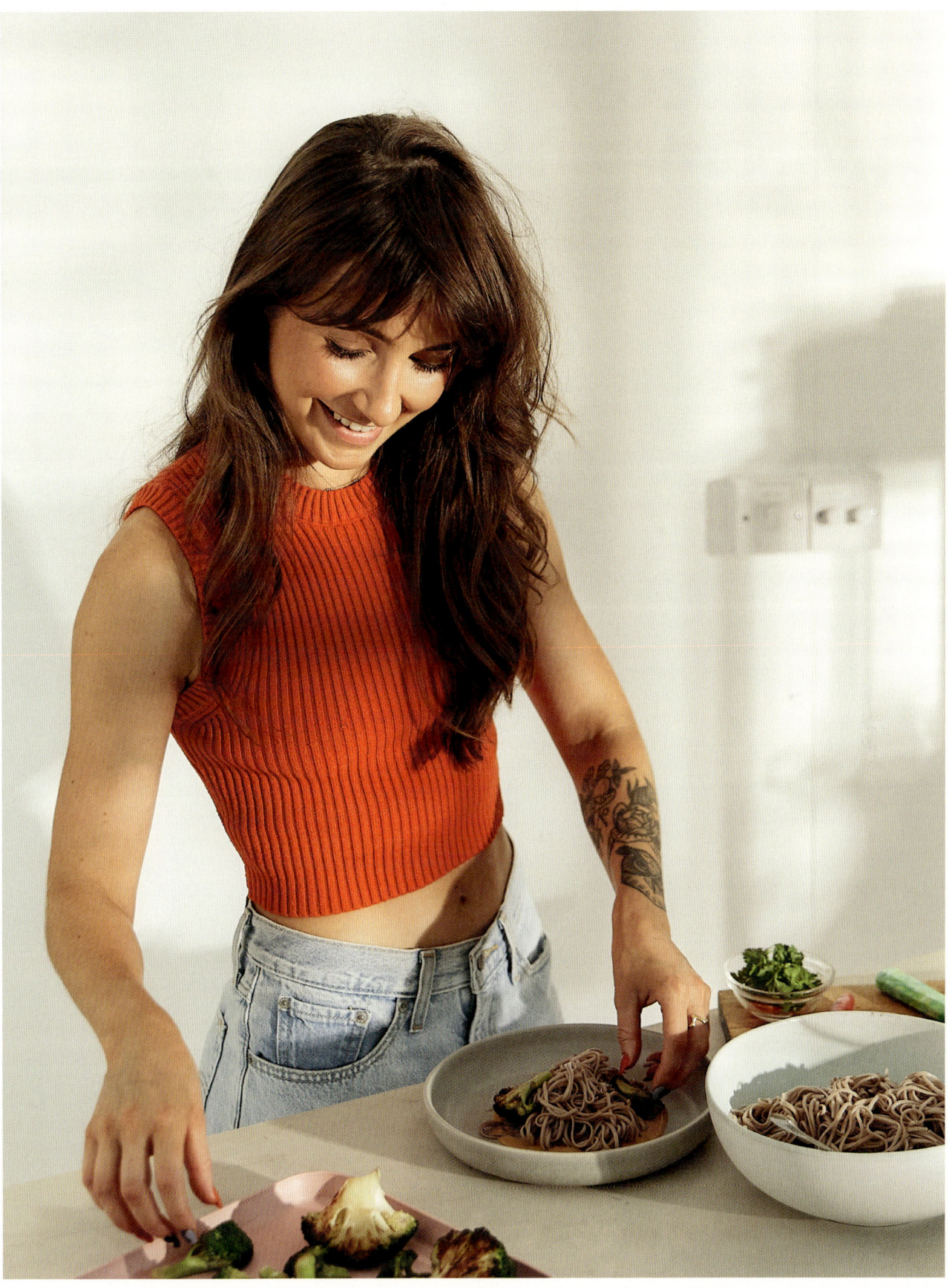

A bit about my journey

When I tell people I've never eaten an animal in my life I'm usually met with some raised eyebrows and some questions – 'How?', 'But ... are you sure?' – and some people who just flat out don't believe me. Fair enough, it is different.

Food is a big part of all our lives and being raised a vegetarian (my mother's choice, later affirmed by myself), as opposed to the default omnivore, caused me to learn to uphold my choices pretty quickly. Often, I'd find myself either served first, or last, at tables. Labelled 'the awkward vegetarian' at friends' houses. But I knew why I'd made the decision and that was enough.

My choice drew attention and, with that, questions. In order to answer these, I grew a virtual FAQ section in my head, I was so well versed in my responses. Occasionally, one would throw me off, such as 'Is your poop green?' or something equally hilarious. It also led me to build a natural interest in nutrition at a young age, as I was asked so many questions about what I ate instead of meat for optimal health. I would sit up straight and attentive in my Biology classes and devour any nutritional literature studies I could get my hands on.

Fast forward to 2017, I decided to take my ethical beliefs one step further and eliminate dairy products from my diet, after learning more about how the dairy industry operates. It's a very personal decision and I'd never expect others to do the same if they didn't want to. I understand it's not easy for everyone to give up certain food groups, for a myriad of reasons, which no-one should ever feel obliged to explain.

After a few years working in a marketing career, I knew my passion lay in food. I am a naturally creative person, preferring Art and English Literature to Maths and Economics at school, but found it a hard, scary prospect to turn my passion into my career. In 2018 however, I did just that, I quit my office job and went to work at a plant-focused cafe in North London, called Miranda. It was there I honed my love for cooking and creating, nurtured by the wonderful owners at Miranda, Francis and Gabriel, who taught me most of what I know, and who I will forever be grateful to. They are both Venezuelan, which is why you may see some Latin American influences in my cooking style.

In late 2019, I started my personal training course after experiencing some of the benefits that weightlifting can offer (I had always been active, but this new style of training added a lot to my life). During the course, the Covid pandemic hit, which really threw things into focus. Some of the people close to me were classified as 'at risk' and I wanted to help. Help more people reap the benefits of resistance training that I had discovered. Help people live longer, happier, healthier lives.

Healthy, active lifestyles require food. Good food. Having a diet that optimises plant variety, adequate protein, fibrous wholefoods and complex carbohydrates is a solid foundation on which to build more activity into your life. More importantly, it's got to taste good. Life is about enjoyment, as much as it is optimisation. I used to think you couldn't have both a 'fit' body and enjoy tasty food, but gosh, was I wrong, and these recipes prove it.

8

Life is about enjoyment, as much as it is optimisation

(and the two are not mutually exclusive)

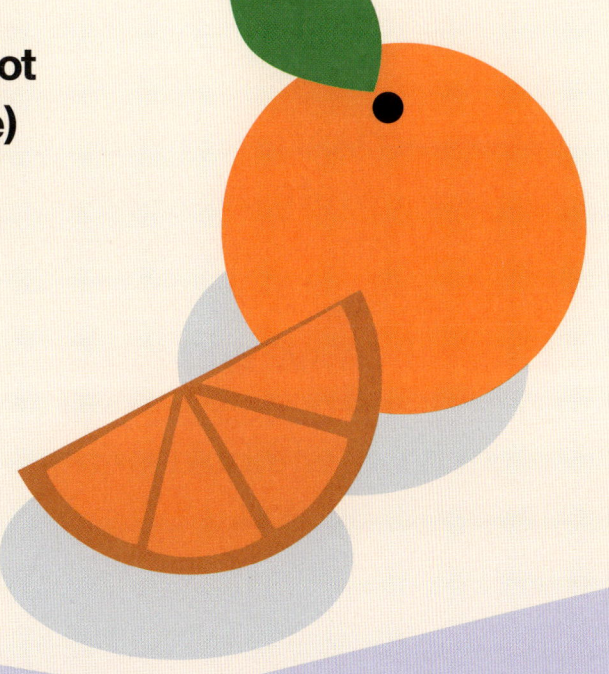

Let's get started

Wherever you're at right now, don't worry, this book and these recipes will meet you there. If you've just picked this up, had a flick through and are thinking 'Wow, this way of eating is quite far removed from my current diet', or 'What on earth is silken tofu and NOOCH?', I've got you.

I encourage you to use this book in a way that applies to you and your dietary choices. Tofu Feta and Cashew Parmesan, for example, can always be swapped for their normal cheese counterparts. You do not have to make an overnight switch, replacing every animal protein with legumes and, similarly, I don't expect you to become an instant tofu fanatic, however, do go into the recipes with an open mind, and never doubt that they will always be delicious!

These pages are full of easy-to-digest facts, takeaways and insights that you can start implementing straight away. I don't press tofu for hours, rarely marinate things for over an hour and use canned legumes for convenience. If I'm honest, this is because I'm a disorganised human and I'm always in a rush! So, over the years I've honed a style of cooking using flavours that give big bang for their bucks, so I have more freedom to try new hobbies, meet new people and enjoy my life.

If you're worried cooking wholefoods from scratch may be lengthy and arduous, have no fear. As you and I know, our modern lives just get busier and busier, so to help, I've added a mini batch-cook chapter, whereby you can prepare food for the week ahead and not have to worry. All other recipes are mostly done and dusted in under an hour, with the under 30 minutes chapter full of quick and satisfying weeknight winners.

You might be thinking, 'But I'm not into fitness. I don't train, so this book isn't for me' or 'Gosh, why the focus on protein? Protein, protein, protein is all I hear nowadays'.

Let me be clear, this is not a 'fitness food' book.

Wherever you are in your journey, I wrote this book with the intention of being easy, accessible and comprehensive enough to answer any questions you might have, without boring the pants off you.

10

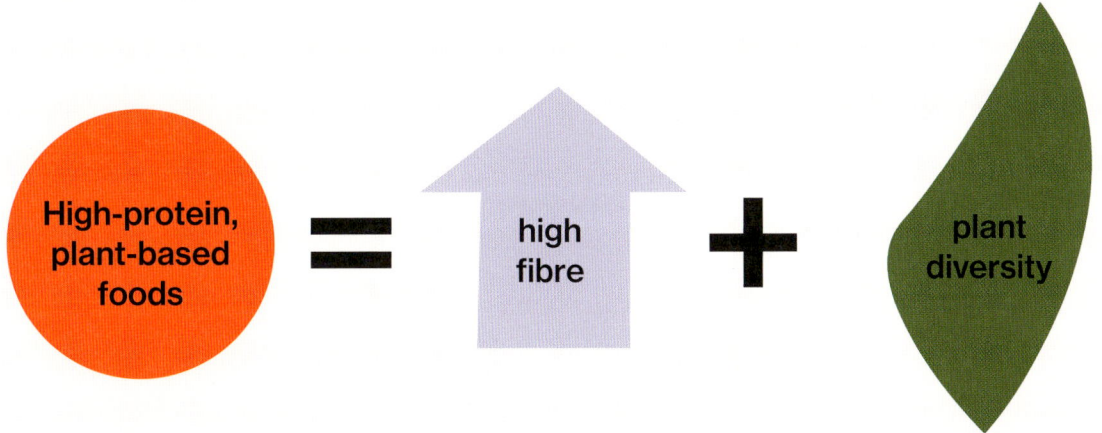

High-protein, plant-based foods = **high fibre** + **plant diversity**

If this is fitness food, what is 'normal'? Plates of food devoid of protein? Food that is lacking certain nutrients? I've lost count of the times I've looked at a restaurant menu and found that not a single plant-based option contains a decent protein source. It's not uncommon for plant-based folk to be served a cauliflower steak or a mushroom burger, both of which are simply not protein rich enough to support a healthy lifestyle. Regardless of your activity status, protein should be consumed in every meal, which is fairly normal in omnivorous diets, meaning it's not really considered an issue.

The reality is that there are bountiful plant-based protein sources (find most of these on page 22), but when people think about plant-based diets they often think of low-protein options such as salads, rendering it necessary to highlight plant protein sources and displace these myths. By enjoying more sources of plant protein, you're diversifying your diet and trying new foods, which in turn, helps support a healthy gut. Many of these protein-rich plant foods are also high in fibre, meaning by proxy, you'll be hitting or exceeding your recommended fibre intake without even trying.

And, lastly, if you're thinking, 'Oh heck, I am not the most confident person in the kitchen. All this is new to me' or 'Oh my god, I need loads of new equipment' – do not fear. You'll find most recipes follow the same sort of pattern, which isn't dissimilar to cooking animal proteins and is (I hope) well explained, without being daunting. For example, tofu is seasoned and fried, just like chicken. The cheeses, smoothies and sauces can

all be made in the same blender. I've included a list of useful equipment on pages 30-31 and my own weekly shopping list on page 25.

Once you try a few of these recipes, your plates will be filled with colour, texture, variety and lip-smacking deliciousness. You'll realise that good, healthy food isn't about restriction, or taking things away from your diet, because that's stealing. It's about enriching it, adding to it, experiencing new tastes, flavours and ultimately enjoying the journey at your own pace.

On the beauty of food, you'll notice the recipes are intricate collages, with many layers and patterns. Cooking, in my opinion, is a form of art. Probably abstract art, but the good kind. It's a chance to create something magical and reap the rewards. It's instant gratification, perfect for people like me who are impatient.

The chances are, if you create a beautiful bowl of food, it's going to taste absolutely incredible, too. So, take this as your sign to unleash your inner artist and have fun with it! Don't worry about getting things perfect, just enjoy every step and know I'm right here with you. So, let's get into it!

Important note: The information in this chapter does not intend to prescribe solutions, or treat any specific medical conditions. It is for general information purposes only.

Where references are given, you can find the numbered source on my website: www.sophsplantkitchen.co

Protein 101

Get ready for some science! Dip into this as much or as little as you like. I know that some of you prefer a light touch, so I've included a takeaway box at the end of each section. Perhaps you already know most of this, or maybe the way I've explained some bits will make something else click. Some of you might want to get into the nitty gritty, so I've included all sources on my website (see page 11).

WHAT IS PROTEIN?

Let's take a step back from the idea that protein is just a fitness trend for bodybuilders. Through a more scientific lens, protein is:

- Found throughout the body, in bone, skin, hair, organs, muscles, of course, and virtually everywhere else.

- Essential for the structure, function and regulation of our body's systems.

- One of the three essential macronutrients, the other two being fats and carbohydrates.

- An energy source.

- Made up of amino acids, the building blocks of proteins. Of the 20 amino acids that make up the proteins found in the human body, 11 of these can be made by the body, nine cannot. This means we must consume adequate sources of these in our diets.

WHY IS EATING A HIGH-PROTEIN DIET IMPORTANT?

- Protein helps us build, maintain and repair strong, healthy bodies.

- It's the most satiating macronutrient, meaning enjoying a higher-protein diet could lead to improved body composition (less fat, more lean muscle) and therefore improved health, when paired with exercise.

- Protein deficiency is rare, but dietary protein optimisation is important for certain people.

LET'S GET STARTED

PROTEIN INTAKE IS ESPECIALLY IMPORTANT FOR:

- Those following a predominantly plant-based or vegan diet.

- Over 65s. As we age, we lose muscle mass, which can increase the overall risk of adverse health outcomes.

- Children.

- Pregnant and breastfeeding women.

- Those looking to improve our ratio of fat to lean muscle through exercise and resistance training (which should be most of us, if our health allows).

- Those who are looking to lose fat, as protein is the most satiating of macronutrients; 'shifting to a high-protein, plant-based diet can be a great way to lose weight, and keep it off.' (Greger M. 'A Whole Food Plant-Based Diet Is Effective for Weight Loss' 2020).

HOW MUCH PROTEIN SHOULD I BE EATING?

- The current recommended daily allowance (RDA) for the average healthy adult for protein is 0.8g (1.7lbs) per kg of bodyweight.

- It's important to note that this data is not based on those eating a plant-based diet, older demographics, or anyone looking to lose fat and gain lean muscle in a training environment.

A study investigating protein intake more specifically (2013), found that certain groups of people should be consuming more than the RDA advises.

- Over 65s: 1–1.2g (2.2-2.6lbs) protein per kilogramme of bodyweight per day.

- Pregnant women: 1.1g (2.4) protein per kilogramme of bodyweight per day.

- Those looking to optimise muscle growth through resistance training: 1.6g (3.5lbs) protein per kilogramme of bodyweight per day.

- Those experiencing or at risk of age-related muscle loss: 1.2–1.5g (2.6-3.3lbs) protein per kilogramme of bodyweight per day.

AGE-RELATED MUSCLE LOSS

- Begins at around 30 years old. Given the huge impact healthy muscle mass has on health and longevity, it's extremely important to build and maintain a healthy, strong body throughout our entire lives, so we minimise any adverse health effects in later life, and uphold our independence.

- Eating healthy, nutritious, high-protein foods to support activity can set you up for success now, and in the future.

Animal protein vs. plant protein. How different is it?

Many people love to pit animal protein against plant protein, often cherry picking information to confirm their own biases. The real truth, of course, is nuanced.

COMPLETE VS. INCOMPLETE PROTEINS

- You may have heard that plant proteins are 'incomplete' or of lower quality, compared to animal protein. This complete vs. incomplete argument refers to the amino acid profile of plant proteins, as it was often thought that plants lack a full 'set' of the nine amino acids the body cannot make, whereas animal protein does not. The truth is all plants contain all nine essential amino acids (EAAs), just in different quantities. This means some have lower amounts of some amino acids and others higher. In order to get a 'complete' source of plant protein, you have to combine different sources.

- This only becomes a health issue if an individual is eating one plant food alone. If you are combining plant foods throughout the day as part of a normal balanced diet, there's nothing to worry about here.

- The great thing about plant protein is it comes with fibre, which animal protein does not.

14

Takeaway

All plant proteins contain all nine essential amino acids, and if you're eating a varied balanced diet, the protein quality is the same as animal protein, but with added fibre.

CAN MY BODY USE PLANT PROTEIN AS EFFECTIVELY AS ANIMAL PROTEIN?

- The short answer is yes, it can. Many older studies say the opposite, because the scoring systems are based on one source of plant protein alone. In these studies, the parameters were not set up effectively to imitate real life situations, so are not to be valued highly.

- Minor fluctuations may occur, but in the long-term, they are negligible, when plant protein amino acid sets are matched to animal proteins.

- Overall, the bulk of the evidence from more recent, human studies points towards there being little to no difference in efficacy from animal to plant protein, when amino acid sets are matched like for like. Minor fluctuations may occur, but these are negligible and nothing to be worried about.

Can plant protein be as effective as animal protein for gaining muscle?

This page is not just for the bodybuilders, but also those looking to optimise body composition (lose fat, gain lean muscle) in a general sense. If you want to get into the nitty gritty, the only thing (on top of hitting your protein targets) that I advise my plant-based clients to be aware of is ensuring you're eating enough of the essential amino acid Leucine.

Leucine is an essential amino acid that's important for overall healthy muscle tissues, as it stimulates protein synthesis and helps reduce muscle breakdown, especially after strenuous workouts.

So for those of you resistance training regularly in the gym, to maximise your progress on a plant-based diet you'll want to aim for 2–3g of leucine per meal. This is usually contained in vegan/PB protein shakes, and can also be found in the following plant foods:

Firm tofu, seitan, beans (black beans especially), seeds (pumpkin seeds especially), oats, lentils, quinoa.

Great news is, my recipes include lots of these ingredients, minus Seitan as it's not my favourite flavour, but please do feel free to sub in various recipes (you'll see notes suggesting if appropriate).

An example of a varied, balanced, protein (including 2–3g of leucine per meal) rich day on my plate:

BREAKFAST

Berry Cacao Overnight Oats, topped with berries and soy milk (see page 54)

LUNCH

Lazy Lentil Chimichurri Pasta Salad (see page 86)

SNACK

Blue Zones Smoothie (see page 77)

ON ANTINUTRIENTS

Antinutrients are natural defence mechanisms within plants, designed to protect them from bacterial infections and being eaten by insects. Some believe these defensive properties act inside the human body when plants are eaten, damaging our ability to absorb nutrients from the food we eat.

Here's the lowdown:

- Contrary to what some internet sensationalist content may tell you, 'antinutrients' are actually good for you. They are a group of polyphenolic compounds, which carry strong anti-inflammatory, antibacterial and antifungal properties and can lower your risk of disease, promote gut health and boost cognitive performance.

- Although studies have shown that typically, the amount of these 'antinutrients' consumed are too small to have any significant impact on nutrient absorption, it's helpful to know that the normal cooking processes involving heat, such as boiling, will destroy these, anyway, so nothing to worry about!

BOOSTING NUTRIENT ABSORPTION

In a similar vein, there are some easy ways to naturally boost the nutrient absorption of certain foods like lentils, beans and nuts, involving soaking or sprouting. I often soak nuts for recipes as you'll see, and buy sprouted seeds on occasion from the supermarket, but it's not essential. A healthy, balanced diet is all you need, and that's what this book contains.

DINNER

Black Bean and Sweet Potato Hotpot with Charred Sweetcorn Salsa (see page 174)

ON PROTEIN POWDERS

An isolated source of plant protein like soy, pea, rice or hemp, or a blend of these, combined with a varied plant-based high-protein diet is a great insurance policy for ensuring your body is getting all the protein it needs for your strength goals, if that's what you're optimising for. I do not consider it 'cheating' or unhealthy. When purchasing, always look for good-quality ingredients on the label, minimising any additives and fillers if possible. I tend to use unflavoured varieties in baking, as I like to add my own form of unrefined sweetener and flavourings.

This daily meal plan example has a total of six plant protein sources, including nuts, legumes, wholegrains, a portion of soy and some protein powder.

Can swapping animal protein for plant protein improve my health?

Long-term studies suggest that yes, it could. However, when looking at your overall health, it's important to consider the whole picture.

Here's a quick glance at two landmark studies looking at the effects of consuming animal and plant protein on long-term health outcomes.

A 2020 study published in JAMA Internal Medicine analysed over 400,000 people over a 16-year period, found that replacing just 3% energy from animal protein with plant protein was associated with longevity, particularly when substituting egg and red meat protein for plant protein.

In summary:

'Higher plant protein intake was associated with small reductions in risk of overall and cardiovascular disease mortality. Our findings provide evidence that dietary modification in choice of protein sources may influence health and longevity'

A 2024 study published in the American Journal of Clinical Nutrition found that women who ate more plant protein in midlife were 46% more likely to age healthily. The study analysed data from over 48,000 women who participated in the Nurses' Health Study between 1984 and 2016.

Additionally, those who ate more protein from meat and dairy products were 6% less likely to stay healthy as they got older.

So, why is this?

The studies concluded that the benefits of plant protein could be because plants are full of a variety of beneficial elements such as

- **Higher dietary fibre**
- **More micronutrients, such as polyphenols, that animal-based foods typically lack**

whilst lower in:

- **Saturated fat**
- **Dietary cholesterol**

Look at the whole picture. Remember that optimal health is dictated by more than diet alone. For example, you could be getting everything right with diet, and have a lot of stress in your life, leading to poor sleep and recovery, and experience low-energy as a result. 'Health' is the whole picture, not just protein.

Takeaway

Swapping even a small amount of animal protein for plant protein is associated with an increase in overall health, but this alone is no magic bullet.

Nutritional information

I have chosen to focus on three indicators of nutrition in this book:

• **Protein counts**
• **Fibre counts**
• **Plant diversity scores**

Omitting calorie counts has divided people online. This decision follows a number of reasons. I myself have struggled with disordered eating, and in the past would avoid the nutrient dense foods (carbs, healthy fats) my body needed. This underfuelling led to a plateau in my training, problems with my hormones, hair loss, and a perpetual feeling of tiredness, grumpiness and general unhappiness.

Learning about calories and food, along with tuning into my body really helped me to turn that around, so I'm sharing what I've learned in this section.

WHAT IS A CALORIE?
A calorie is defined as: 'the amount of heat required to raise the temperature of one kilogramme of water one degree Celsius.'

Calories in our food are calculated using the Atwater factors, developed in the late 19th century. These use a system based on a single energy value (factor) for each macronutrient – proteins, fats and carbohydrates – regardless of the food it is found in. The energy values per gram are:

These are used to calculate every calorie count you see on foods today.

But how do we know they are accurate?

• Recent findings have proven that we don't, really. Inaccuracies have been found during scientific trials, for example, in almonds the calculations resulted in a 32% overestimation of their calorie content. (14)

• So even if you are weighing your food to the gram, the inaccuracy of calories themselves mean your calculations could be wrong.

• Additionally, many people will often over or underestimate their daily calorie consumption.

It's also important to note that our bodies will process and absorb energy (calories) in different ways and, in some cases, this can be vastly different, due to age, genetics, metabolism, lifestyle factors and so on.

THE FOOD MATRIX
You might have heard 'food is food, it all goes in the same way', but this isn't always true. For example, a 2007 study (15) found that in participants consuming whole peanuts versus peanut butter, peanut oil or peanut flour, those consuming the whole peanuts absorbed less calories than the alternatives. This suggests that despite the labels showing the same calorie value, the energy absorbed can be different.

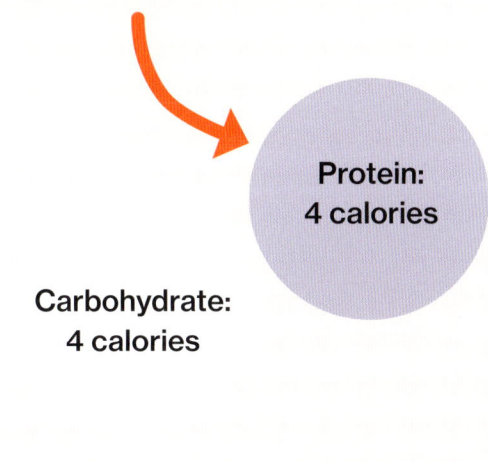

Carbohydrate:
4 calories

Protein:
4 calories

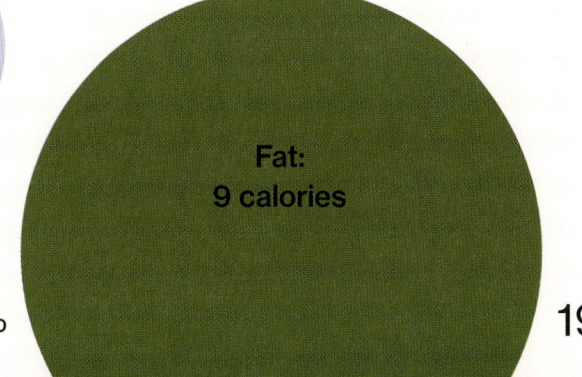

Fat:
9 calories

CALORIE COUNTING ISN'T ALL BAD

As a trainer, I do see some value in calorie counting for people who are starting to take more of a mindful approach to their diet, typically those who are looking to lose fat and gain lean muscle, or those looking to put on weight. It's definitely a short-term solution, almost like having the sides up at a bowling alley, or stabilisers on a bike. It can help you get a good handle on how energy-dense foods really are, and how much you should be eating, so you can work towards a goal of not tracking calories and counting nutrients instead.

In this book, to help you to tune into your body and to shield anyone who might experience a negative response to calorie counts, I have decided to omit them, keeping protein counts alone. Although me doing the work of giving your calorie counts might seem attractive in the short-term, it may hold you back from taking an active role in your diet.

WHY IS COUNTING PROTEIN IMPORTANT?

As mentioned on page 12, for those following a predominantly plant-based diet, wanting to maximise lean muscle mass to live longer, happier, healthier lives, keeping an eye on overall protein content is important. While I understand calculating fat and carbohydrates is necessary for those with some health conditions and can be advantageous for those with purely aesthetic goals, eating a varied, plant-based diet rich in protein, fibre and healthy fats is generally a less invasive and an easier way to live, rather than aiming for a specific target number.

I have also observed that some people can be deterred from eating energy-dense healthy foods due to their carb or fat counts, however, in the long-run, complex carbohydrates and healthy fats are a key part of a healthy, balanced diet.

The bottom line is that you are the best person to decide whether or not you're counting calories or macros. If I provided this information, I would be making that choice for you, which could potentially cause more harm than good. If you do want to track information not included here, the extra five minutes spent calculating should not cause too much of an inconvenience.

NUTRITIONAL INFORMATION IN THIS BOOK

I've calculated the nutritional information using professional culinary software, but please be advised this is still just a rough guide, so try not to get hung up about it. If you do use another app, you might get a slightly different result. Protein count will depend on brands and ingredients used, and also your serving sizes. My servings are calculated with healthy, active lifestyles in mind.

I've included fibre counts, too, although a wholefood, plant-based diet is very naturally high in fibre (you will see this!). Choosing meals higher in fibre makes us feel fuller for longer, helps with digestion and provides a low, sustained energy supply to the body. There is also strong evidence to show that eating plenty of fibre is associated with a lower risk of disease, including heart disease and some cancers.

For plant diversity scores, these are calculated simply. Each type of plant on your plate counts for one point, with herbs and spices counting for ¼ of a point. The more plant points, the more diverse your diet is, and the more diverse your gut microbiome is. A healthy, diverse gut microbiome has been linked to a myriad of health benefits, including a healthier immune system and increased brain function. The latest research shows we should all be aiming for 30 different plant sources per week.

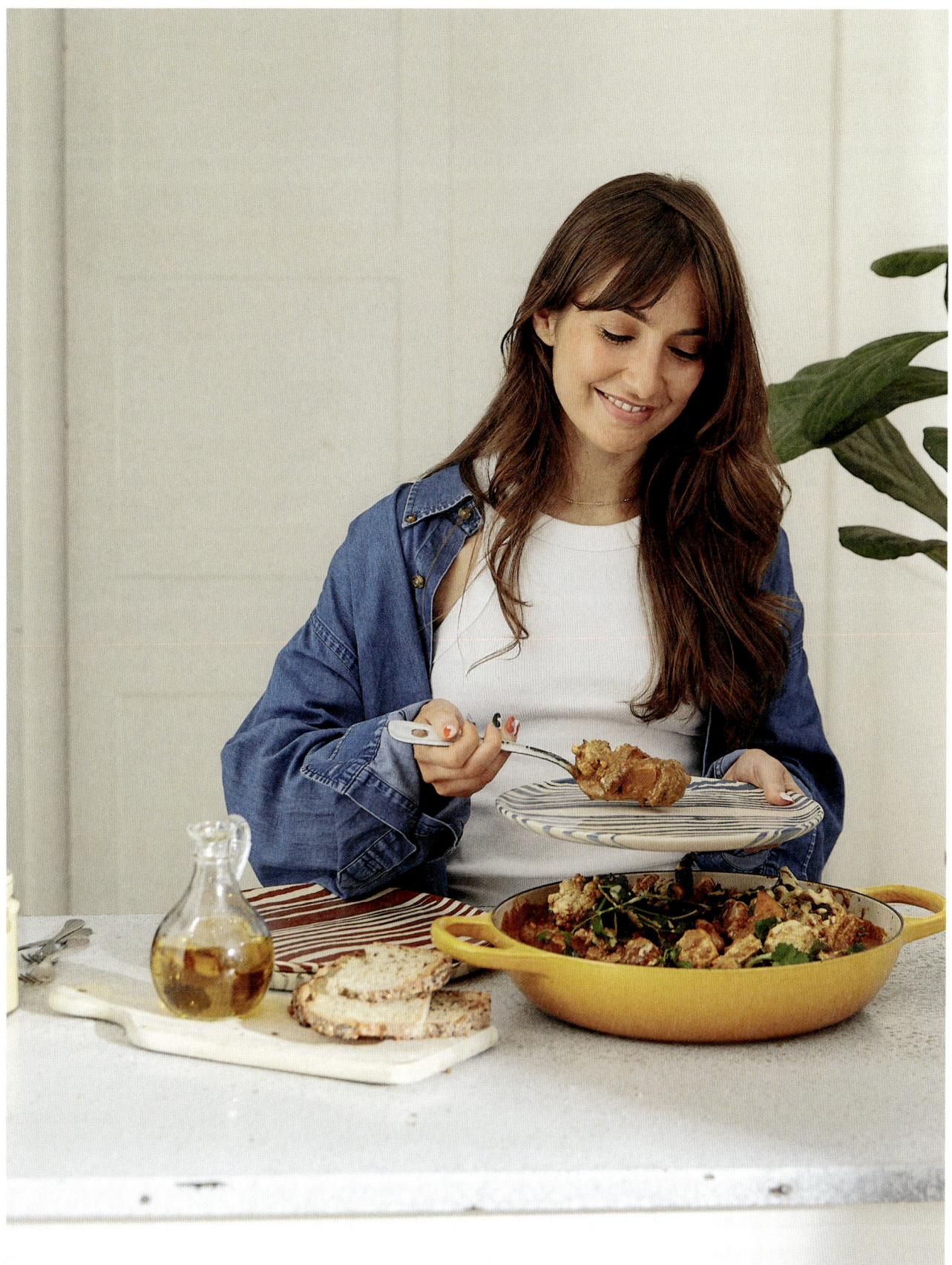

Plant protein sources

This is a non-exhaustive list of plant protein sources (prepared and cooked weight). As you can see, there's plenty to choose from!

Food	Protein content (g/100g/100ml)
Beans (butterbeans, haricot, black, kidney, pinto, borlotti)	6–9g
Split peas	8.3g
Red lentils	7.6g
French green lentils (cooked)	8.8g
Puy lentils	10.6g
Quinoa	4.4g
Buckwheat	3.4g
Wholemeal pasta (uncooked)	5.2g
Lentil pasta	12.6g
Chickpea pasta	17g
Lentil sprouts	9g
Pea sprouts	8.8g
Alfalfa sprouts	4g
Couscous	7.2g
Wild rice	5.3g
Brown rice	3.6g
Buckwheat (soba) noodles	5.1g
Nutritional yeast	50g

Food	Protein content (g/100g/100ml)
Extra-firm tofu	13–15g
Silken tofu	7.1g
Tempeh	20.7g
Edamame beans (boiled)	10.9g
Soy milk	2.4g
Oats	10.9g
Pumpkin seeds	24.4g
Sunflower seeds	19.8g
Flaxseeds	18.3g
Sesame seeds	18.2g
Tahini	18.5g
Hemp seeds	31.6g
Chia seeds	16.5g
Cashew nuts	17.7g
Almonds	21.1g
Pine nuts	14g
Walnuts	14.7g
Pistachios	20.3g
Peanut butter	24.9g
Almond butter	21g
Cacao powder	25g
Green peas	6.7g
Sweetcorn	3.6g
Mushrooms	1.4g
Broccoli	3.3g

The truth about soy

WHAT IS SOY?

Tofu, tempeh, miso, edamame, soy yoghurt, soy milk and more; all are made from soybeans. They're one of the most versatile, nutritious and affordable food sources, eaten worldwide for thousands of years.

WHY DO SOME PEOPLE CONSIDER SOY TO BE DANGEROUS?

- Soybeans contain isoflavones, often referred to as phytoestrogens, which are similar in structure to human oestrogens so some people speculate that eating too much soy will cause a hormone imbalance, disease, or even make men grow boobs.
- It's important to note that these phytoestrogens do not affect the human body in the same way as human oestrogen.
- According to research, phytoestrogens are in the region of $\frac{1}{100}$–$\frac{1}{1000}$ of the strength of human oestrogen, in other words, much, much weaker.

THE EVIDENCE

- When analysing the data, it is clear many of these concerns stem from individual case studies, animal studies, and extreme cases whereby the individuals are consuming such a large amount of soy that it is all they are eating.
- These studies have been debunked by multiple observational research and randomised control trials in humans, offering significantly more reliable data.
- In fact, many reliable studies have shown that eating soy products as part of a balanced diet can reduce the risk of certain cancers, reduce cholesterol, promote hormonal health and reduce menopausal symptoms in women.

An extract from a 2019 study reads: 'Generally, soy and isoflavone consumption is more beneficial than harmful. The results herein support promoting soy intake as part of a healthy diet.'

Personally, I consume soy products at least twice per day. I recognise everyone is different, so if you want to include soy as part of a healthy balanced diet, there are some very well-documented health benefits. I understand some are allergic or might be unable to consume soy for other reasons, so rest assured, your protein needs can still be met on a balanced plant-based diet without soy.

Takeaway

- Soy is one of the healthiest, cheapest, most accessible, convenient and versatile plant protein sources.

- Some of the negative myths about soy come from the fact it contains a compound (phytoestrogen) that mimics human oestrogen. However, this has much, much weaker effects than human oestrogen and would only be an issue if soy was the only thing you consumed.

- Eaten as part of a varied diet, soy has been scientifically proven to reduce the risk of many diseases.

Living on legumes

Beans, beans, the wonderful fruit, the more you eat... the longer you'll live (what did you think I was going to say?) If you're not a big bean fan already, you're about to become one, not least because most of my recipes contain some form of legume, but also because they are incredibly nutritious. They're rich in fibre, protein, carbohydrates, B vitamins, iron, copper, magnesium, manganese, zinc and phosphorus, naturally low in fat, practically free of saturated fat and cholesterol free.

Average anatomy of a bean:

21% protein, making them hearty and satisfying

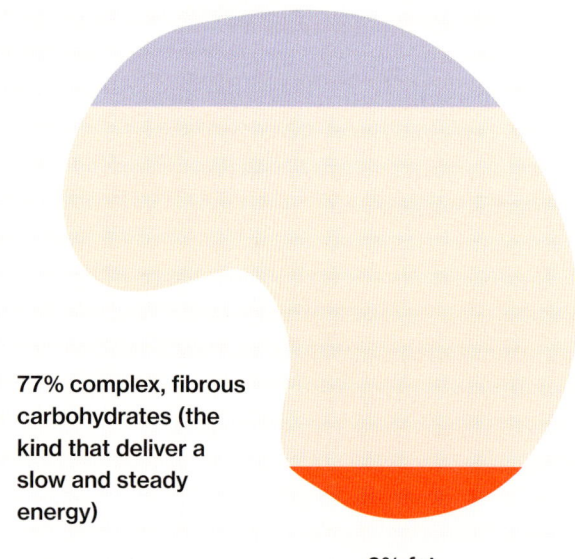

77% complex, fibrous carbohydrates (the kind that deliver a slow and steady energy)

2% fat.

You might have heard of the Blue Zones, regions in the world with the highest concentration of centenarians (people who live to be over 100 years in age). Beans are a common theme in Blue Zone diets, dubbed the 'cornerstone of every longevity diet in the world'. Blue Zoners are said to eat at least a large handful of beans every day!

TYPES OF BEANS
Adzuki beans, black beans, black-eyed peas, cannellini beans, borlotti beans, fava beans, chickpeas, green beans, butter beans, mung beans, haricot beans, pinto beans, red kidney beans, soybeans.

WHY I LOVE BEANS, AND YOU SHOULD, TOO
They're accessible, cheap and incredibly versatile. When cooked, they have a creamy, mild flavour. Blend them into sauces, soups (see Healing Greens and Beans Soup, page 116), Stewed Apple and Sweet Chickpea Protein Bread (see page 72), bake them in cookies (Chunky Chickpea Cookies, see page 233) or crunchy meal toppers (see page 78 [Crispy Roasted Legumes]) or simply enjoy them in the social media famous Bean Bowl (see page 135).

Shopping list

This is a pretty comprehensive list of what I usually have in my fridge or cupboard, though not all are necessary to enjoy the recipes. I tend to go for the same ingredients every week, switching things up seasonally. You'll see certain ingredients have an asterisk, because I go for a specific version. See overleaf for why, and where to buy.

FRESH INGREDIENTS

- Lemons and limes
- Apples
- Bananas
- Blueberries
- At least one other seasonal fruit (I try to pick things I don't usually eat)
- Tomatoes – salad and cherry
- Gem lettuce
- Kale
- Spinach
- Carrots

- Celery
- Red peppers
- Onions, red and brown
- Shallots
- Garlic
- Ginger
- Fresh red chilli
- Avocado
- Seasonal veg (carrots, broccoli, cauliflower, celery, aubergine, etc)
- Sweet potatoes (purple if available)

- Fresh herbs (flat-leaf parsley, coriander, chives, basil)

Chilled or frozen Ingredients
- Tofu – extra-firm (plain and smoked) and silken*
- Tempeh*
- Fortified soy milk*
- Barista style oat milk for coffee
- Soy yoghurt
- Frozen peas and edamame beans
- Frozen berries

STORE CUPBOARD INGREDIENTS

- Tins or jars of beans – butter beans, kidney, black, chickpeas
- Tins of good-quality plum tomatoes
- Whole jumbo oats*
- Sourdough bread*
- Dried lentils – split red, beluga, brown and green
- Packets of pre-cooked Puy lentils*
- Pastas – 100% durum wheat semolina and legume*
- Nuts – almonds, cashews, Brazils, pine, walnuts etc
- Nut butters – almond, peanut*
- Rice – wild and brown, or a mix*
- Flour – spelt, buckwheat and chickpea (gram)*
- Quinoa (tricolour)*
- Buckwheat (soba) and spelt ramen noodles*

- Dried fruit – apricots, sultanas, Medjool dates
- Seeds – sesame, sunflower, pumpkin, hemp, chia
- Coconut milk
- Couscous
- Vinegars – apple cider, red wine, white wine, rice wine and balsamic
- Ground spices – cumin, coriander, turmeric, smoked paprika, nutmeg, oregano, garam masala, curry powder, cayenne chilli pepper, medium chilli powder, ras el hanout, Lebanese 7-spice, kasuri methi (fenugreek leaves)
- Whole spices – cumin and coriander seeds, cardamom pods
- Vegetable bouillon powder and stock cubes
- Coffee beans

- Mustard – Dijon and wholegrain
- Plant-based mayo
- Gochujang paste
- Sriracha sauce
- Harissa paste
- Sesame oil
- Mirin
- Tomato purée
- Nutritional yeast*
- Miso paste – sweet white and brown/red
- Marmite
- Protein powder – unflavoured, chocolate and vanilla
- Creatine powder*
- Vanilla extract
- Cacao nibs and powder
- Dairy-free dark chocolate - chips and bars

Key ingredients

Why I buy these ingredients, where you can get them from, how to cook them and any substitutes you can use.

BUCKWHEAT (SOBA) NOODLES AND SPELT RAMEN NOODLES

Apparently, eating a bowl of buckwheat noodles before midnight on New Year's Eve is an old Japanese tradition that is supposed to bring long life and prosperity to the year ahead. Japan is a country that's at the top of my bucket list; the culture and food has always fascinated me.

I go for 100% buckwheat soba noodles, which are naturally gluten free and a great source of protein. They're usually sold in thick, stout spaghetti type packages, in bundles of three.

Spelt ramen noodles are higher in protein and iron than their refined counterparts and should be easy to find in health stores and larger supermarkets. Sub wholewheat ramen noodles if you can't find them.

CREATINE POWDER

Creatine is one of the most widely studied, safe and reliable sports performance supplements. It works by supplying extra energy to your muscles when you're performing high intensity exercise, such as interval sprints or heavy lifting.

Our bodies make a limited amount of creatine, and it's also found in red meat and seafood, meaning omnivores can top it up from their diet. If you're following a predominantly plant-based diet, it may be a good idea to take 2–4g of creatine powder to optimise bodily function.

Recent research has shown it's not just athletic performance that can benefit, as creatine has also been linked to improved brain health, heart health and may protect against age-related muscle loss.

Creatine monohydrate is a synthetic form of creatine powder suitable for those following a plant-based diet. I take mine before my workout, mixed into my water with a little pinch of sea salt to help replenish my electrolytes, along with a slice of pre-workout toast with peanut butter and berries to get those carbs and sugars into my body pre-training.

EDAMAME BEANS

Edamame are young soybeans! These little beans taste fresh and almost 'buttery' at the same time and are loaded with nutrients.

I buy mine frozen, as they're cheaper and retain their bright green colour more. Find them in the frozen sections of larger supermarkets.

FLOUR (SPELT, BUCKWHEAT AND CHICKPEA/GRAM)

I opt for spelt flour over regular white flour as, generally, I find it tastier (it has a mild, nutty flavour) but it's also rich in iron, magnesium and zinc, and has a slightly higher protein content.

I use buckwheat flour in my banana bread recipe, it's a gluten-free, protein and fibre-rich flour with antioxidant and anti-inflammatory properties, great for muscle repair post exercise. You should be able to find this and spelt flour in larger supermarkets, failing this, wholewheat or plain flour will do just fine!

Chickpea (gram or besan) flour is made from ground chickpeas. It's high in protein and fibre, making it a great choice for frittatas, pancakes and more. Find it in the 'world foods' aisle of the supermarket, often in the Indian food sections.

There are other flours such as vital wheat gluten, hemp, peanut and soy, some of which I've experimented with, some I have not been able to get hold of easily, which makes spelt, buckwheat and chickpea the best options in terms of health, taste and accessibility.

FORTIFIED SOY MILK

Soy milk is the plant milk with the highest amount of protein, so is preferable for those looking to maximise their protein intake on a plant-based diet. I try to buy brands which say the milk is fortified with calcium, vitamin D and iodine to optimise my nutrition.

I also buy oat milk in a barista edition for my coffee but tend to stick to soy for other uses. Larger supermarkets or online are the best places to find plant milks. Bulk buying long-life will save you some cash.

MISO PASTE (SWEET WHITE AND BROWN)

The word 'miso' means 'fermented beans' in Japanese and is a staple in Japanese cooking. It's made from fermented soybeans, meaning it's high in protein and fibre.

The colour of the miso refers to how long it's been fermented for. The lighter the miso, the less fermenting, and vice versa. Some of the darker varieties have been fermenting for years!

Miso is one of my favourite flavour hits – it has a rich umami depth, perfectly salty and a little sweet at the same time. It goes really well with tofu and aubergine, although I've experimented with it in soups, bean bowls and cheesy sauces.

You should be able to find it in small glass pots or pouches at your local supermarket, probably the larger supermarkets for the sweet white miso. If not, check out your local health food store or order online. With darker miso, a little goes a long way. With the lighter varieties, don't be shy! Be mindful of how much extra sea salt you add during cooking if you know miso is going to be added later.

Always stir in miso at the end of cooking, when your dish has just come off the heat. This will ensure the flavour doesn't fade.

NUT BUTTERS (ALMOND, CASHEW, PEANUT)

I prefer minimally processed brands with shorter ingredients lists, avoiding any added sugar and oils. I'm team crunchy!

NUTRITIONAL YEAST

Nutritional yeast (also known as nooch) is a dried, deactivated form of Saccharomyces cerevisiae, an ancient species of yeast. It starts as wild yeast, which grows naturally, and is picked, rinsed and heat-dried to destroy any live cultures, deactivating the yeast and stripping it of its leavening properties.

It has a natural umami flavour which tastes a little cheesy and nutty, making it the perfect ingredient for DIY plant-based cheeses and dressings, and adds a little flavour boost in curries, soups, stews and more. It's also a great source of protein, thiamine, riboflavin, niacin, folic acid, vitamin B6 and often fortified with vitamin B12.

I use it liberally in this book and buy it in bulk! Check online for stockists near you.

Unfortunately, there's no real like-for-like swap for nooch. The closest would probably be sweet white miso paste, but you wouldn't be able to use this for Cashew Parmesan (see page 221), or any other recipes using nooch where the key ingredients need to be dry.

PACKETS OF PRE-COOKED PUY LENTILS

I do use dried lentils, however, the darker varieties take a while to soak and cook, so having a few pouches or cans of these in the cupboard is a must. They're so easy to throw into salads for work lunches or into pasta sauces to bump up the protein content.

PASTAS (100% DURUM WHEAT SEMOLINA AND LEGUME)

I opt for these varieties because they're naturally higher in plant protein than others. Look for lentil, chickpea and other bean pastas in larger supermarkets or health stores.

Legume pastas like red lentil and black bean often have a super-high protein content, so are a weekly staple at ours. They have more of an earthy taste and can be a bit softer when cooked, so I like to cook them until very al dente and add a light, creamy sauce and seasonal veg instead of weighing them down with a heavy, rich sauce.

You should be able to find these at larger supermarkets. They are often red, green or darker in colour.

PROTEIN POWDER (UNFLAVOURED AND CHOCOLATE SALTED CARAMEL)

Protein powders are a great way of getting closer to your protein target without filling up too quickly. I do not consider it cheating. If consumed as part of a healthy balanced diet, they are perfectly safe to consume every day. I prefer to blend mine into smoothies with oats and fruit – or bake it into banana bread or brownies. Please be aware that protein powders are not meal replacements and should not be considered a fat-loss tool. Read more about my take and what protein powders to go for on page 17.

QUINOA (TRICOLOUR)

Apart from just looking sexier on your plate, tricolour quinoa is tastier, nuttier and more satiating due to its higher protein and fibre content. It's not a must have, white quinoa is fine, but if you do see it, try it out!

RICE (WILD AND BROWN, OR A MIX)

I once had a back-and-forth in the comment sections of one of my Instagram recipes, where a man was telling me by using brown rice I was 'sucking all the joy out of life'. 'I actually prefer the taste of brown rice,' I said, not to mention it has a higher protein and fibre content than white refined rice.

I don't blame him, of course, refined carbohydrates can be more palatable, but it did make me reflect on how my taste buds had changed substantially over time, as I didn't always feel this way.

If you're not a fan of brown or wild rice, try introducing it slowly. According to science, taste buds regenerate around every two weeks, so stick with it!

SOURDOUGH BREAD

Arguably the best part of my social media videos is my signature sourdough bread tear, so unsurprisingly, sourdough is a key ingredient! If you weren't part of the sourdough baking lockdown crew, that's fine, you were probably too busy perfecting your banana bread, or screaming into the void.

As sourdough undergoes a long fermentation, this can improve vitamin and mineral bioavailability, compared to conventional bread. It also has a lower glycaemic index, meaning any spike in blood sugar is normally lower than with conventional bread, and it is generally digested more easily.

I buy mine from a local bakery if I'm near one. Some supermarkets do sell sourdough but it's never quite the same. In the future, I'd love to learn how to make it myself.

If you can't find sourdough, normal wholegrain, buckwheat, rye or spelt bread are good options.

TEMPEH

Tempeh is a traditional Indonesian food made from fermented soybeans. The fermentation increases the nutrient density, making tempeh a very healthy and high-protein alternative to animal products. It has a slightly nutty, earthy flavour. I love crumbling it and cooking with plenty of tamari/soy or garlic to enhance its natural taste.

You should be able to find tempeh in the refrigerated aisles of larger supermarkets but if you can't, use tofu instead.

TOFU, EXTRA-FIRM (PLAIN AND SMOKED) AND SILKEN

Tofu can seem like a bit of a minefield if you haven't used it before. There are many brands and textures, extra firm being at one end of the scale and silken at the other. The 'firmness' of the tofu you buy refers to the time it's been pressed for. The longer it's been pressed, the firmer it is, as the pressing reduces the water content.

Generally, the firmer the tofu, the better the texture for using as a meat replacement, and the less prep work you have to do before it's holding flavour and tasting great. Some people boil or freeze their tofu to make it even firmer or change the texture slightly. I haven't tried these methods as it seems like an unnecessary extra step for a minimal gain in taste, when the sauces are the real star of the show in my tofu dishes.

I generally opt for extra-firm tofu, but I'll use firm at a push. When I use it, I'll drain off the water and give it a good squeeze, wrapped in two pieces of kitchen paper or a dry tea towel, before chopping or tearing it apart. If you don't use a whole block at a time, make sure to take it out of the packet, drain off the water and pop it into a sealed food container, back in the fridge. Consume within two days.

Silken tofu is very soft and delicate, you'll see I use it mostly for sauces. There is no need to 'press' silken tofu. It should be available to purchase in most larger supermarkets, usually in the ambient (dry goods) isles, and sometimes in the 'world foods' aisles as it's used regularly in Southeast Asian cooking.

VEGETABLE BOUILLON POWDER AND STOCK CUBES

I prefer vegetable bouillon powder or organic cubes over stock pots or ready-made liquid as I find it tastes better, and I have more control over the sodium content. The stock pots are often full of gelling agents to keep them stuck together and ready-made liquid never goes far, or tastes as potent, in my opinion.

Of course, the best stock is the stock you make yourself, using vegetable scraps. There are some great online recipes for this.

WHOLE JUMBO OATS

Whole jumbo oats release energy slower and steadier than their porridge or rolled oat counterparts, making these my oats of choice. You should be able to find these in most medium–large supermarkets.

Kitchen equipment

Here's a list of some of my favourite kitchen equipment. Not all of this is essential, but it will often make food prep a lot quicker and easier!

CAST IRON OVENPROOF SHALLOW CASSEROLE PAN, 30CM (12IN)
The question I get asked the most on social media is where is your big circular pan from! Often an investment but so versatile and will last a lifetime. The great thing about these is you can start by cooking on the hob and then pop them straight into the oven to grill veg.

My grandmother kindly gifted me my first pan as a graduation gift many, many years ago and I've had it ever since. Just be sure not to use any metal utensils on the surface, as these will scratch.

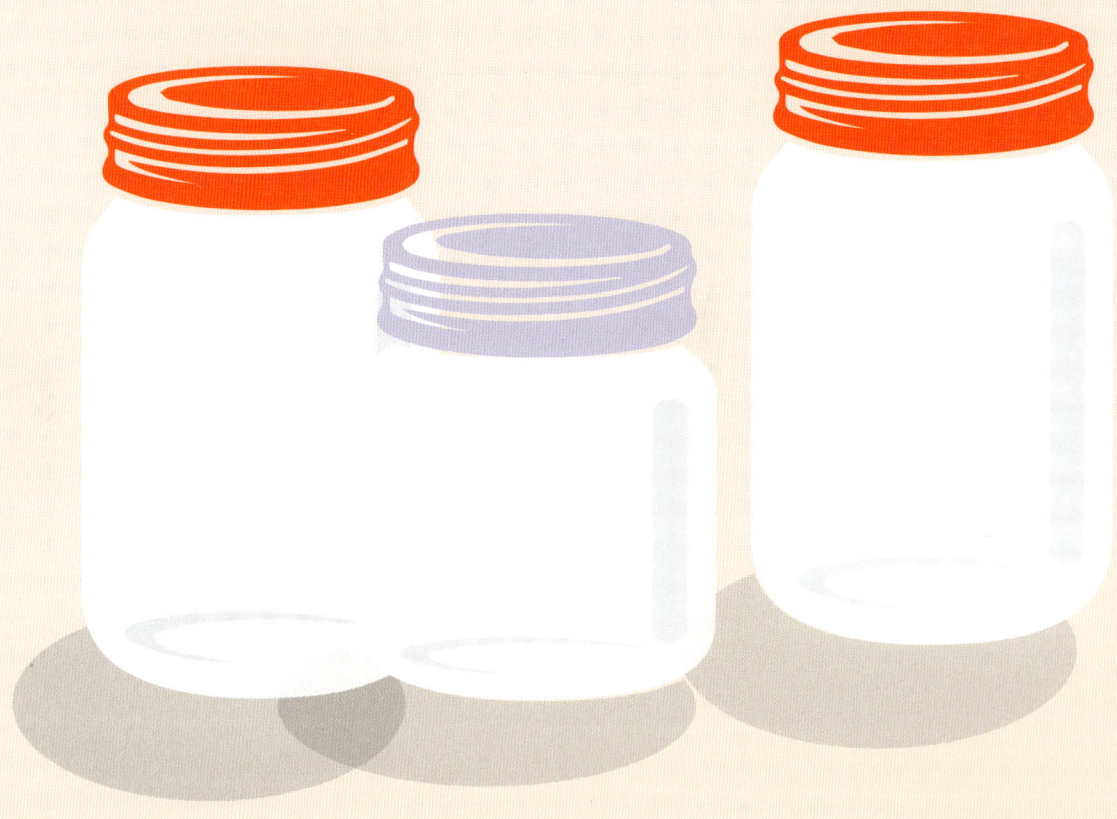

SMALL 900W BULLET BLENDER

I use this daily, from whipping up quick protein smoothies to making creamy sauces, pesto, ground nuts, garlicky breadcrumbs and more. The higher-powered models are better and break down ice or blend nuts into creamy sauces. A definite kitchen essential.

FOOD PROCESSOR

This will save you lots of time during food prep and help make recipes like my Homemade 'Sausages' (see page 224) and Homemade 'Meatballs' (see page 225), not to mention desserts, such as the high-protein Decadent Dark Choc and Orange Pud (see page 236)!

A REALLY GOOD KNIFE

I often find when you buy a nest of knives that you only really use one (or I do anyway) and maybe the paring knife occasionally. As I don't eat meat, I have no need for bigger knives, so I tend to stick to my Santoku knife for most prep. Keep it nice and sharp, so prep becomes easier and quicker.

SILICONE SPATULAS

More hygienic and convenient than your typical wooden spoon, they make scraping sauces out of blenders easy and waste less.

GLASS FOOD STORAGE CONTAINERS

You can never have too many.

WIDE MOUTH MEAL PREP JARS

Great for meal prep salads to take to work, easy to get the food out into a bowl! I like 950ml (32oz) capacity.

WAX WRAPS

Sustainable food storage.

PLENTY OF NATURAL FIBRE TEA TOWELS

Rotate every couple of days.

MICROPLANE GRATER

I use mine for grating aromatics and zesting citrus.

FLAT WHISK

For dressing and marinades.

A GOOD NON-STICK FRYING PAN

Easy to clean, fuss free.

A GOOD NEST OF HEAVY-BOTTOMED SAUCEPANS

For pastas, sauces, stews and more.

STAINLESS-STEEL MIXING BOWLS

Handy and always needed.

WOODEN CHOPPING BOARD

Let's banish those plastic wibble-wobble ones, and glass too while I'm at it. They're not safe enough when using sharp knives and the glass can blunt the knives over time. Not to mention, plastic cutting boards degrade and result in the ingestion of a credit card's worth of plastic over the course of a year.

DOUGH CUTTER/SCRAPER

You'll see foodie content creators use these a lot on social media as they're very handy for scooping things off chopping boards and also for cutting Tofu Gnocchi (see page 163) and naan dough (see page 206).

PESTLE AND MORTAR

Great for sauces, grinding nuts and whole spices.

SERVING PLATES AND BOWLS

I love pottering around local independent pottery shops and homeware stores wherever I travel. Taking home a nice bowl, plate or mug is always my souvenir of choice. Makes a great dinner party story!

Planning and storing food

There's a lot of tips online about how to save money and time and reduce your environmental impact by storing your food correctly. I don't profess to be a food waste expert and I could always do more. Here's a few things I find help me the most:

PLAN YOUR MEALS

On a Sunday, take a minute to plan realistically for the week ahead. Which days are you planning to be out and which days will you be cooking? I know when I worked in an office, Thursdays and Fridays were generally spent out, straight from work.

STAGGER YOUR SHOPS

Buy all your non-perishables, other long-life items and fresh items for your imminent 2–3 meals from home in one shop, avoiding buying too much fresh stuff all at once. Top up with fresh items like bagged salads, ripe avocados, fruit and herbs during the week, when you know you'll need them.

ORGANISE

The one I'm worst at. It sounds like a faff, but Marie Kondo-ing your kitchen so you can see exactly what you already have, including the fridge, store cupboard and drawers, will stop you from duplicate purchasing.

I try to decant dried goods like legumes, flours, nuts and seeds into glass jars, as they look pretty and you can see what you're running low on. Just don't leave them in direct sunlight as this can speed up the spoiling process.

REUSABLE CONTAINERS AND CLIPS

The golden rule here is always seal any open packages from direct air. If food is left out or unsealed, air gets in, the food oxidises faster and spoils quicker.

Store leftovers in reusable glass containers (I prefer glass as it's BPA free and microwave safe), check out IKEA for good, cheap glass containers.

Use clips on plastic packages of things like nuts, seeds, spices and crackers.

FRIDGE LIFE

You'll notice most recipes don't specify how long something lasts after cooking. The rule of thumb is generally 4 days, for something that's been stored in the absence of air (sealed correctly) in the fridge, if necessary.

If this isn't the case, don't worry, the recipe will clearly state this.

If you're ever unsure, your senses are best placed to guide you. Use sight, smell and taste to determine if something is fit for consumption. A tiny little teaspoon of soup probably won't hurt you, even if it is off!

32

FREEZER

If you're anything like me and suffer somewhat with object permanence, the freezer might be your worst enemy. I tend to refrain from freezing too much as I do forget it, so first things first, some tape and a marker pan for labelling contents before freezing is essential.

Some foods I like to freeze are:
• Sliced sourdough
• Bulk-made sauces like ragù and tomato sauce
• Soups
• Lasagnes (portioned out)
• Lentil pie fillings
• Ice-cube trays of chopped garlic, ginger and chilli
• Whole chillies (grate them from frozen)
• Cookie dough portions
• Banana bread (whole)
• Cakes

Some recipes like cheese sauces, cooked pastas, bean bowls don't make it into the freezer, because they keep for less time and on defrosting can turn mushy and unappetising. Instead, I take them with me for lunch the next day or use the leftovers in a meal the following night. We often have mix 'n' match dinners, where various small portions of meals are served up as tapas or picky bits with bread or a fresh salad.

I often make a large batch of lentil ragù (see page 160) if I know I'm going away for a week and won't fancy cooking on my return.

Generally, I keep things in the freezer for no longer than 6 weeks, but some can last for up to 3 months. By that point, I've probably frozen newer portions and forgotten, so it's all about organising, thinking 'when will I use this?' and factoring it into one of your weekly meal plans. Be realistic, so as to not overcrowd your freezer.

LOVE YOUR LEFTOVERS

Don't shun your leftovers! Something that looks a bit sad can be given a new lease of life with a squeeze of fresh lemon juice, a new dressing, a sprinkle of nutritional yeast flakes or even a little more stock to pump up the flavour.

Sprinkle over some fresh herbs, a dollop of soy yoghurt and some roasted seeds (see page 209) to add some texture.

Before you start ...

- Specific olive oil amounts are not listed in many of the recipes, unless key to the overall quality of the dish in question. The general amounts for sautéing or frying are for you to decide but do bear in mind that olive oil is a great flavour carrier of the main base of many dishes (onions/shallots, garlic and spices) so limiting it may affect the final taste.

- If a recipe looks long, try not to be deterred. Although I've tried to reduce the words in many places, I want you to have a smooth and enjoyable cooking experience with me, and for that I need to explain things properly. Rest assured, even the longest of recipes are actually fairly easy once you get going. One of my most popular Instagram recipes, my Winter Veg Curry (page 171) seems daunting if you look at the steps, but it's actually one of my most made, and I constantly receive positive feedback for the end result.

- I have tested all these recipes with sea salt, not regular table salt or iodised salt. For best results, I recommend doing the same.

- Black pepper refers to freshly ground cracked black pepper, unless stated otherwise.

- Season recipes to your own taste, making sure to taste the ingredients throughout, as some brands of items may have different salt quantities (especially jarred/canned beans).

- All beans, unless otherwise stated, come from a can or jar, for convenience, but you can always use beans cooked from scratch if you desire.

- Serving sizes are suggestions only. The amount you eat will depend on your goals, activity levels, routine and more.

- Serving sizes will alter the amount of protein in your dish, so do be aware of this and recalculate the nutrient contents if you desire.

- Cook with care, attention to detail and love. It may sound silly, but rushing through a long recipe when you really can't be bothered will end with a sub-par result. Always read the cooking times and choose something appropriate!

- Please read through the entire recipe before starting, so you know when and what to prepare.

- Keep a small bowl beside you for discarding onion skins and other bits as you cook, this will make the clean-up a lot easier.

- Use a nice sharp knife (always be careful) this will help speed up prep times and enable you to get cleaner, smaller cuts on veg and aromatics, which will boost the overall flavour of a dish.

- Make sure to check on oven bakes regularly, as each person's oven may yield different results, due to hot spots or other features.

- Don't be afraid to substitute ingredients for what you already have, or what you can find. If you think it might work, it probably will. Trust your intuition! For example, any leafy greens can more or less be subbed for another leafy green, squash for sweet potato, and so on.

- Lastly, enjoy it! Put your favourite tunes on, dance around the kitchen, and enjoy the creative practice that cooking is.

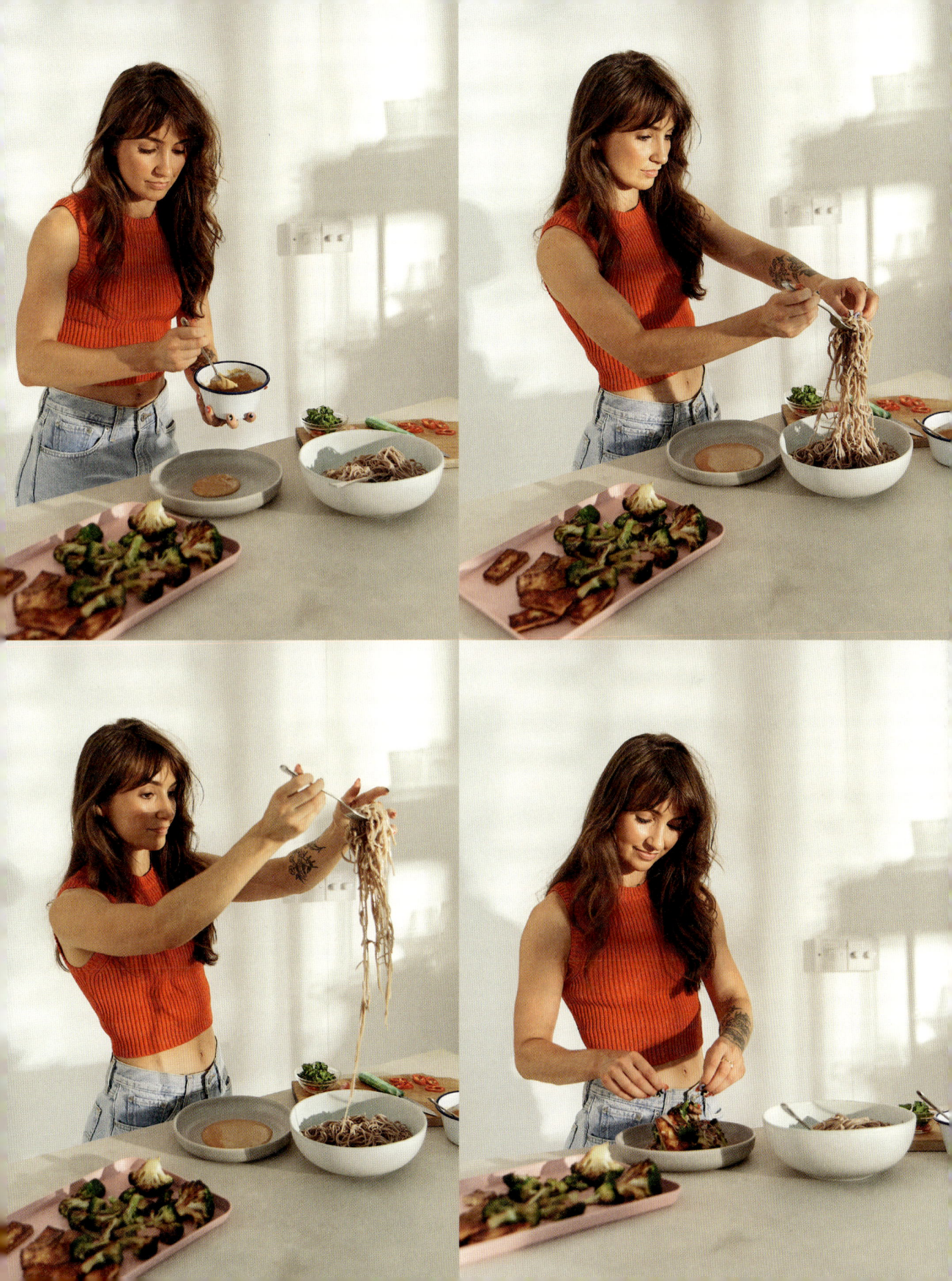

Building an active lifestyle

If you're an avid exerciser already, this section may not be relevant to you (but might be to a friend or family member). Now that we've covered why high-protein diets are important, and found delicious recipes to put the principles into practice, let's look at the second (but no less important) part of creating a long and healthy lifestyle.

WHAT IS AN ACTIVE LIFESTYLE?
We all know what activity can look like, whether it's something as simple as a brisk walk in the morning before work, a gym class with friends, or enrolling in a physical challenge like a run, swim, cycle, or hybrid workout. However, the cornerstone of maintaining an active lifestyle isn't just the exercise itself, it's also about your 'mindset to move'. Integrating activity into your daily routine can add a lot to your life, whether that's social connection, and associated health benefits, including:

+ Lower risk of disease

+ Improved mood

+ Healthy ageing

+ Improved sleep quality

+ Better self-esteem

+ Less stress

Source: NHS UK

HOW CAN I SHIFT MY MINDSET?

Mindset shifts can be hard and it depends on where you start from. Everyone has different schedules and exercise preferences. If you don't know where, or how, to start, I encourage you to think about your why.

Why do you want to start bringing more mindful activity into your life? What benefits would you like to gain? Here are a few ideas:

'I want to be able to run around with my grandkids.'

'I want independence in my later years.'

'I want to maximise my lifespan.'

'I want to meet like-minded people.'

'I want to feel happier.'

'I want to feel less bodily pain.'

You'll notice that not one of these focuses on physical appearance. This is because, although it's a nice side effect of an active lifestyle in some cases, it's more of a short-term goal and is unlikely to be conducive to long-term health and happiness. Looking 'good' (which is often conflated with bodyweight) doesn't always mean someone is feeling good or living a healthy life. For so many years, exercise has been viewed as just a way to burn calories. We have become obsessed with 'losing weight' and 'burning fat'. It's important to note that throughout our lives,

our bodies will change. Our weight will fluctuate and that's totally normal. If we want to create lasting, impactful change in our lives, we have to move away from aesthetic goals, and use real markers for longevity and joy, like the above mentioned.

As a trainer, I have my own opinions about exercise and although we are all wonderfully different and unique, we are all humans, with similar skeletons, muscular and nervous systems. This leads me on to my next point ...

The importance of resistance training

WHAT IS RESISTANCE TRAINING?

'The performance of physical exercises that are designed to improve strength and endurance. It is often associated with the lifting of weights. It can also incorporate a variety of training techniques including variations of bodyweight exercises, such as jumping or static holds.'

Resistance training, or strength training, has often been viewed as dangerous, male-dominated, and unimportant. For decades, many women have avoided lifting weights for fear of instantly growing huge, bulging biceps (I wish!). When I first started posting my lifts on social media, my mother viewed one of these Instagram stories and later that day I received a phone call lecturing me about 'damaging my spine', 'hurting myself' and saying 'you'll get huge muscles'. None of that came true true – growing big strong muscles is hard!

Ironically, four years later, my mum started to experience lower back pain. I explained the role of resistance training in pain prevention and how training her legs, back and abdominal muscles to encourage better posture would help. A year later, after working with a local trainer, she is pain-free, mobile and happy.

Our muscles are the largest organ in our bodies, making up around 40% (17) of our total weight, and for good reason. Thousands of years ago, our ancestors relied on muscular builds to gather food, make shelter and go about their daily activities in order to survive. Not using their muscles was not an option.

Fast forward to the present day and we have machines that take care of washing, cooking, sometimes cleaning, and we are more sedentary than ever. It's become an option as to whether we utilise our muscle mass each day, and this is a key factor in the global rise of many diseases. A 2020 study found that 'one-third of the global population aged fifteen years and older engages in insufficient physical activities', and 'Sedentary behaviours have wide-ranging adverse impacts on the human body including increased all-cause mortality, cardiovascular disease mortality, cancer risk, and risks of metabolic disorders.' (19)

It has never been more important to act now and take care of our bodies throughout our lives.

A 2012 study revealed that 'Inactive adults experience a 3% to 8% loss of muscle mass per decade, accompanied by resting metabolic rate reduction and fat accumulation. Ten weeks of resistance training may increase lean weight by 1.4 kg, increase resting metabolic rate by 7%, and reduce fat weight by 1.8 kg.' (18)

I remember sitting in one of the lectures for my personal training qualification and our tutor thanked us all for being there, saying, 'It's never been more important to train more people in this field, as we are experiencing a global health epidemic, and you have a crucial role to play'. That has stayed with me ever since, along with the fact that after the age of 30, we start to gradually lose our muscle mass. This is why I encourage everyone, especially women, of all ages, to take care of their skeletal muscle mass throughout their lives, not just when muscle loss occurs. This will ensure maximum quality of life.

We live in a society that often treats the symptoms, not the cause. If you have a strong body composition (a favourable lean muscle to body fat ratio), your starting point will be higher than someone who has not trained, so your rate of decline, and therefore risk of disease, will be lower.

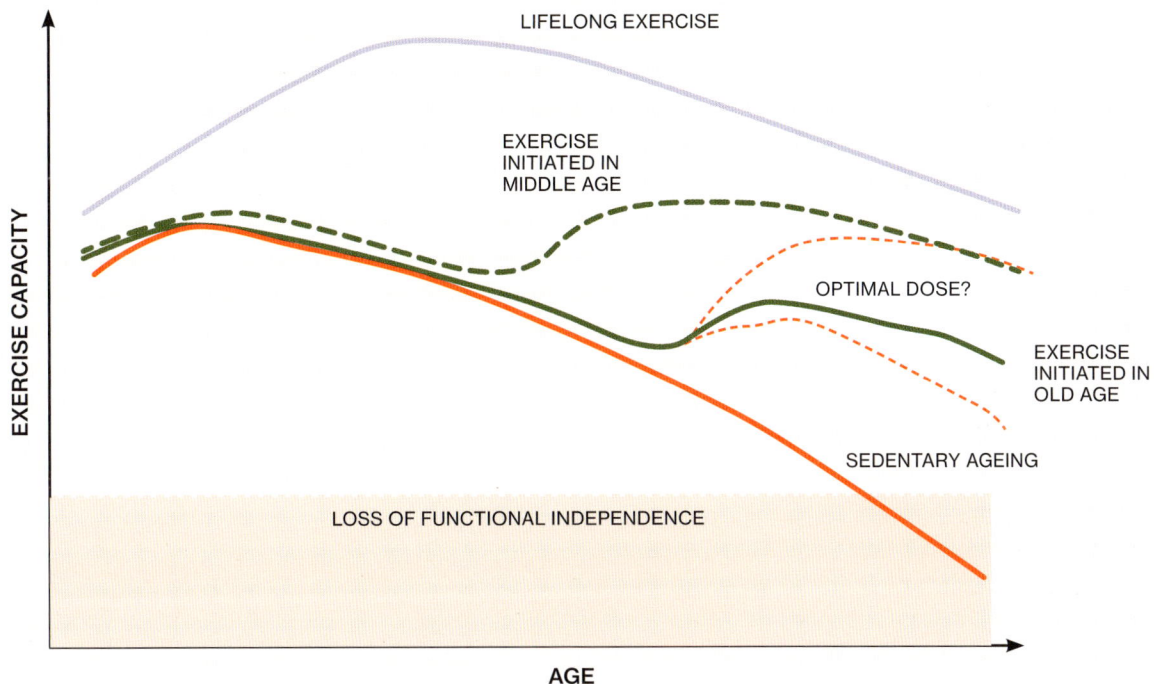

LIFELONG EXERCISE

EXERCISE
INITIATED IN
MIDDLE AGE

OPTIMAL DOSE?

EXERCISE
INITIATED IN
OLD AGE

SEDENTARY AGEING

LOSS OF FUNCTIONAL INDEPENDENCE

EXERCISE CAPACITY

AGE

Everyone, if they can, should be engaging in some form of resistance training weekly.

If we prioritise training our muscles over burning calories we will:

- Burn more energy and therefore improve our body composition (muscle tissue demands more energy at rest).

- Reduce our risk of disease and injury (as resistance training strengthens our bones).

- Improve cognition. (16)

- Improve proprioception (awareness of space in the body).

- Improve posture.

- Improve heart health.

- Boost metabolism.

- Improve confidence.

- Improve mental health.

- Decrease risk of disease.

- Help with fat loss.

- Enhance our overall quality of life.

It's refreshing to see in recent years that the tides are starting to turn, but we still have a long way to go in terms of getting the people who need it most into resistance training.

HOW CAN I START?

This will depend on your current level of activity, mobility and health. For complete beginners, I recommend investing in a personal trainer for at least a month. In my opinion, the investment is worth its weight in gold. Learning how to move well in the beginning will set you up for success in the long-term. If you're unsure, think of the opportunity cost of risking your health and come back to your 'why'. Gym classes are also a great way to introduce yourself to resistance training in a safe environment, and you can meet some like-minded people, too.

I recognise this can be a privilege, so if you have access to the internet on your phone, there are many great free beginner workouts on YouTube you can try any time. If nothing else, a nice brisk walk up a hill will work wonders!

It's also worth noting that some GP surgeries can refer you for specialised, subsidised group exercise classes if you suffer from certain disease risk factors, as some personal trainers will be unable to legally train you. A personal trainer should ask you to fill in a questionnaire before getting started (ParQ), so do be honest with your answers otherwise you could put yourself at risk. Most personal trainers are not qualified to train someone with cardiovascular disease or diabetes, for example.

Some key things to remember:

- Everyone starts somewhere, and everyone was a beginner once.

- Despite what you may think, it's very likely no-one is looking at you in the gym; they're too focused on themselves.

- Start hydrated, stretch after your workouts and rest when you need it.

- Motivation will come and go, so make it easier for yourself to exercise regularly by preparing everything you need so you're ready to go. Making some high-protein snacks (examples on page 65) and even arranging to meet a friend (so you're less likely to bail!).

- There will be days when you don't get to exercise, and that's fine – life happens! The best thing you can do is not berate yourself and get back on track as soon as you can.

- Hydrate well; add a tiny pinch of sea salt to your water to help replenish electrolytes.

- If you're a woman of reproductive age, it's a good idea to eat something before you work out, even if it's just a snack. This will ensure you are not exercising in what's called a 'low energy' state and under-fuelling your workouts for positive adaptation.

The quality and enjoyment we get from our lives is correlated with the health of our muscles.

Breakfast

I've structured this chapter to work for everyone. We've got small snacks for those eating early before working out as well as larger shakes or bowls for a post-workout protein boost. I have both sweet and savoury ideas, things that can be thrown together in a pinch, prep-ahead ideas to take to work and some larger brunch ideas for weekend breakfasts.

I'm a huge fan of oats, which is why you'll see them in a fair few of these recipes. They're super versatile and are a great source of complex carbs (the slow energy releasing ones), fibre and protein. Great for a pre- or post-workout meal.

Loaded Sourdough Toast, 3 Ways

There's something elegant about an artfully loaded slice of sourdough, the textures just seem to jump off the plate. Love at first sight, and bite.

I'm always asked how to find good sourdough, and unless you're baking it yourself, your best bet is a local bakery, or even a larger supermarket.

Peanut Butter, Banana and Cacao Nibs

SERVES 1
TOTAL TIME: 5 MINS

1 slice of sourdough
2 tbsp crunchy or smooth natural peanut butter
½ banana, sliced
Sprinkle of cacao nibs
Sprinkle of hemp seeds
Drizzle of maple syrup (optional)

Slice and toast your bread, generously spread the peanut butter all over, layer the sliced banana, sprinkle the cacao nibs and seeds, then drizzle over the maple syrup (optional).

Peanut butter, banana and cacao nibs:
14g protein, 7g fibre, plant diversity score 5

Pesto butter beans and kimchi:
11g protein, 7.7g fibre, plant diversity score 6

Tofu cream cheese, sun-dried tomatoes and chives:
11g protein, 4g fibre, plant diversity score 4

Pesto Butter Beans and Kimchi

SERVES 1
TOTAL TIME: 10 MINS

120g (3½oz) butter beans, (roughly half from a 400g/14oz can or jar)
2 tbsp Hemp Seed Pesto (see page 216)
Squeeze of fresh lemon juice (optional)
1 slice of sourdough
Extra virgin olive oil
Sea salt
1 heaped tbsp kimchi

Drain and rinse the beans, then add to a bowl with the pesto sauce and mix well. Season to taste, I like to add a little more freshly squeezed lemon. Slice and toast your bread, then drizzle over a little extra virgin olive oil, a small pinch of sea salt, then layer over the beans and finish with the tablespoon of kimchi on top.

Tofu Cream Cheese, Sun-dried Tomatoes and Chives

SERVES 1
TOTAL TIME: 5 MINS

1 slice of sourdough
2 tbsp Tofu Cream Cheese (see page 220)
2 large sun-dried tomatoes, from a jar
1 tbsp finely chopped fresh chives
Extra virgin olive oil
Flaky sea salt
Black pepper

Slice and toast your bread, then drizzle over a little extra virgin olive oil, a small pinch of sea salt, then generously slather the tofu cream cheese all over the toast. Cut the sun-dried tomatoes into small-ish pieces and arrange these on the toast. Finish with the finely chopped chives, a little more flaky salt and black pepper.

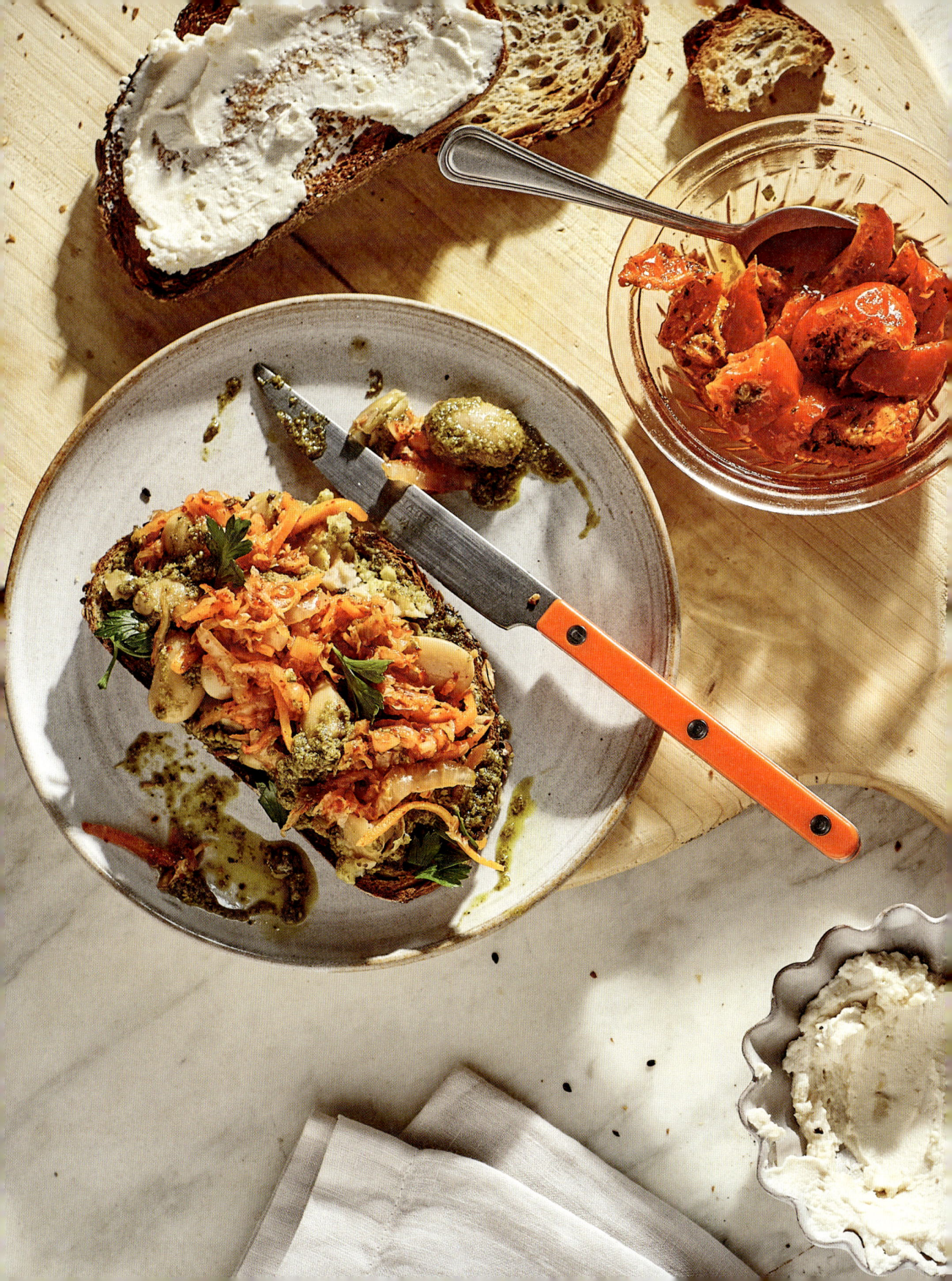

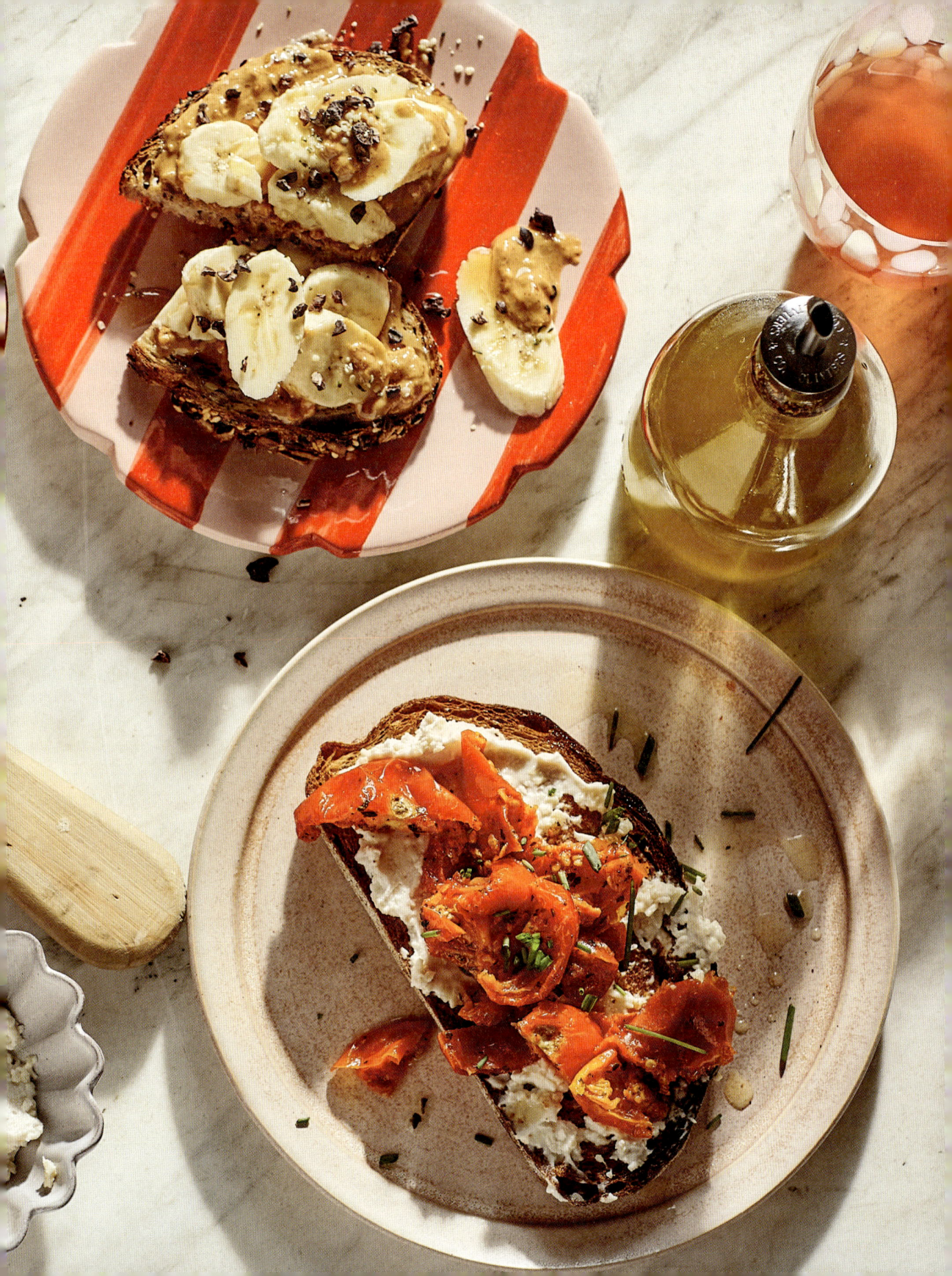

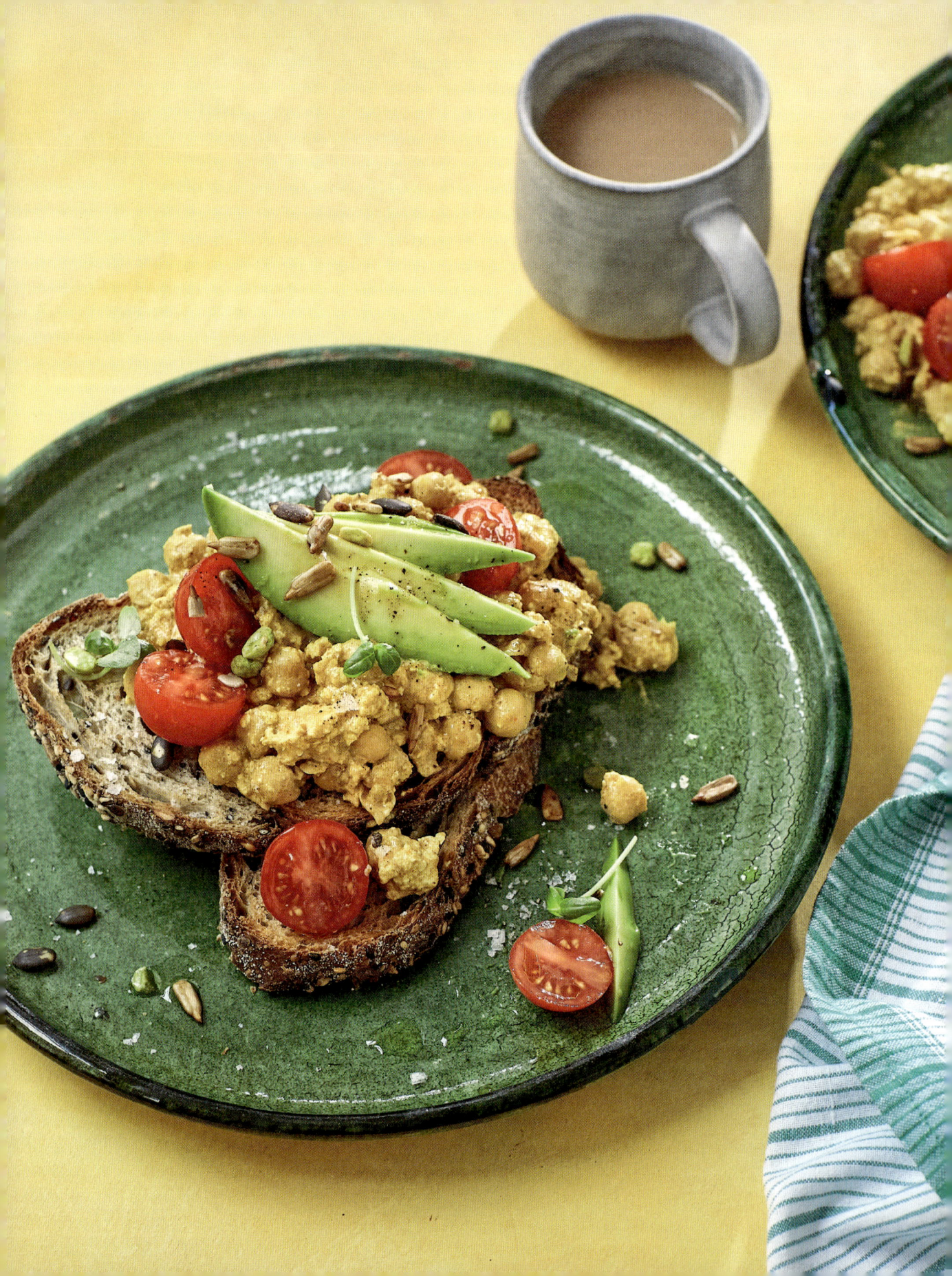

Easy Spiced Scramble

MAKES 2 LARGE PORTIONS
TOTAL TIME: 20 MINS

**My favourite way to make scrambled tofu, with a
little more texture and bite from the addition of
chickpeas, and of course, plenty of spice.**

1 shallot, finely chopped
2 garlic cloves, minced
1 tsp ground cumin
1 tsp ground coriander
1 tsp smoked paprika
½ tsp ground turmeric
¼ tsp kala namak (Indian black salt, optional)
200g (7oz) extra-firm tofu, crumbled into small pieces
240g (8½oz) chickpeas, from a jar or can, plus 2 tbsp
  of their liquid
200g (7oz) silken tofu
4 tbsp nutritional yeast
Extra virgin olive oil
Sea salt
Black pepper

TO SERVE
Toasted sourdough bread
Omega-3 Boost (see page 209)
Small handful of cherry tomatoes
Avocado slices
Fresh coriander leaves (optional)

In a medium non-stick saute pan, on a medium heat,
heat olive oil and fry the chopped shallot for
5 minutes, with a small pinch of sea salt. Add the
garlic and fry for 2 minutes more, then add the spices
and fry for a further 1 minute, adding more oil if you
need to.

Add the crumbled tofu and chickpeas, plus 2
tablespoons of their canning liquid. Stir well and
cook down for 5 minutes, until the chickpeas begin to
soften and you can gently squish a few of them down
into the pan.

Whilst that's cooking, whizz up the silken tofu and
nutritional yeast with ½ teaspoon sea salt in a small
bullet blender. Pour that all in, mix well and season
to taste. Cook for 3–5 minutes, until a desired 'eggy'
consistency is reached (cook longer for a drier mix).
Season to taste.

Serve over toasted sourdough bread with a handful of
chopped cherry tomatoes, Omega-3 Boost, avocado
slices and coriander.

Protein per serving: 36g
Fibre: 16g
Plant diersity score: 9

Tahini, Coconut and Cinnamon Crunch Granola

MAKES 6–8 SERVINGS
TOTAL TIME: 25 MINS

When I was testing this, my partner Will was eating it faster than I could make it. The tahini balances perfectly with the juicy sultanas, sweet cinnamon and toasted coconut flakes. It's absolutely heavenly and won't last long in your kitchen.

200g (7oz/1½ cups) jumbo oats
135g (4¾oz) mixed nuts and seeds (I used almonds, walnuts and pumpkin seeds – although any would work)
20g (¾oz/½ cup) coconut flakes
30g (1oz) hemp seeds
30g (1oz/¼ cup) sultanas
3 tsp ground cinnamon
1 tbsp coconut sugar
60g (2¼oz) good-quality runny tahini
50ml (2fl oz/3½ tbsp) maple or agave syrup
1½ tbsp coconut oil, melted

Preheat the oven to 160°C fan/180°C/gas mark 4 and line a large baking tray with baking parchment.

In a mixing bowl, combine the oats, mixed nuts and seeds, coconut, hemp seeds, sultanas, cinnamon and coconut sugar.

In another small mixing bowl, combine the tahini, maple or agave syrup and melted coconut oil with a small whisk until runny and creamy.

Pour the wet ingredients into the dry and combine well with a rubber spatula. Spread the mix out in an even layer on the lined tray and press down firmly.

Bake for 16–18 minutes. Once baked, leave on the counter to cool completely before breaking it up loosely. Pour it into an airtight jar, keep at room temperature and eat within 14 days.

Per serving if divided into 8:
Protein: 8g
Fibre: 5.5g
Plant diversity score: 9

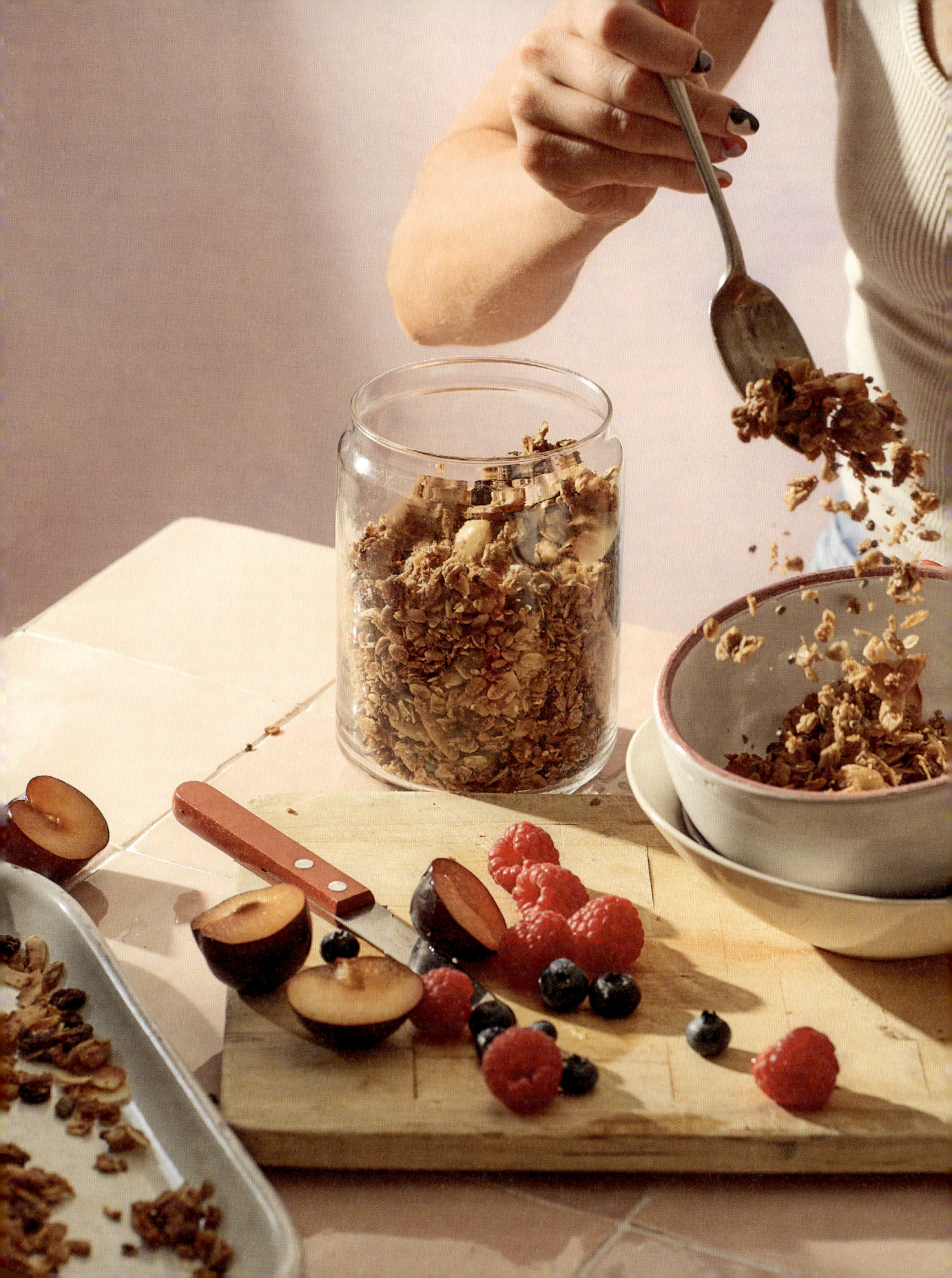

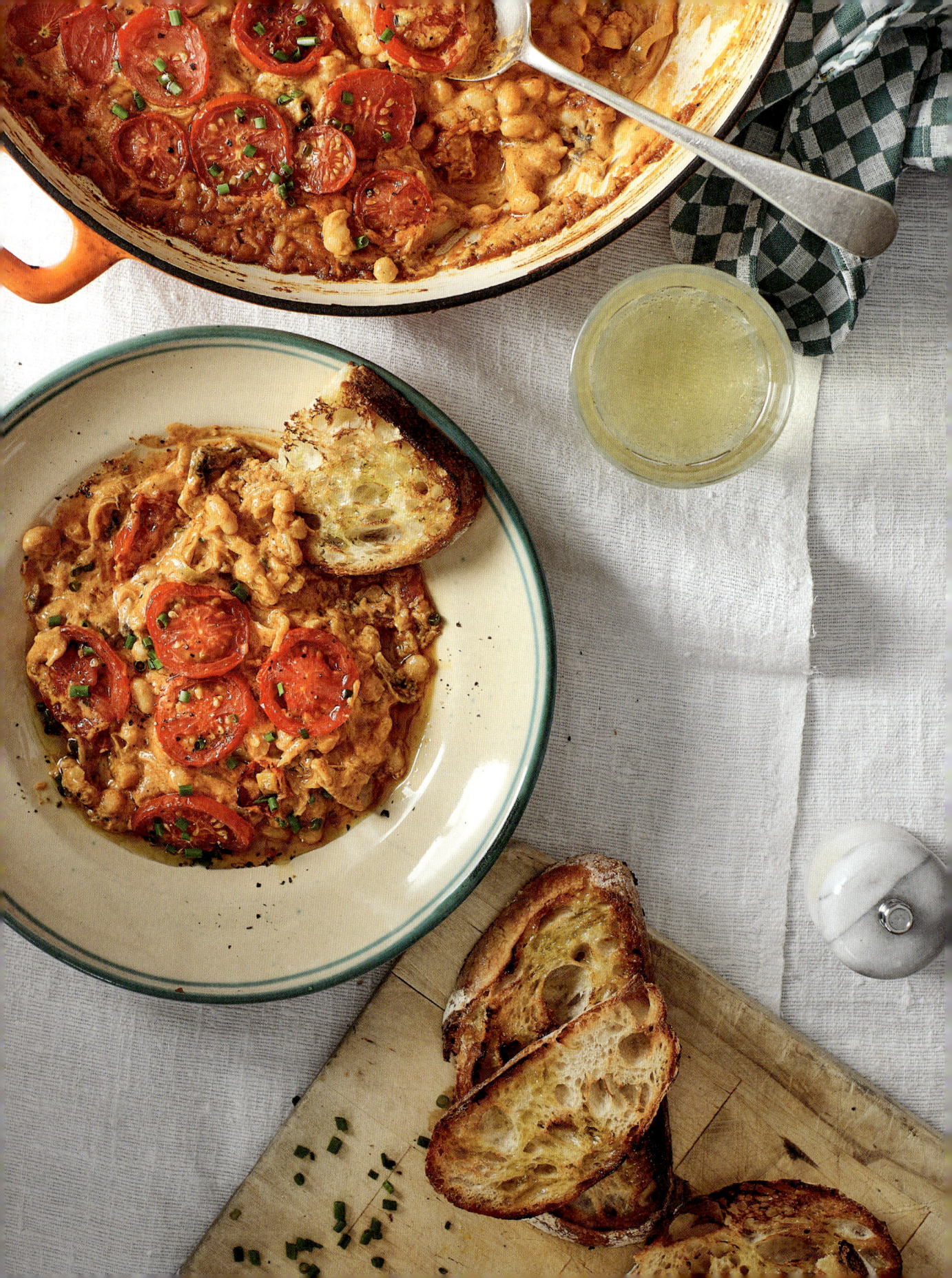

One-pan 'English Breakfast' Beans

MAKES 3 PORTIONS
TOTAL TIME: 30 MINS

Ever wanted to make a full English, but the thought of many pans to wash up put you off? Enter these gorgeous, one-pan cannellini breakfast beans. Get those plant points in nice and early by cooking leeks and mushrooms in oil and spices, followed by plenty of beans for protein and fibre, topped with grilled tomatoes for juicy goodness.

1 white onion, sliced
1 leek, white and light green parts sliced into half-moons
4 tbsp extra virgin olive oil, plus more if needed
250g (9oz) chestnut mushrooms, finely chopped
5 garlic cloves, minced
2 tsp smoked paprika
1 tsp ground cumin
1 tsp ground coriander
700g (1lb 9oz) canned white beans, plus their juices (if the bean juice is not salted, add ½ vegetable stock cube, crumbled)
3–4 medium tomatoes, sliced
Salt and black pepper

FOR THE SCRAMBLE SAUCE
35g (1¼oz) cashews or sunflower seeds
280g (10oz) silken tofu
20g (¾oz) nutritional yeast
1 garlic clove or 1 tsp garlic powder
1 tsp smoked paprika
1 tbsp sweet white miso
1 tbsp lemon juice
1 tsp Dijon mustard

TO SERVE
Freshly chopped chives
Homemade 'Sausages' (see page 224, optional)
Sourdough toast

Start by soaking the cashews in boiling water for 10 minutes. Drain and set aside.

In an ovenproof casserole dish on a medium heat, fry the onion and leeks in plenty of extra virgin olive oil with a pinch of salt and lots of black pepper for 8 minutes until caramelising. Add the mushrooms, more salt, and fry until the water has evaporated (you'll see the steam from the mushrooms subsiding). Add the garlic and spices, and more oil if you need it. Fry for another 2 minutes until aromatic.

Add the beans and their juices. If you don't want to use the bean water, replace it with 100ml (3½fl oz/ scant ½ cup) hot water, with the veg stock cube dissolved in it. Stir to combine and season to taste.

In a small blender cup, blend all the ingredients for the scramble sauce. Add a little water if needed to loosen the sauce slightly so it's a pourable consistency. Add to the pan. Stir well and season to taste, adding a little more lemon juice, salt or pepper if you think it needs it.

Heat the grill to its top setting, then arrange the tomatoes on top of the dish, drizzle with olive oil and add a little salt, then transfer to the top rack and grill for around 6–10 minutes, or until the tomatoes start to catch a small char. This will vary greatly depending on your pan, strength of your oven and grill placement, so do keep an eye on it as the tomatoes can burn very quickly.

Top with fresh chives and serve with my homemade wholefood sausages and sourdough toast, if you like.

———

Protein per serving: 30g
Fibre: 13g
Plant diversity score: 9

Overnight Protein Oats, 2 Ways

SERVES 1 (I RECOMMEND TRIPLING
THE MIX FOR MEAL-PREP)
TOTAL TIME: 10 MINS

What's a high-protein, plant-based cookbook without a solid overnight oats recipe? Although it might seem an easy recipe, these little jars of goodness actually took me quite a while to develop and get 'right'. I want them to be something I would genuinely make every day, something which doesn't overdo sweetness and has enough nutrients to be a weekday staple. Bookmark this one, you're going to need it!

Berry Cacao

50g (1¾oz/⅓ cup) jumbo oats
1 tbsp chia seeds
Small pinch of sea salt
200ml (7fl oz/¾ cup) soy milk
1 Medjool date, pitted
30g (1oz) chocolate vegan protein powder
1 tbsp cacao powder
1 serving of creatine (optional)
Small handful of frozen or fresh strawberries, blueberries or raspberries (I often use the frozen mixed bags)

FOR THE TOPPINGS (OPTIONAL)
Fresh berries, quartered or halved
Cacao nibs
Soy yoghurt

In a mixing bowl, combine the oats, chia seeds and salt.

In a blender cup, blend the soy milk, date, protein powder, cacao powder and creatine (if using). Pour over the oats and seeds, mix well. It should be a runny consistency, very easy to pour. Different protein powders will yield different results, consistency wise, so if the mix is too thick, add more soy milk or water.

Pour into a meal-prep container or jar, then scatter or mix in the frozen berries. Leave overnight in the fridge, covered, then enjoy in the morning with your choice of toppings.

Banoffee Pie

50g (1¾oz/⅓ cup) jumbo oats
1 tbsp chia seeds
Small pinch of sea salt
200ml (7fl oz/¾ cup) soy milk
30g (1oz) vanilla vegan protein powder or 1 tsp vanilla extract
1 serving of creatine (optional)
1 Medjool date, pitted
15g (½oz) crunchy or smooth natural peanut butter
½ banana, sliced
1 tbsp creamy soy yoghurt
Cacao nibs, for topping (optional)

In a mixing bowl, combine the oats, chia seeds and salt.

In a blender cup, blend the soy milk, protein powder, creatine (if using), date and peanut butter. Pour over the oats and seeds, then mix well. It should be a runny consistency, very easy to pour. Different protein powders will yield different results, consistency wise, so if the mix is too thick, add more soy milk or water.

Layer in a glass or jar, starting with the oats, then the sliced banana, yoghurt dollops, and repeat until you have no mix left.

Leave overnight in the fridge, covered, then enjoy in the morning with cacao nibs on top, if you like.

54

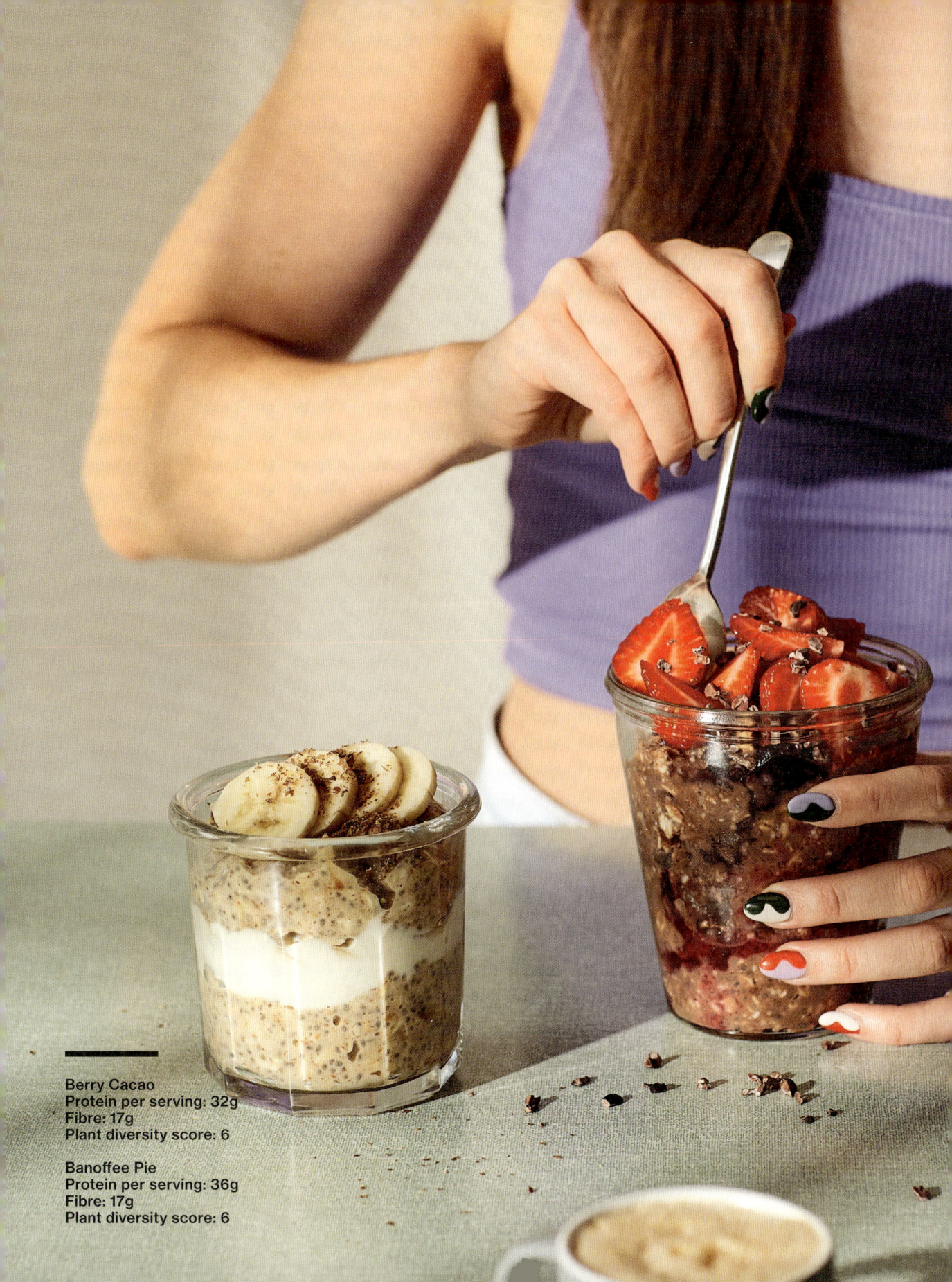

Berry Cacao
Protein per serving: 32g
Fibre: 17g
Plant diversity score: 6

Banoffee Pie
Protein per serving: 36g
Fibre: 17g
Plant diversity score: 6

Spiced Black Bean Breakfast Burrito

MAKES 4 SMALL BURRITOS
TOTAL TIME: 30 MINS

100g (3½oz/½ cup) quinoa
3–4 wholemeal wraps or roti

FOR THE BLACK BEANS

4 spring onions, white parts finely chopped
½ red chilli, finely chopped
Large handful (about 15g/½oz) of fresh coriander,
  leaves and stalks separated, stalks finely chopped
1 tsp ground coriander
1 tsp ground cumin
2 tsp smoked paprika
½ tsp cayenne pepper
Pinch of ground cinnamon
3 garlic cloves, minced
1 tbsp tomato purée
2 x 400g (14oz) cans black beans, plus their juices
2 tbsp smooth peanut butter
Extra virgin olive oil
Squeeze of lime juice
Salt and black pepper

FOR THE GUACAMOLE

1 large ripe avocado
1 tbsp chopped red onion
½ tbsp chopped red chilli
2 garlic cloves, minced
Juice of 1 lime or lemon
1 tbsp olive oil, plus more to taste
½ tsp salt, plus more to taste
Small handful chopped cherry tomatoes (optional)
Small handful very finely chopped fresh coriander
  leaves (optional)

TO SERVE

2 tbsp per burrito of Cashew Queso (see page 219) or
  you can use shop-bought cheese
1 tbsp per burrito of Quick-pickled Red Onion (see
  page 206)

This was an instant hit on social media, so it seemed rude not to include it here. I eat a version of these beans at least once a week, with lots of guacamole and tangy pickled onions, on plenty of sourdough toast.

This is another breakfast recipe I will happily chow down for dinner.

Cook the quinoa according to the packet instructions and set aside with a tea towel over the lidded saucepan to help it fluff up.

Now, start the beans. In a frying pan on a medium heat, fry the spring onions, chilli and coriander stalks in some olive oil with a pinch of salt for 5 minutes. Add all the spices and garlic, and some more olive oil here if you need to, making sure everything is fragrant and the spices aren't burning. Your kitchen should be smelling lovely at this point! Now add the tomato purée, mix to combine, then add the beans and their juice, the peanut butter, mix everything very well, bring to a bubble, then reduce to a simmer and cook down on a medium heat for 10–15 minutes, stirring occasionally, until reduced and thick (the consistency you're looking for should slowly fall off a spatula). Season to taste. Take off the heat and squeeze over the juice of about half a lime. Mix and leave to one side.

In a mixing bowl or on a chopping board, mash all the guacamole ingredients bar the cherry tomatoes and fresh coriander (if using) together with a fork. Season to taste, adding more salt, lime or lemon or olive oil to your liking. I like mine super salty and citrussy! Once happy, stir through the cherry tomatoes and the very finely chopped coriander leaves.

Layer the burrito, starting with the cashew queso, then the cooked quinoa, the black bean mix, the guac and the pickled onions. Roll up and cut in half, then drizzle with some more queso, if you like!

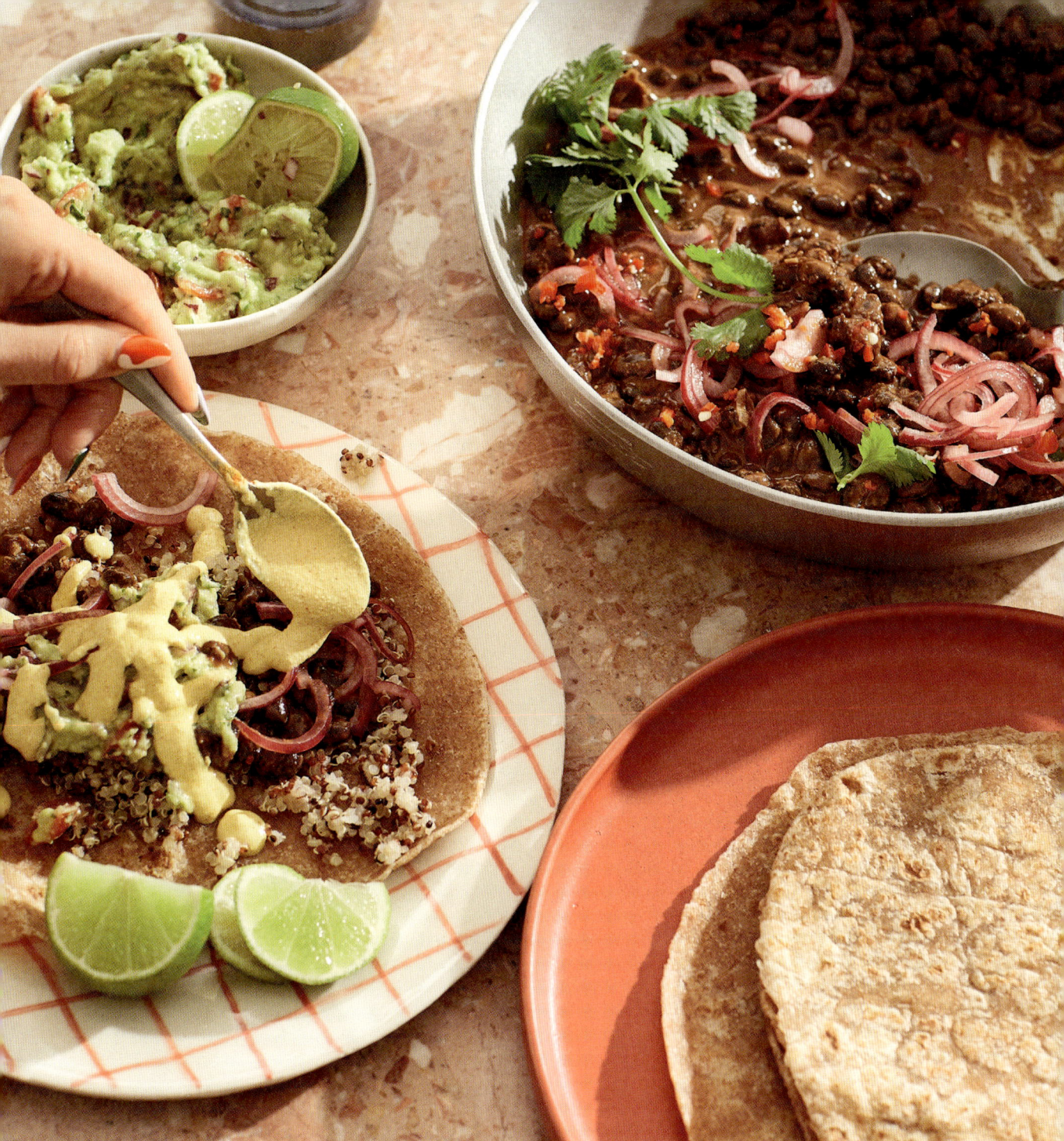

Protein per burrito: 16g
Fibre: 16g
Plant diversity score: 11

NOTES
If you'd rather not use the bean water, you can drain and rinse the beans and replace the liquid with 100ml (3½fl oz/ scant ½ cup) warm water mixed with a pinch of stock powder or salt.

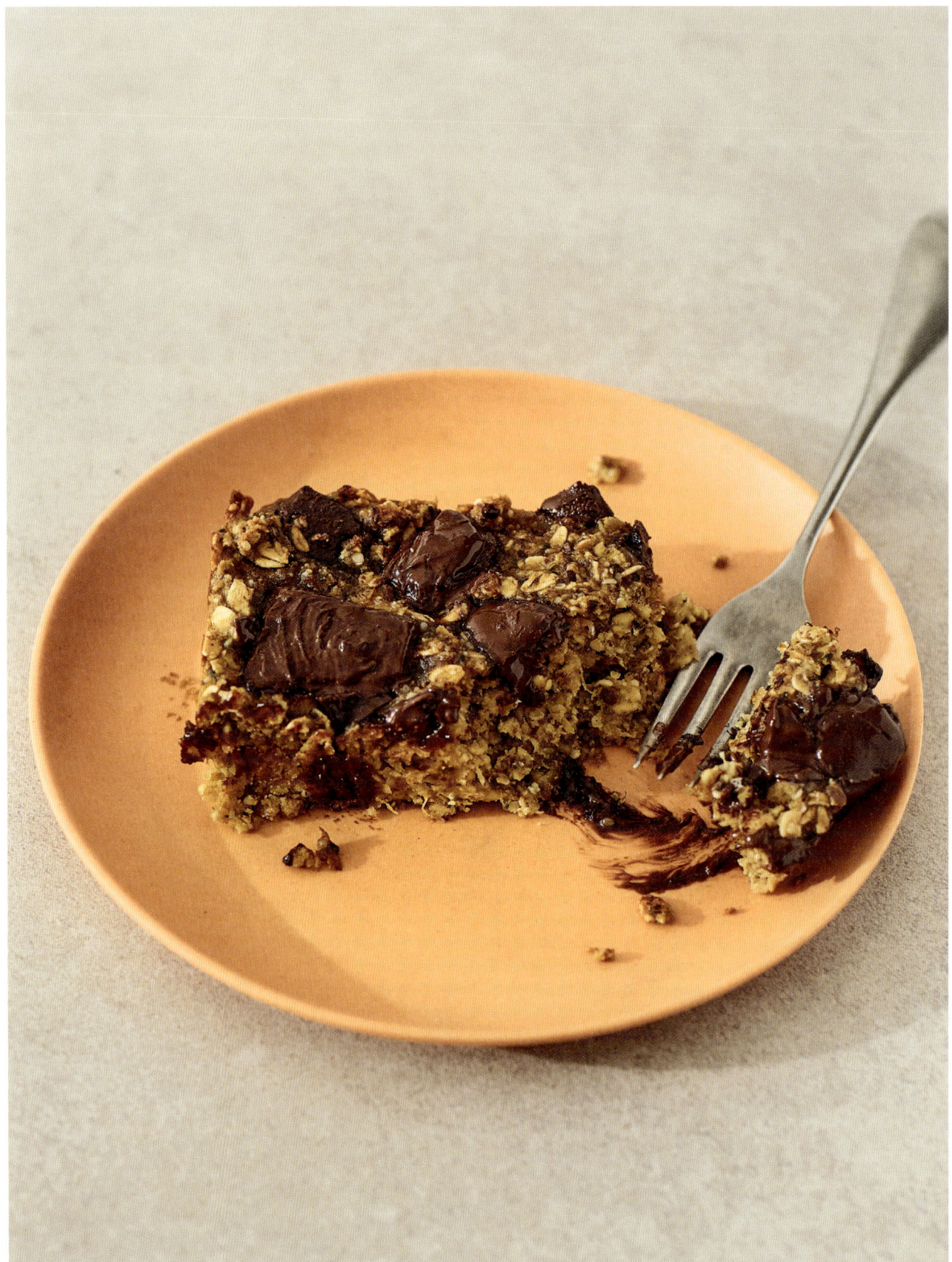

Lemon Drizzle and Dark Chocolate Baked Oats

MAKES 6 SQUARES
TOTAL TIME: 30 MINS

These oats really will make breakfast the best meal of the day – they might be slightly naughtier but will provide great fuel for training hard! Inspired by my favourite flavour combination in a chocolate bar, lemon and dark chocolate is not to be slept on!

4 tbsp coconut sugar
Zest of 2 unwaxed lemons, plus more to serve
1 large ripe banana
200g (7oz/1½ cups) jumbo oats
60g (2oz/½ cup) ground almonds
50g (1¾oz) hemp seeds
2 tbsp ground flaxseeds
½ tsp sea salt
1 tsp baking powder
1 tsp ground cinnamon
2 scoops (60g/2oz) vanilla or unflavoured vegan protein powder
350ml (12fl oz/scant 1½ cups) soy milk
2 Medjool dates
150g (5½oz) dark chocolate (check the label for hidden milk if you're PB/vegan!), broken into irregular pieces

Preheat the oven to 160°C fan/180°C/gas mark 4.

In a 22 x 22 cm (9 x 9in) lined baking dish, measure the sugar, grate the lemon zest, and rub together with your fingers, so the oils infuse. Add the banana and mash it in with a fork, combining it with the sugar and lemon zest mix. Add all the other ingredients minus the milk, dates and chocolate, then in a blender whizz up the milk with the dates, then pour over and combine well. Fold in half the chocolate pieces and stir to combine. Scatter the rest of the chocolate on top, and bake for 18–20 minutes until the top turns golden brown.

Leave to cool, then divide into 6 portions and seal in an airtight container.

Lasts for up to a week in the fridge.

Protein per serving: 18g
Fibre: 10g
Plant diversity score: 10

Pre- and Post-training Smoothies:

One of these is my go-to morning smoothie, one of these is my partner, Will's. Can you guess who's is who's?

Will is fully plant-based and has been for over three years now. He's an avid exerciser and has this spinach, almond, oat chocolate shake every day, after he trains.

I prefer something brighter and lighter, as I like to eat before I train. This apple, beetroot and berry smoothie is my go-to for a quick energy boost at breakfast.

Interestingly, studies have shown the consumption of beetroot has been linked to a boost in athletic performance.

If you're eating pre-training, I'd go for half the apple, beet and berry, saving half for after to have with a bowl of oats. I wouldn't advise going for the Hulking, Bulking, pre-training, as the oats will take longer to digest and could affect performance.

Apple, Beetroot and Berry Smoothie (pre-training)

1 cooked beetroot (I use the ones in packets you can get from the supermarket)
1 small apple, chopped
Handful of frozen mixed berries
½ scoop (30g/1oz) vanilla vegan protein powder
1 serving of creatine
100ml (3½fl oz/scant ½ cup) soy milk
100ml (3½fl oz/scant ½ cup) filtered water

In a blender cup, blend all the ingredients until very smooth, transfer to a glass and enjoy.

———

Apple, Beetroot and Berry Smoothie
Protein per serving: 26g
Fibre: 11.5g
Plant diversity score: 4

Hulking, Bulking, Breakfast Smoothie
Protein per serving: 38g
Fibre: 17g
Plant diversity score: 5.5

Hulking, Bulking, Breakfast Smoothie (post-training)

100g (3½oz/¾ cup) jumbo oats
3 nests of frozen spinach
2 heaped tbsp almond or peanut butter
1 scoop (30g/1oz) chocolate vegan protein powder
1 serving of creatine
½ tsp ground cinnamon
1 tbsp soy yoghurt
3 ice cubes

In a blender cup, add all the ingredients and pour over enough filtered water to cover the mixture by 2.5cm (1in). Blend until all the ingredients are very smooth – you may need to do this in bursts, shaking the ingredients here and there to make sure it all gets blended. If it's really not blending, add more water to help. Pour into a glass or transfer to a transportable cup to enjoy on the go.

NOTES
Neither of us are huge fans of banana in smoothies, as we find it tends to dominate the taste. If you prefer, you can add ½ a frozen banana to both of these!

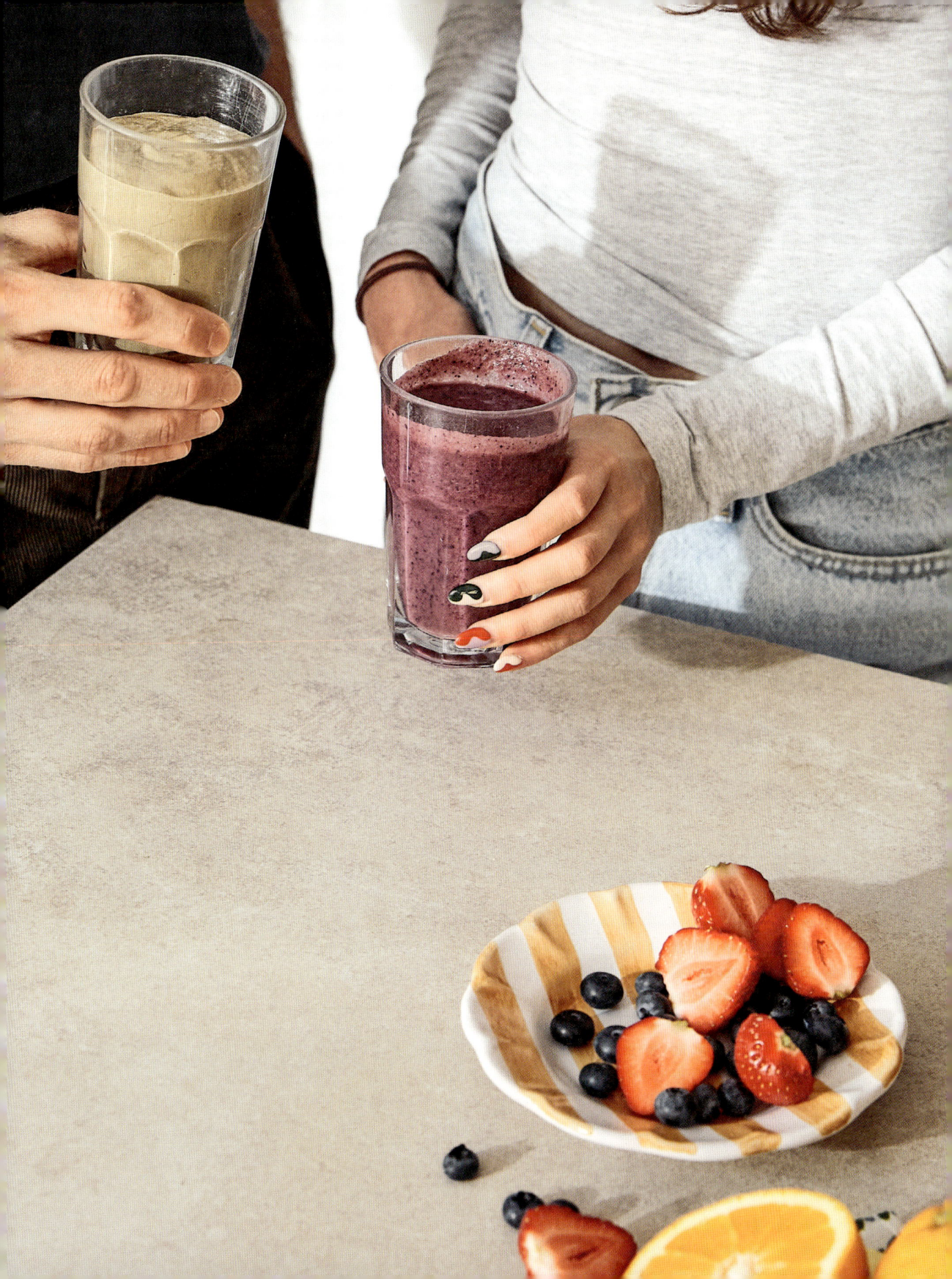

Feeling Snackish

These are all suitable for any time of day and excellent for a pre- or post-workout energy boost. I prefer my snacks less sweet and more fibrous so they're more satiating. If you prefer a sweeter snack, I've added a few pointers in the notes so you can adjust quantities of ingredients where appropriate. Most of these travel well, so you can make ahead and take on hikes, walks, days out at the park or beach and even on flights (where plant-based options are scarce!).

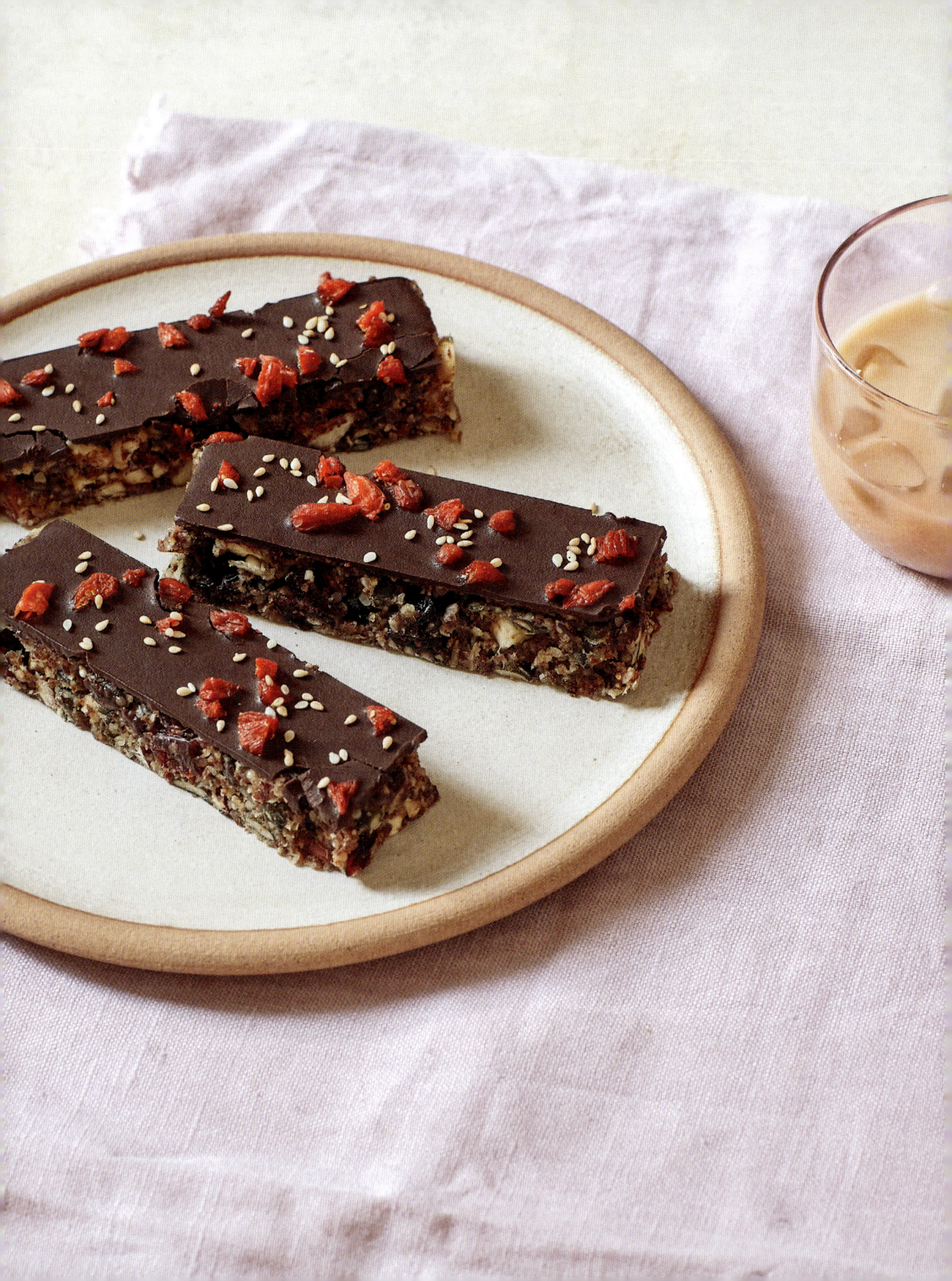

Superfood
Energy Bars

MAKES 8 BARS
TOTAL TIME: 50 MINS

In another life, I worked in a shopping centre for 3 years. On delivery days, we had to open the store super early, so grabbing a granola bar from the nearest coffee chain became a habit and a little treat to get me through. These are my healthier, high-protein versions.

8 large Medjool dates, pitted
60g (2¼oz/⅓ cup) cashews, roughly chopped
60g (2¼oz/⅓ cup) almonds, roughly chopped
60g (2¼oz/scant ½ cup) pumpkin seeds
50g (1¾oz) oat flour
50g (1¾oz) hemp seeds
50g (1¾oz) ground flaxseeds
Pinch of salt
Small handful of cranberries
1 tsp vanilla extract
3 tbsp maple syrup

FOR THE TOPPING
50g (1¾oz) 70% dark chocolate
1 tsp coconut oil
Goji berries or freeze-dried berries such as
    raspberries, cherries or strawberries (optional)

In a small bowl, soak the dates in boiling water. Leave for 5 minutes while you measure out the dry ingredients and cranberries, and add them to a mixing bowl.

Drain and add the soaked dates to a small blender, along with the vanilla, maple syrup and 1 tablespoon of warm water. Blend until a thick paste forms, adding a little more water if you need to.

Add the date paste to the nut and seed mix and combine well with your hands until a ball forms.

Line a 23cm (9in) square baking tray or silicone tray with baking parchment. Press the mixture down very firmly, using the bottom of a heavy glass, a cup measure, or the back of a large spoon to help. Pop this in the fridge to firm up for at least 30 minutes.

Once firm, cut it into bars with a sharp knife and place the bars on a clean piece of baking parchment.

Melt the dark chocolate with the coconut oil in a bain-marie (a heatproof bowl placed over a saucepan of boiling water, without touching the water's surface) or in a microwave in 15–20-second bursts, stirring each time it comes out (be careful to not let the chocolate burn!). It's ready to take off the heat when there are some smaller lumps left, as the residual heat will melt these.

Pour the melted chocolate over the top of the granola bars, use as much or as little as you like here! Then sprinkle over some roughly chopped goji berries or freeze-dried berries if you like.

Store in an airtight container in the fridge for up to 1 week.

Protein per bar: 10g
Fibre: 7.2
Plant diversity score: 10

Cookie Dough
Bliss Balls

Little balls of goodness to get you through busy days, and the perfect pre-gym snack if you're a particularly early riser and can't stomach much food first thing.

50g (1¾oz/⅓ cup) cashews
80g (2¾oz/⅔ cup) oat flour
1 scoop (30g/1oz) vanilla vegan protein powder
20g (¾oz/¼ cup) ground almonds
Pinch of salt
1 tsp ground cinnamon
1 tbsp chia seeds
2 tbsp smooth peanut butter
2 tbsp maple or agave syrup
1 tsp vanilla extract
4 tbsp soy milk
Small handful of dark chocolate chips

In a small bowl, soak the cashews in boiling water for 15 minutes. Drain.

Meanwhile, add the oat flour, protein powder, ground almonds, salt, cinnamon and chia to a medium mixing bowl and stir to combine.

To a small blender cup, add the soaked cashews, the peanut butter, agave or maple, vanilla and milk. Blend. Add this to the dry ingredients, along with the chocolate chips. Mix with your hands until a sticky ball forms. Add a little water if it's too dry.

Roll into 10–12 balls and pop into the fridge for 20 minutes to firm up.

Protein per ball: 4.5g
Fibre: 2g
Plant diversity score: 11

FEELING SNACKISH

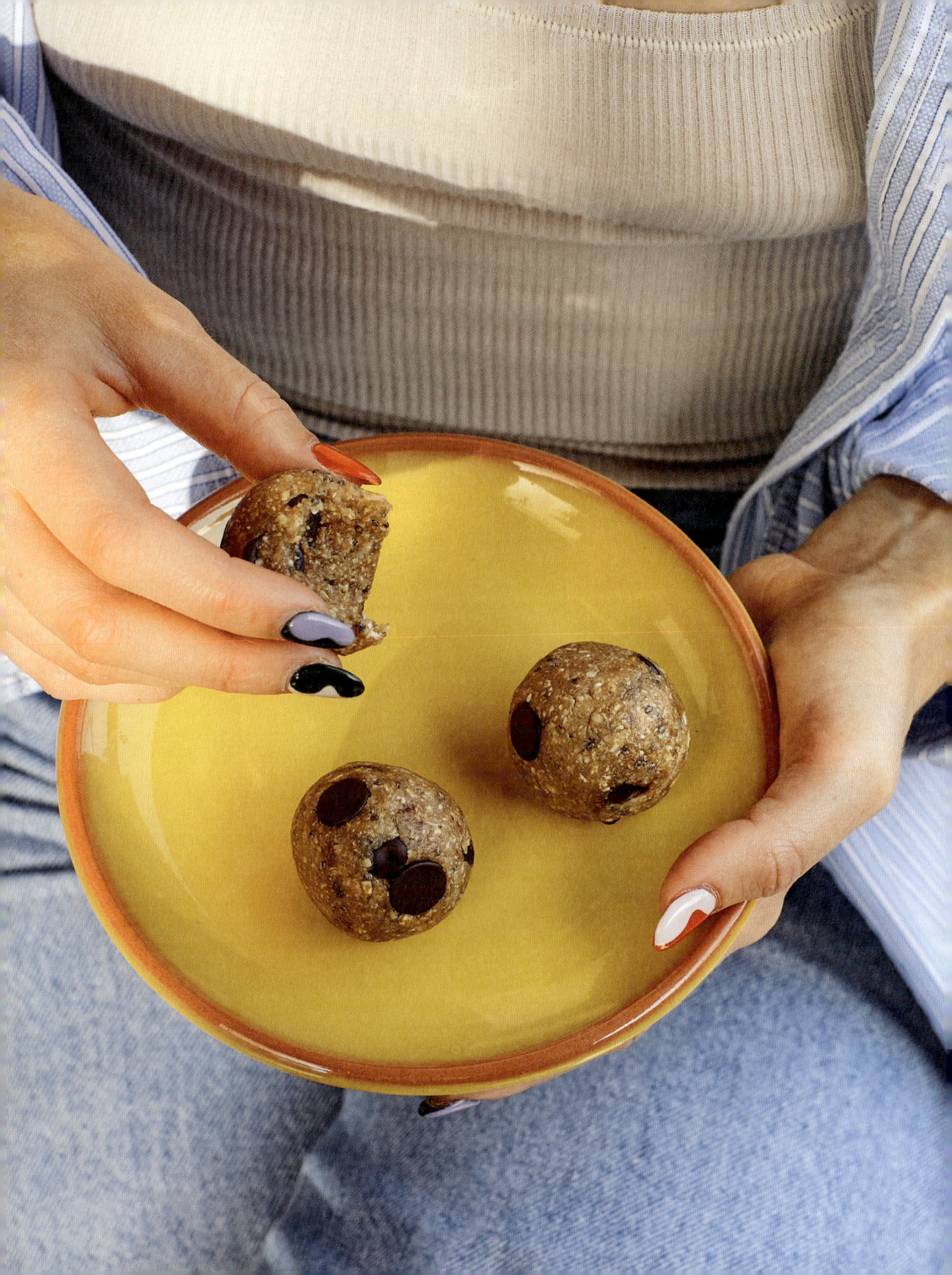

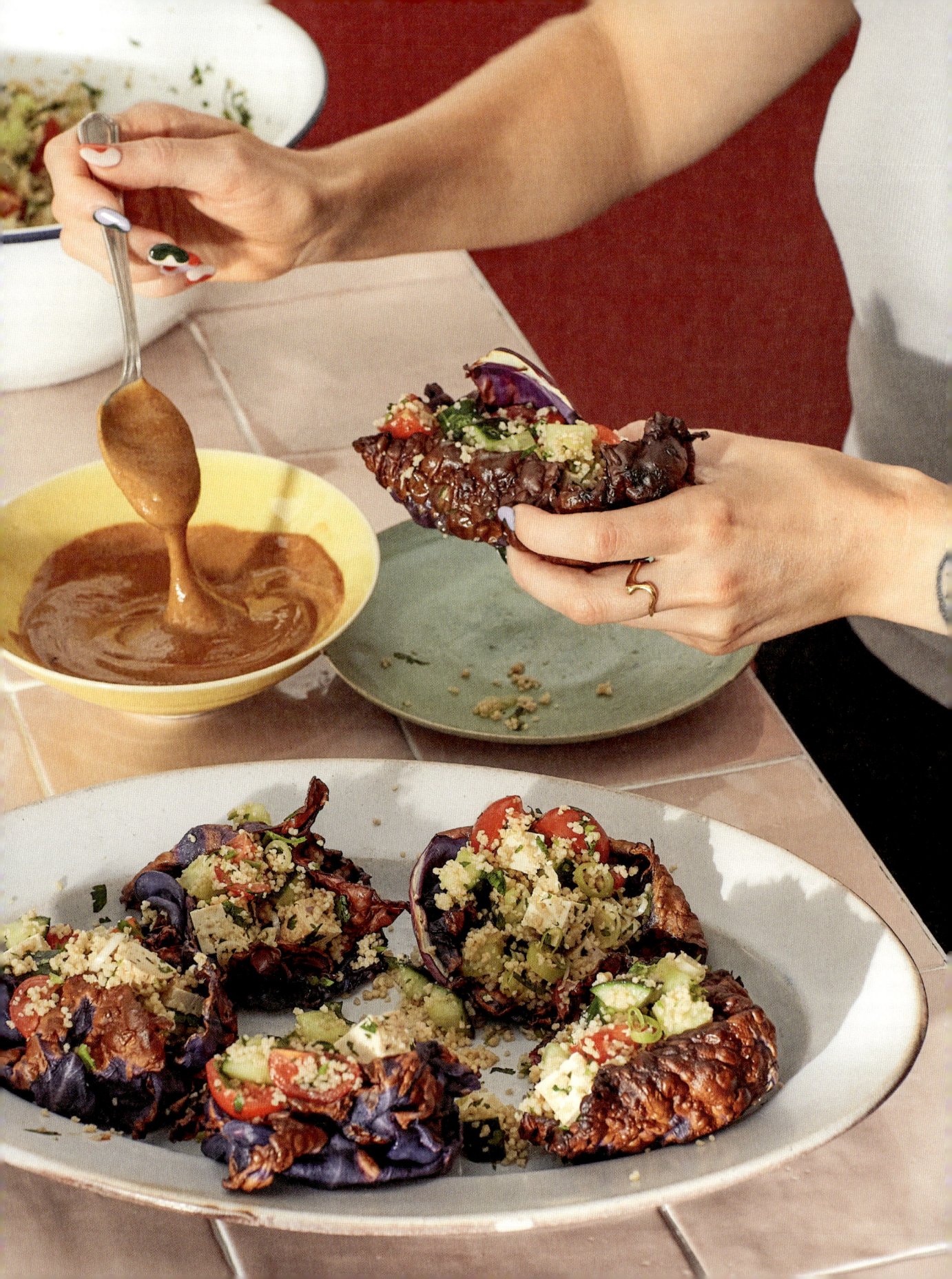

Crispy Red Cabbage Cups with Peanut Sauce

MAKES 3 SERVINGS
TOTAL TIME: 25 MINS

Red cabbage cups are the new lettuce cups. You heard it here first.

They crisp up at the top and add a beautiful texture to these snacks, which are also a great way of using any leftover salad bits you've got in the fridge.

Olive oil
6–8 red cabbage leaves
Salt

FOR THE FILLING
100g (3½oz) extra-firm smoked tofu, cut into small cubes
50g (1¾oz/⅓ cup) cooked wholemeal couscous
3 spring onions, white parts finely sliced
½ small cucumber, cut into small cubes
Small handful of cherry tomatoes, cut into quarters
Small handful of fresh coriander leaves, finely chopped
½ tbsp olive oil
Juice of ½ lemon
Pinch of sea salt

FOR THE PEANUT SAUCE
2 tbsp peanut butter
1 tbsp tamari
1 tbsp rice vinegar
1 tbsp warm water

Preheat the oven to 170°C fan/190°C/gas mark 5.

Oil the red cabbage leaves lightly, sprinkle with salt and roast for 15–20 minutes, until the ends start to crisp up (keep an eye on them). They will shrink considerably, this is normal!

In a mixing bowl, combine the filling ingredients and mix well. Season to taste.

In another, smaller bowl, combine the peanut sauce ingredients.

Serve the filling in the crispy cabbage cups and dip into the sauce before eating.

Protein per serving: 10g
Fibre: 6g
Plant diversity score: 11

Cheesy Flax Crackers and Smoky Red Lentil Dip

Great for lunchboxes, snacks or travelling! I love using the smoky red lentil dip as a sandwich spread, thinning it out into a soup, or even as a pasta sauce.

Cheesy Flax Crackers

MAKES AROUND 12 CRACKERS
TOTAL TIME: 30 MINS

80g (3oz) ground flaxseeds
50g (1¾oz/5 tbsp + 2 tsp) pumpkin seeds
30g (1oz/¼ cup) sesame seeds
2 tbsp nutritional yeast
⅓ tsp sea salt
6-7 twists of freshly ground black pepper
2 tbsp olive oil
50ml (2fl oz/3½ tbsp) warm water

Preheat the oven to 160°C fan/180°C/gas mark 4.

In a medium mixing bowl, combine the ground flax, pumpkin and sesame seeds, nutritional yeast, sea salt and black pepper.

Add the olive oil and water and mix together so it forms a rough dough. It should not be too sticky to hold or roll out, but not too dry that it's super crumbly. If it's too crumbly, add a touch more water; too wet, add a little more ground flax.

———

Cheesy flax crackers
Protein per serving: 3g
Fibre: 3g
Plant diversity score: 6

Smoky red lentil dip
Protein per serving: 5g
Fibre: 6g
Plant diversity score: 9

On a clean, flat surface, lay out a sheet of baking parchment, add the cracker mix on top, push it down a little, then add another sheet of parchment on top. Gently roll out the cracker mixture until it's about 2mm (⅛in) thick. If you want uniform crackers, lightly cut them into squares but don't pull them apart; they will snap easily after baking.

Bake for 18–20 minutes, or until the edges turn a shade darker.

Allow to cool completely, then snap into squares. Store in an airtight container at room temperature for up to 1 week.

Smoky Red Lentil Dip

MAKES 3 SERVINGS
TOTAL TIME: 45 MINS

1 shallot, finely chopped
Olive oil
3 garlic cloves, minced
1 tsp smoked paprika
1 tsp ground cumin
125g (4½oz/½ cup) split red lentils, drained and rinsed
3 sun-dried tomatoes
250ml (9fl oz/1 cup) vegetable stock
2 large roasted red bell peppers, from a jar
1 tbsp lemon juice
2 tbsp red wine vinegar
Sea salt and black pepper

In a medium saucepan on a medium heat, sauté the chopped shallot in olive oil with a pinch of sea salt for 5 minutes. Add the garlic, spices and a little more olive oil. Cook for another 3 minutes, then add the lentils. Cover the lentils really well in the aromatics, then

70

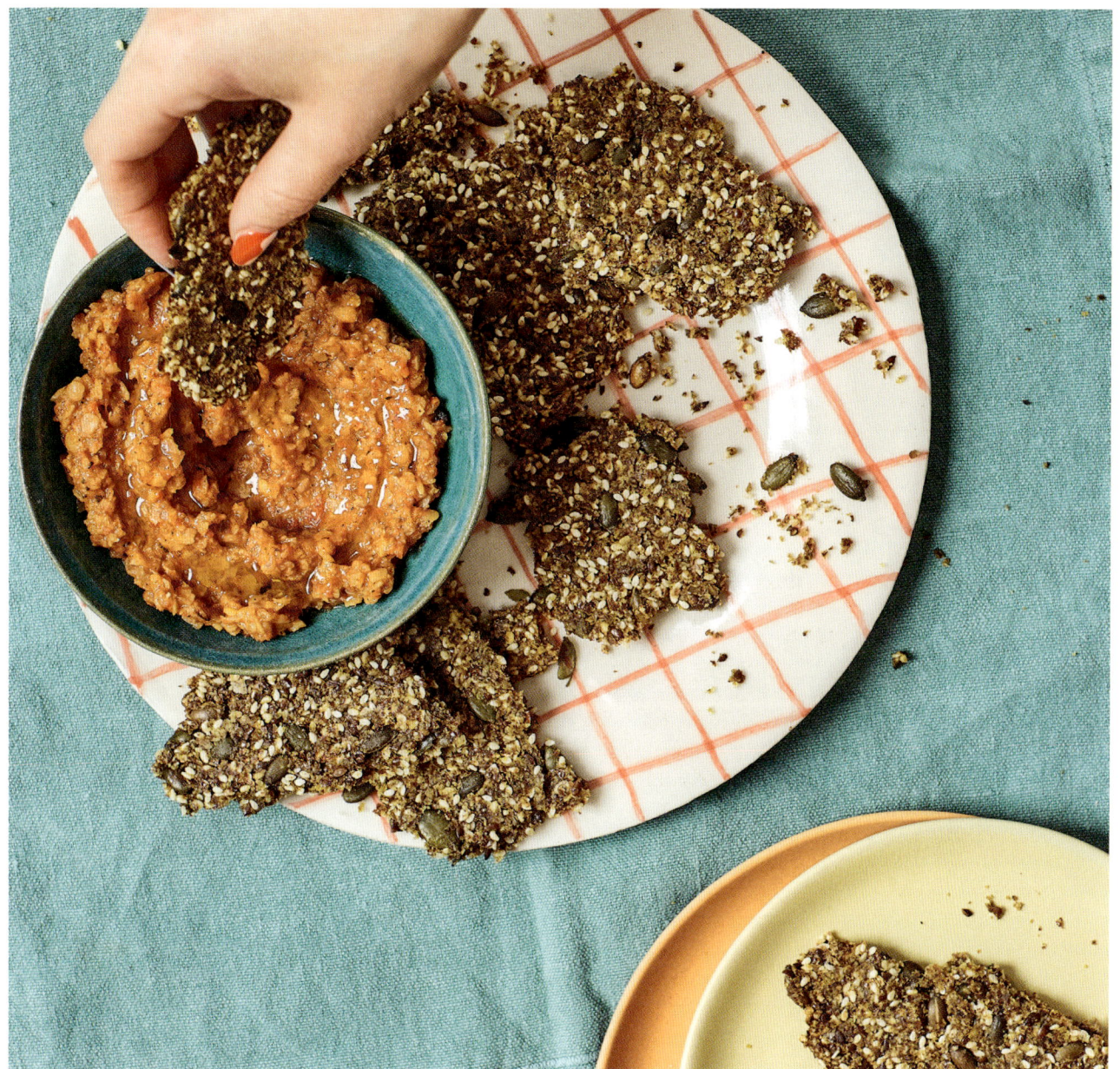

add the stock. Turn the heat up until the mix starts to bubble, stir well, then reduce the heat and simmer for about 15 minutes until the lentils are soft, and the water has been absorbed. Once cooked, take them off the heat and allow to cool.

Add the cooked and cooled lentil mix, the sun-dried tomatoes, the jarred red peppers, lemon juice, vinegar, ⅓ teaspoon of salt and some black pepper, then blend until a chunky texture is achieved. Drizzle a little olive oil while blending to help emulsify. Season to taste, pulsing again after adding more seasoning.

Serve with the crackers, veg sticks, or as a spread. You can also use this as a relish for barbecued veg.

NOTES
If you have some dip left over, use it for a sandwich spread, it goes really well with lettuce and smoked extra firm tofu slices!

Stewed Apple Protein Bread

MAKES 6 SLICES
TOTAL TIME: 20 MINS

A lighter protein snack, great for early mornings or a post-workout energy boost.

Feel free to sub any stewed fruit; get creative with what's in season! The basic mix should work with most drier fruits.

2 large Bramley apples
1 tsp ground cinnamon
80g (3oz/¾ cup) chickpea (gram) flour
50g spelt flour
1 tsp baking powder
Pinch of salt
1 scoop (30g/1oz) vanilla or salted caramel protein powder
200ml (7fl oz/¾ cup) soy milk
2 tbsp agave syrup
Small handful of walnuts, roughly chopped
2 tbsp hemp seeds
Small handful of sultanas
Sprinkle of coconut sugar, or light or dark brown sugar

Preheat the oven to 160°C fan/180°C/gas mark 4 and line a loaf tin or silicon mould with baking parchment.

Chop most of the apples into small 1–2cm (½–¾in) chunks. In a small, heavy-bottomed saucepan, slowly cook the apple with a splash of water and the cinnamon for around 10 minutes, until soft.

In a mixing bowl, add the flours, baking powder, salt and protein powder. Mix together, then add the soy milk and agave syrup and mix until combined. Stir through the walnuts, hemp seeds, sultanas and stewed apples.

Pour into the lined tin and sprinkle with the coconut sugar. Bake for 18–20 minutes, or until the sugar starts to caramelise.

Take out the oven and leave to cool completely, before cutting into slices. Keeps for up to 4 days in an airtight container in the fridge.

Protein per slice: 9.5g
Fibre: 5g
Plant diversity score: 9.5

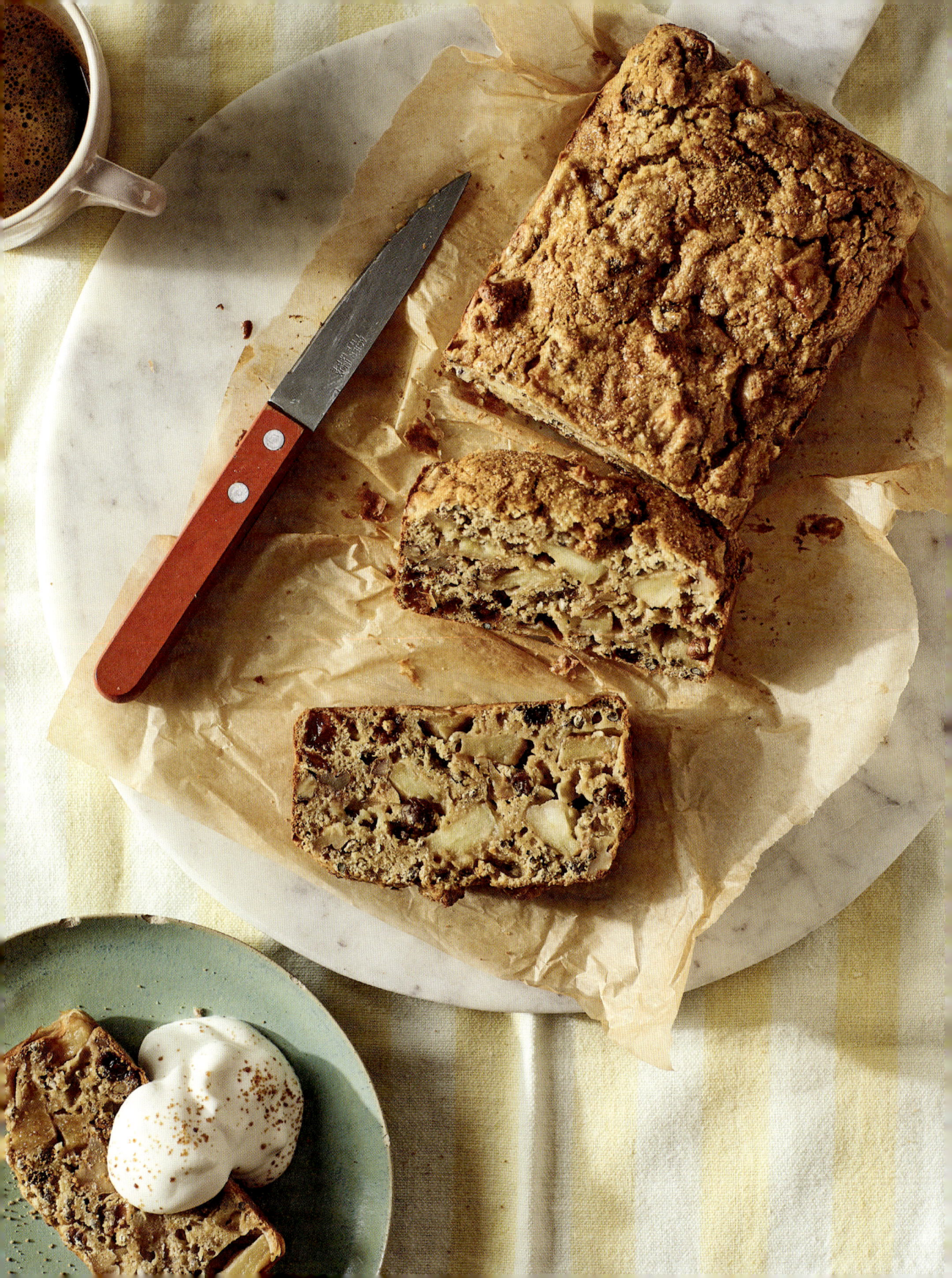

Banging Buckwheat Banana Bread

MAKES 6 SLICES
TOTAL TIME: 50 MINS

Without doubt, I always have a variation of this loaf on the go and keep some in the freezer for emergencies. It's extremely satiating, travels well and tastes incredible toasted with peanut butter.

We always bring a few slices to airports when flying, to avoid the dreaded plane snack options. So I can confirm, no issues with security.

FOR THE DRY INGREDIENTS
130g (4½oz/1 cup) buckwheat or plain flour
135g (4¾oz/1 cup) rolled oats
1 tsp ground cinnamon
1 tsp baking powder
50g (1¾oz/scant ½ cup) cacao powder
3 tbsp hemp seeds
Large handful of chopped walnuts or almonds

FOR THE WET INGREDIENTS
3 ripe bananas
1 tbsp lemon juice
3 tbsp maple syrup or 3 Medjool dates, pitted
2 tbsp chia seeds soaked in 4 tbsp water
125ml (4½fl oz/½ cup) plant milk
80ml (3fl oz/⅓ cup) melted coconut oil
¼ tsp salt
1 tsp vanilla extract (optional)

TO DECORATE
Sliced banana
Sprinkle of sugar
Hemp seeds

Preheat the oven to 175°C fan/195°C/gas mark 5½.

In a medium mixing bowl, combine all the dry ingredients, except the seeds and nuts.

In a blender cup, measure the wet ingredients and blend until fairly smooth. The mix should be wet enough to fall slowly off a spoon. If it's not, add a little more plant milk.

Pour the wet ingredients into the dry, fold in the seeds and nuts. Mix until just combined, top with sliced banana and sugar, then pour into a loaf tin and bake for 40 minutes, or until a knife/toothpick comes out almost clean.

Serve a thick slice with peanut butter and berries.

It will keep in an airtight container or wrapped for up to 1 week, at room temperature.

Protein per slice: 8.5g
Fibre: 11g
Plant diversity score: 10

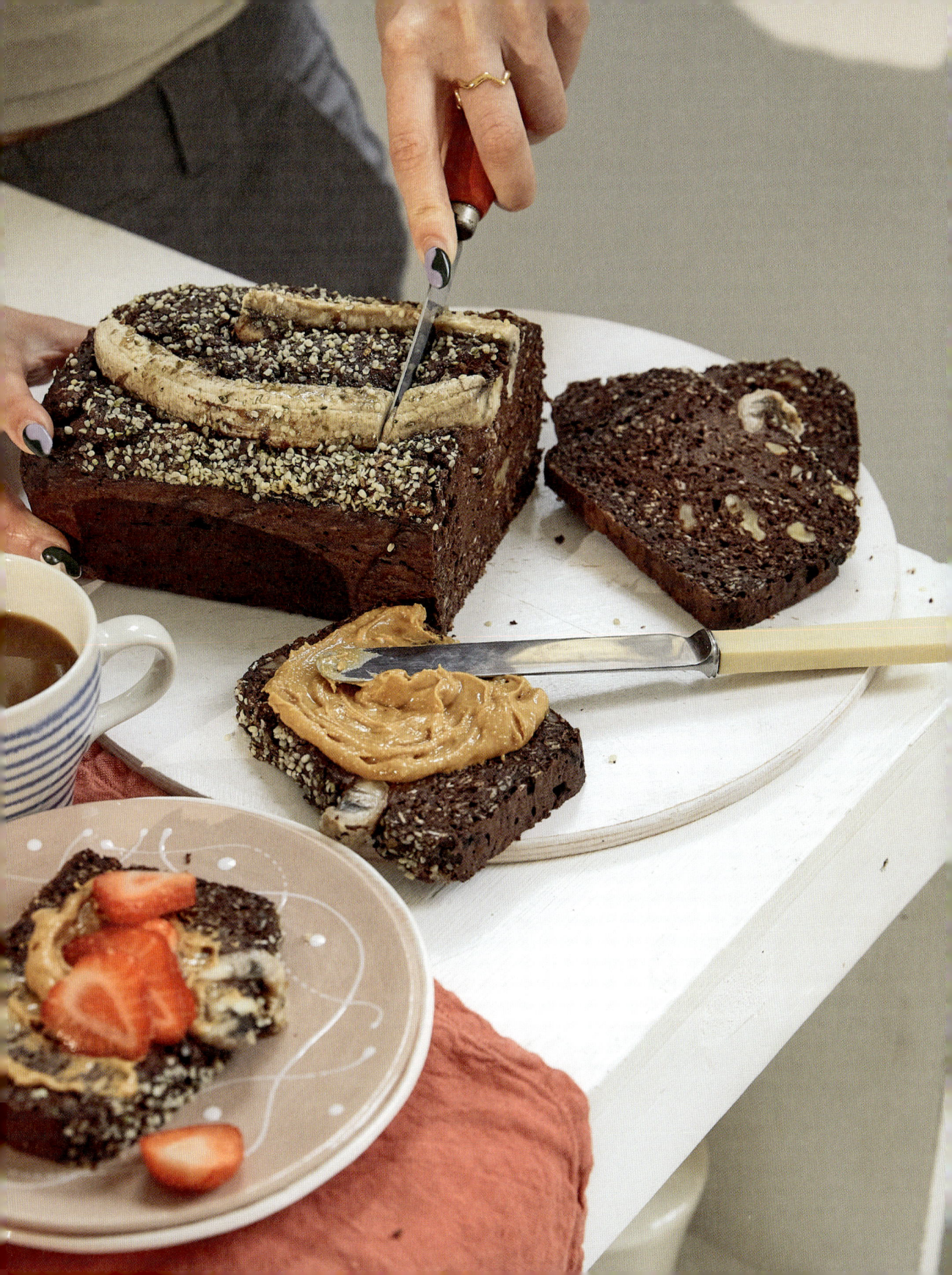

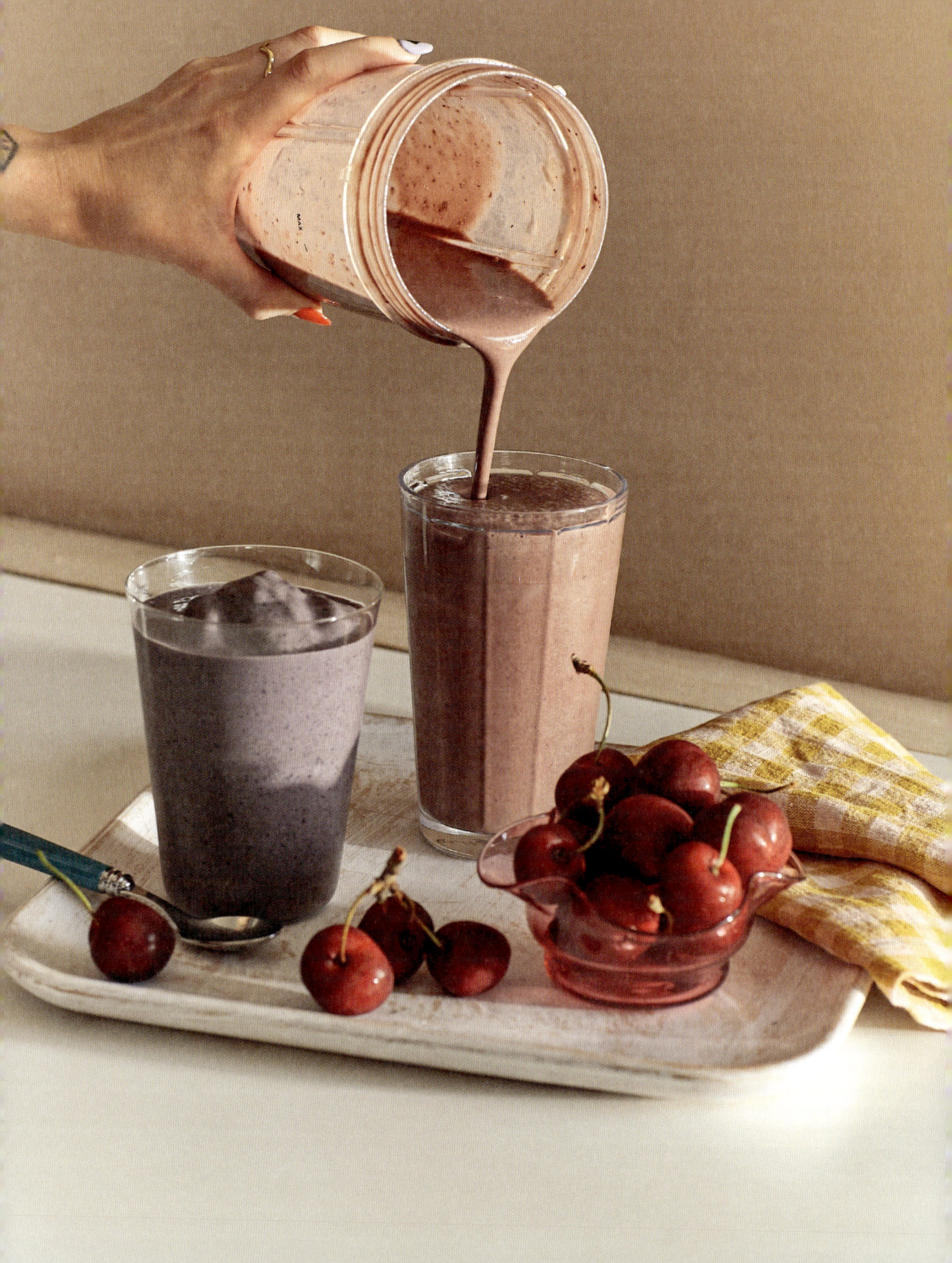

Blue Zone Smoothie

MAKES 1
TOTAL TIME: 5 MINS

Blue Zones are defined as regions of the world where people tend to live longer than the average person, maintaining good health, so naturally there has been some investigation and documentation into how they do this, and what they eat! According to Blue Zone experts, you can't go wrong with spinach and blueberries in a smoothie. Cinnamon adds natural sweetness without added sugar.

I've added a banana and peanut butter to bulk this out into more of a filling snack, but feel free to omit.

½ small banana
2 nests of frozen spinach
Small handful of blueberries
1 scoop (30g/1oz) vanilla vegan protein powder
½ tsp ground cinnamon
½ tbsp crunchy or smooth peanut butter
Juice of ½ lemon
100ml (3½fl oz/scant ½ cup) soy milk
Small handful of ice cubes

Add everything to a blender and blend until super smooth! Pour into a glass and enjoy.

Protein per smoothie: 28g
Fibre: 9g
Plant diversity score: 6

Sweet Cherry Chocolate Smoothie

MAKES 1
TOTAL TIME: 5 MINS

Who doesn't love cherries? They're juicy, sweet, tart, full of vitamins, minerals and more. Get your fix in this delicious cherry chocolate combo.

Handful of frozen or fresh cherries
2 tbsp soy yoghurt
1 Medjool date, pitted
1 tbsp cacao powder
1 scoop (30g/1oz) chocolate vegan protein powder
100ml (3½fl oz/scant ½ cup) soy milk

Add everything to a blender, and blend until super smooth! Pour into a glass and enjoy.

Protein per smoothie: 26g
Fibre: 7g
Plant diversity score: 5

Crispy Roasted Legumes

MAKES 6–10 SERVINGS
TOTAL TIME: 25 MINS

Great crispy snacks to munch on between meals or use as meal toppers! They go especially well on salads.

240g (8½oz) lentils, chickpeas or any other bean, from a can or jar, drained, rinsed and dried very well
1 tbsp olive oil
½ tsp salt
1 tsp spices, such as smoked paprika, ground cumin or coriander (all optional)

Preheat the oven to 200°C fan/220°C/gas mark 7.

Rinse and dry the legumes very well, using a tea towel or kitchen paper. The drier they are, the crispier they will get. Line a large baking tray with baking parchment or a silicone mat, then add the legumes, olive oil, salt and spices (if using) and combine very well.

Bake for 12–20 minutes, or until crispy and turning a shade of golden brown (where applicable). Smaller legumes (lentils) will need less time than chickpeas or butter beans. Don't be surprised if the beans you're roasting start to pop, that's normal. I recommend getting them out halfway through the roasting time and giving them a good toss around so they bake evenly.

When crisped up, let them cool on the side for 30 minutes, then store them in an airtight jar or container at room temperature for up to 10 days.

Protein and fibre per serving (4 servings each legume)

Chickpeas – Protein: 4g Fibre: 4.5g
Puy lentils – Protein: 6.5g Fibre: 4.25g
Beluga lentils – Protein: 3.5g Fibre: 4.25g
Butter beans – Protein: 6.5g Fibre: 4.25g

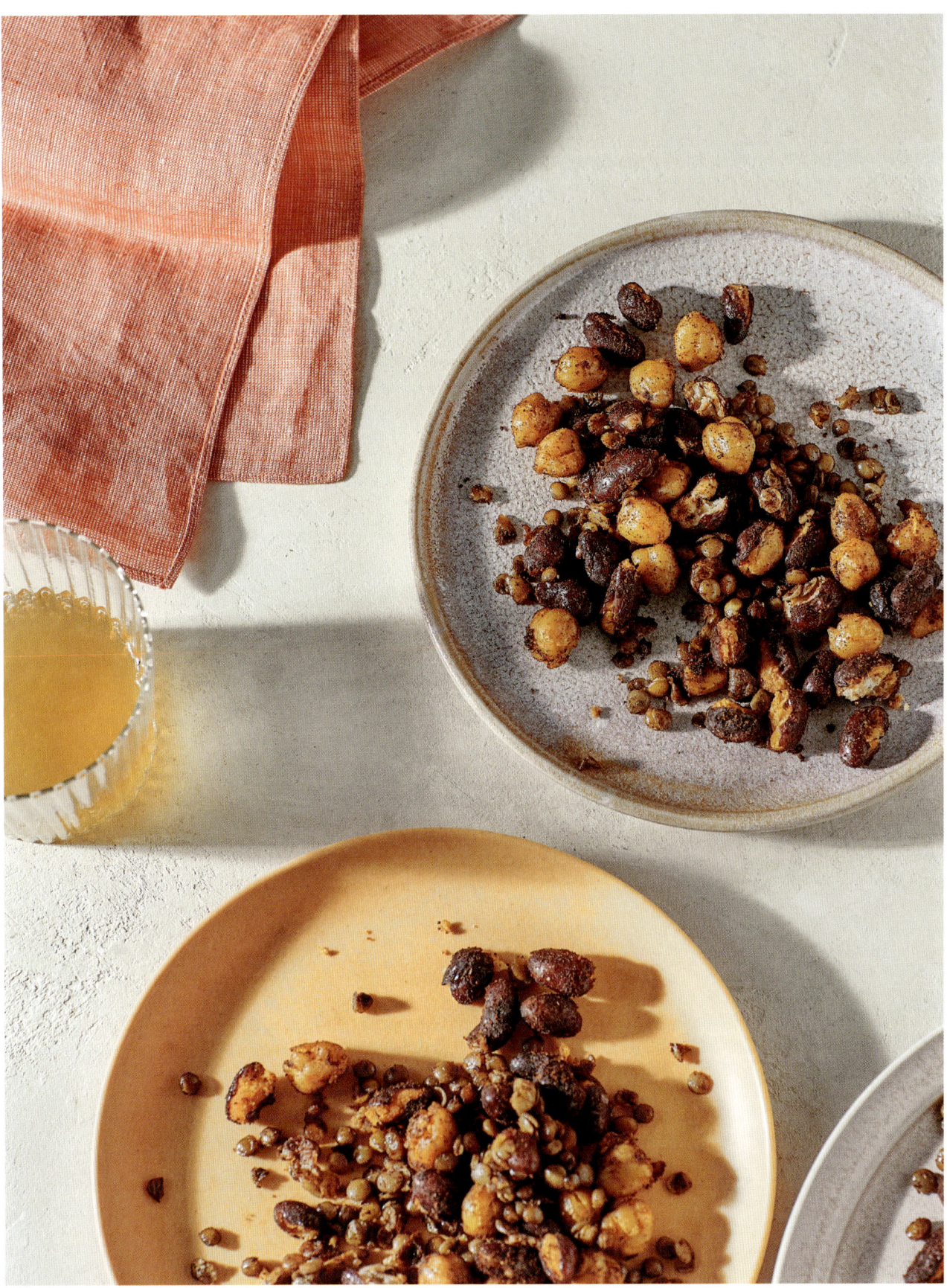

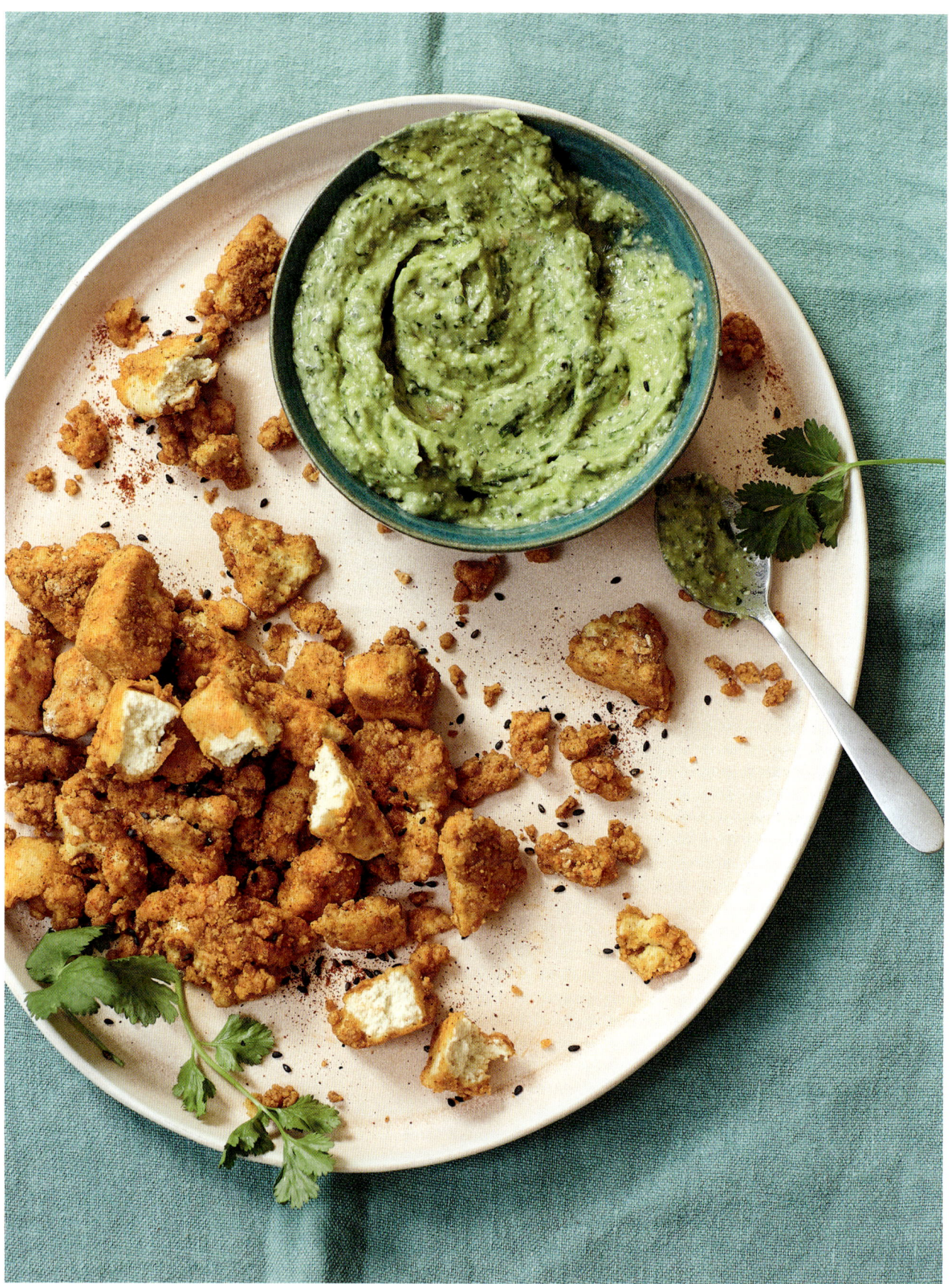

Tofu Nuggets

SERVES 3
TOTAL TIME: 25 MINS

The perfect mix of protein and healthy fats for a midday snack, the nuggets can also go on top of pastas to amp up the protein content.

You can use an air fryer for the nuggets, if you have one!

FOR THE CRISPY TOFU
200g (7oz) extra-firm tofu
Olive oil, for drizzling
30g (1oz/¼ cup) chickpea (gram) flour
1 tbsp cornflour
1 tsp smoked paprika
1 tsp ground cumin
1 tsp sea salt
Black pepper

FOR THE HERBY GREEN AVO SAUCE
1 ripe avocado
30g (1oz) fresh herbs (I used coriander and chives)
2 garlic cloves
2 tbsp hemp seeds
½ tsp sea salt, plus more to taste
1½ tbsp apple cider vinegar or lemon juice
1 tbsp extra virgin olive oil
1–2 tbsp water

Preheat the oven to 170°C fan/190°C/gas mark 5.

Wrap the tofu in kitchen paper and give it a good squeeze to remove any excess water.

In a bowl, tear the tofu into rough 2cm (¾in) pieces with your hands. Drizzle with 1 tablespoon of olive oil and toss to coat.

In another bowl, add the chickpea flour, cornflour, spices and seasoning. Add the tofu and toss to coat, then place on a baking tray, drizzle with a little more olive oil and bake for 20 minutes, or until golden (or spray with olive oil and pop in your air fryer!).

In a small blender, whizz up all the sauce ingredients until smooth. Season to taste.

Serve the crispy tofu on a plate next to the sauce.

Tofu nuggs
Protein per serving: 12g
Fibre: 2.5g
Plant diversity score: 3

Avo sauce
Protein per serving: 4.3g
Fibre: 2.3g
Plant diversity score: 3

Salads and Power Bowls

This chapter is all about meal prep-able, easily transportable bowls of nutrient-dense, protein-packed goodness. Most don't need heating up, or cooking, aside from searing the odd triangle of tofu or tempeh, or batch cooking some grains. On the topic of grains, you'll notice a few common themes. I like to buy wholegrain versions for added protein and fibre.

   I love using super-firm tofu for these recipes – it keeps its shape, is easy to prep and holds flavour really well. You'll also notice I love mixing grains with ready-cooked lentils or beans, as it's a cheap and easy way to bump up your protein intake and keep things tasty and interesting.

Triple Glow Bowl with Walnut Pesto Chickpeas, Quinoa and Tofu Feta

MAKES 4 PORTIONS
TOTAL TIME: 30 MINS
FRIDGE LIFE: 3–4 DAYS

Pesto chickpeas are an instant winner here. Paired with a healthy portion of quinoa and lentils, and a tangy, creamy hit of protein from the tofu feta, this dish is a delight that will get you well on your way to hitting those protein targets.

250g (9oz/1¼ cups) tricolour quinoa
½ tbsp vegetable bouillon powder or ½ vegetable stock cube
240g (8½oz) cooked green or Puy lentils
200g (7oz) extra-firm tofu
Juice of 1½ lemons
4 tbsp olive oil
1 tbsp dried oregano
1½ tsp sea salt
3 tbsp nutritional yeast
50g (1¾oz/½ cup) walnuts
75g (2½oz) kale leaves, stripped from stems
2 garlic cloves
30g (1oz) fresh basil
2 x 400g (14oz) cans chickpeas, drained and rinsed

TO SERVE
Quick-pickled Red Onion (see page 206)
Omega-3 Boost (see page 209)

NOTES
Swap the tofu for fried red lentil or chickpea tofu (page 210-211) to make this soy free!

Protein per portion: 28g
Fibre: 16g
Plant diversity score: 10

Start with the quinoa. Dissolve the vegetable powder or stock cube in boiling water (the ratio of water to quinoa is generally 2:1), then add the quinoa and cook according to the packet instructions. Once cooked, stir in the cooked lentils.

Give the tofu a gentle squeeze in kitchen paper to drain off any excess water. Chop into small cubes, roughly 5mm–1cm (¼–½in). Add to a bowl with 1 tablespoon of the lemon juice, 1 tablespoon of the olive oil, the oregano, ½ teaspoon of the salt and 2 tablespoons of the nutritional yeast and give it a good stir. Set aside in the fridge while you prepare the pesto.

Crumble the walnuts into a dry frying pan with your hands, then toast for 3–4 minutes, moving regularly, until they turn brown and start to smell heavenly. Take off the heat and allow them to cool for a few minutes.

Add the kale leaves to a colander or sieve. Boil some water and pour it over them, then rinse the leaves under the cold tap, squeeze them to remove any excess water and add them to a bullet blender, along with the toasted walnuts, garlic, remaining nutritional yeast, olive oil, salt, lemon juice and basil. Pulse a few times until a chunky texture forms, scraping down the sides as needed and adding a little water to help it blend if necessary. Season to taste.

In a small bowl, combine the walnut pesto with the chickpeas.

Assemble your bowls or meal prep containers, quinoa and lentil mix first, then the walnut pesto chickpeas, then the tofu feta. Top with the pickled red onion and omega-3 seed boost.

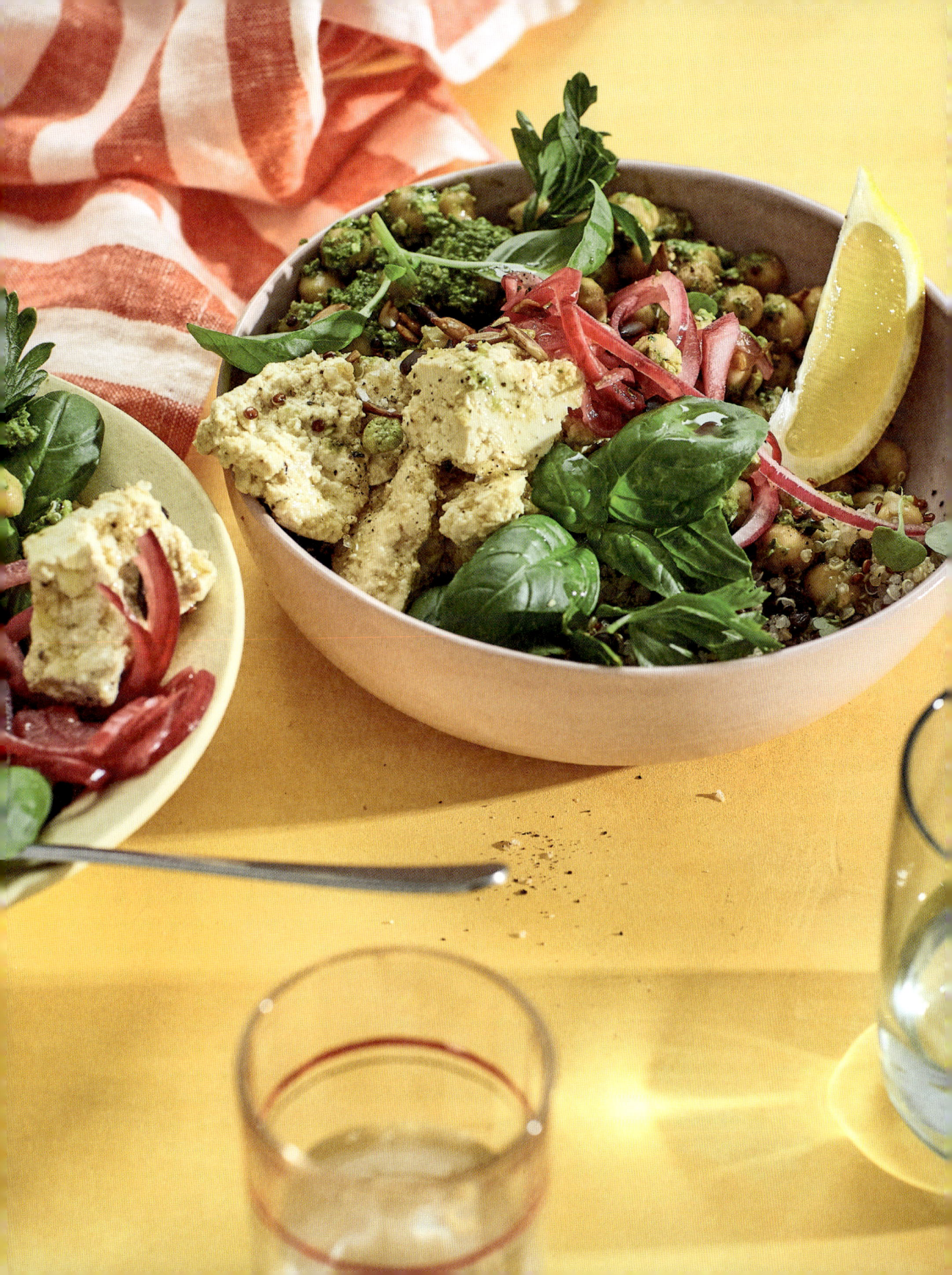

Lazy Lentil Chimichurri Pasta Salad

MAKES 4 SERVINGS
TOTAL TIME: 20 MINS
FRIDGE LIFE: 3–4 DAYS

Originating in Argentina, Chimichurri sauce is usually served with meat. Here, I'm combining it with lentil pasta and puy lentils to make a flavoursome, nutrient dense pasta salad.

There's loads of protein in Puy lentils; I like buying them in ready-cooked pouches for ease. Lentil pasta also packs a punch; you can pick this up from larger supermarkets or your local health food store.

300g (10½oz) dried lentil pasta
60ml (4 tbsp) extra virgin olive oil
2½ tbsp red wine vinegar
3 fat garlic cloves, minced
15g (½oz) chopped fresh parsley
20g (¾oz) chopped fresh coriander
1–2 tbsp finely chopped red chillies (omit or reduce if you don't like spice)
1 tsp salt, plus more to taste
3 large handfuls of rocket leaves (about 80g/2¾oz)
240g (8½oz) cooked Puy lentils
150g (5½oz) cherry tomatoes, quartered
1 tbsp dried oregano

TO SERVE
Omega-3 Boost (see page 209)
Chopped fresh coriander and parsley

Cook the pasta in plenty of salty water for 1 minute less than the packet instructions.

Now, make the chimichurri sauce. In a small/medium bowl, mix the olive oil, vinegar, garlic, fresh chopped herbs, chillies, and salt. Combine well, season to taste, adding a little more vinegar or salt if you think it needs it (I added a touch more salt).

Add the cooked, drained pasta to a large bowl, then tip in the rocket, lentils, tomatoes, and the chimichurri sauce. Toss until well combined, divide between bowls or meal prep containers. Top with the Omega-3 Boost and fresh herbs.

Protein per portion: 20g
Fibre per portion: 9g
Plant diversity score: 8.5

NOTES
Add Tofu Stracciatella-style Balls to bump up the protein and make it creamier (page 222)

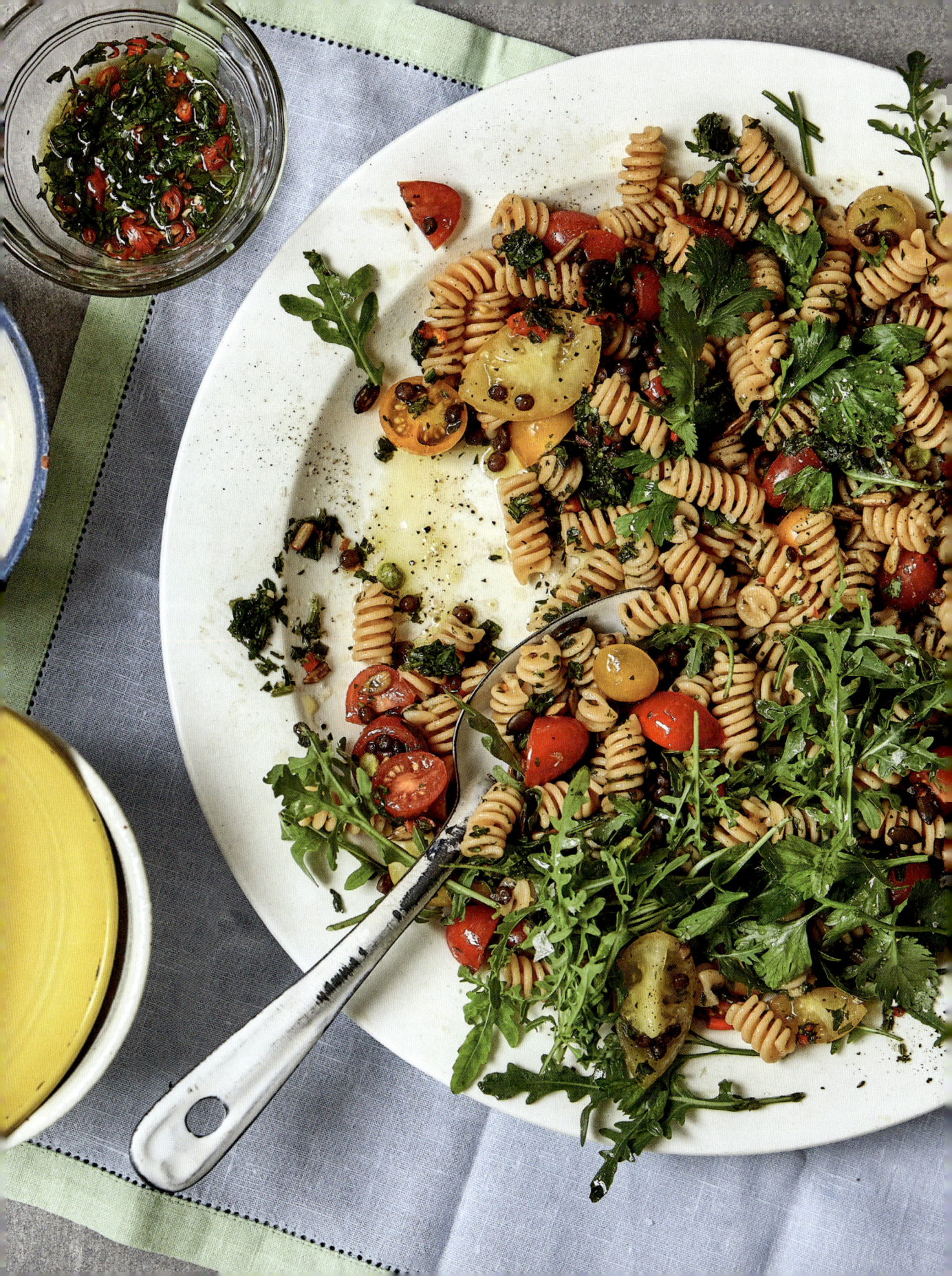

Mango, Avo and Tofu Macro Bowl

MAKES 3 SERVINGS
TOTAL TIME: 35 MINS
FRIDGE LIFE: 3–4 DAYS

Inspired by a Lisbon café, Comoba, this delightful rainbow salad reminds me of hazy summer days in Lisbon, sipping coffee and watching the imperfect sprawl of washed pastel buildings glow against the unusually blue sky.

1 large leek
3 garlic cloves
100g (3½oz/½ cup) quinoa
200ml (7fl oz/¾ cup) vegetable stock
150g (5½oz) red cabbage
Juice of 1 lime
300g (11oz) extra-firm tofu
3 tbsp cornflour
2 tbsp olive oil
2 tbsp tamari
Quick Blender Hummus (see page 214)
3 tbsp sauerkraut or kimchi
1 ripe mango
1½ ripe avocados
Sea salt

FOR THE PEANUT SAUCE
2 tbsp smooth peanut butter
1 tbsp tamari
1 tbsp rice vinegar
Juice of ½ lime

Rinse the leek well, cut in half from top to bottom, and place the halves cut side down and slice into 5mm (¼in) half-moons. Mince the garlic.

In a heavy-bottomed saucepan on a medium heat, fry the leek for 5 minutes until softening, then add the garlic and cook for a further 2 minutes. Rinse the quinoa grains, then add them to the leek and the garlic. Stir well to combine, toast for a further 60 seconds, then add the vegetable stock. Bring to the boil, reduce to a simmer, then cover with a lid, leaving about a 2.5cm (1in) gap until the quinoa is cooked (you'll see the spiral separates from the grain). Take off the heat and set aside whilst you prep the rest.

Slice the cabbage in half, then place one half cut-side down and slice it widthways, very finely, until you have thin strips. Put the strips into a bowl, pour over the lime juice, add a pinch of sea salt and gently massage with your hands until it starts to soften. Set aside while you prep the rest of the bowl.

Press the tofu with kitchen paper to remove any excess water. Slice lengthways into slices around 1cm (½in) in width, then slice these diagonally into triangles. Grab a bowl, add the cornflour, a pinch of sea salt and stir to combine, then gently place each triangle into the bowl one-by-one, making sure the cornflour evenly covers the entire triangle. Lay these out on a plate near the hob, ready to fry.

Once all covered, heat the olive oil in a large sauté pan on a medium-high heat. Shallow-fry the tofu triangles for a few minutes on each side, until golden and crispy. If your pan is not big enough to fit all the triangles, you'll have to cook them in batches. Once lightly golden, drizzle the tamari over the tofu and fry until the darker liquid has almost all evaporated. Remove carefully and place on a plate lined with kitchen paper.

In a small bowl, add all the peanut sauce ingredients and whisk together.

Swoosh 2 tablespoons of hummus into each bowl, then pile in the quinoa and leek mix, the red cabbage, tofu triangles, peanut sauce, tortilla chips, kimchi or sauerkraut, then finely slice both the mango and avocado. Carefully transfer them to a wide knife and slide them onto your plate.

Sprinkle some black sesame seeds on the mango and avocados, garnish with a lime wedge, and enjoy!

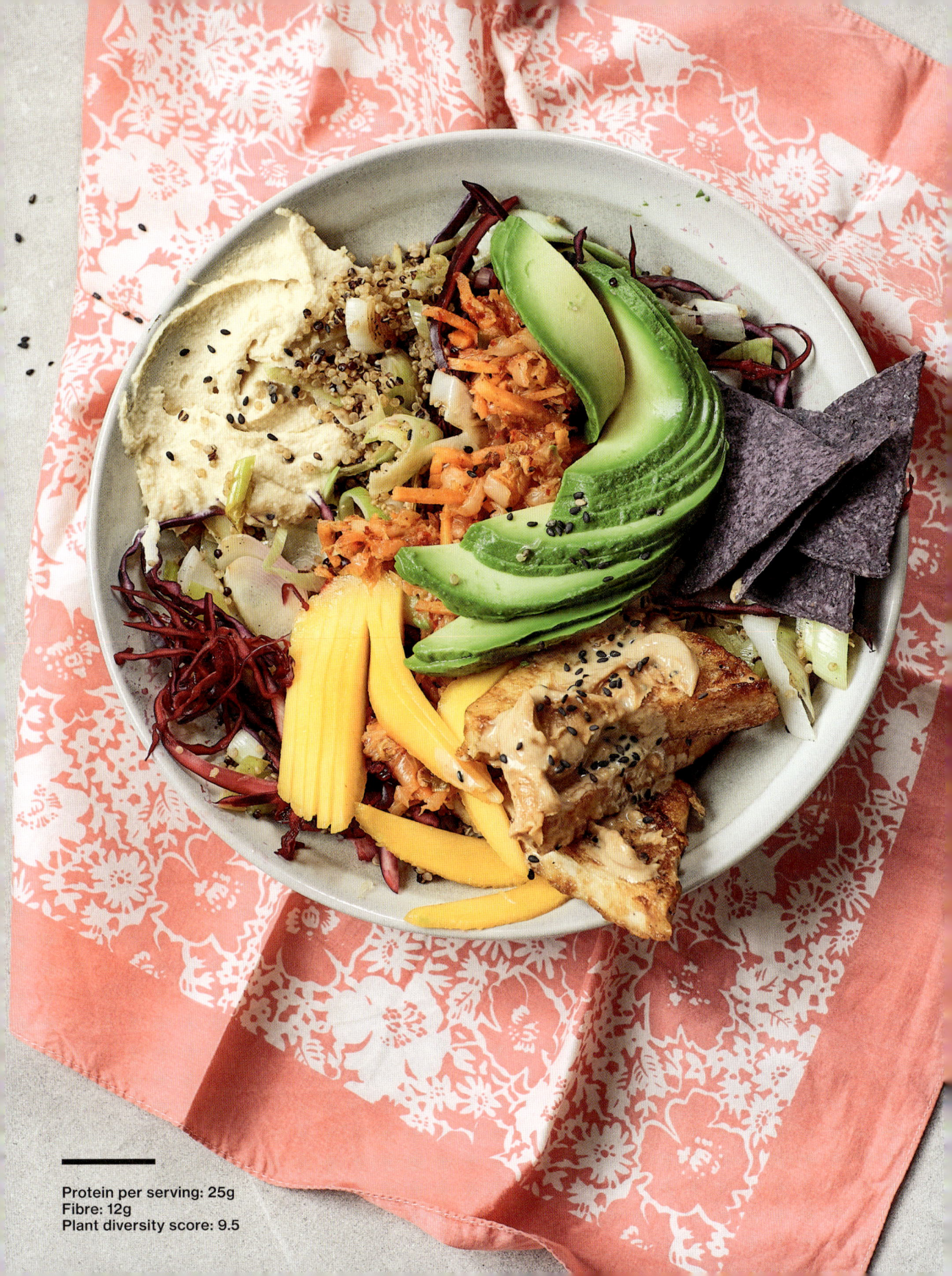

Protein per serving: 25g
Fibre: 12g
Plant diversity score: 9.5

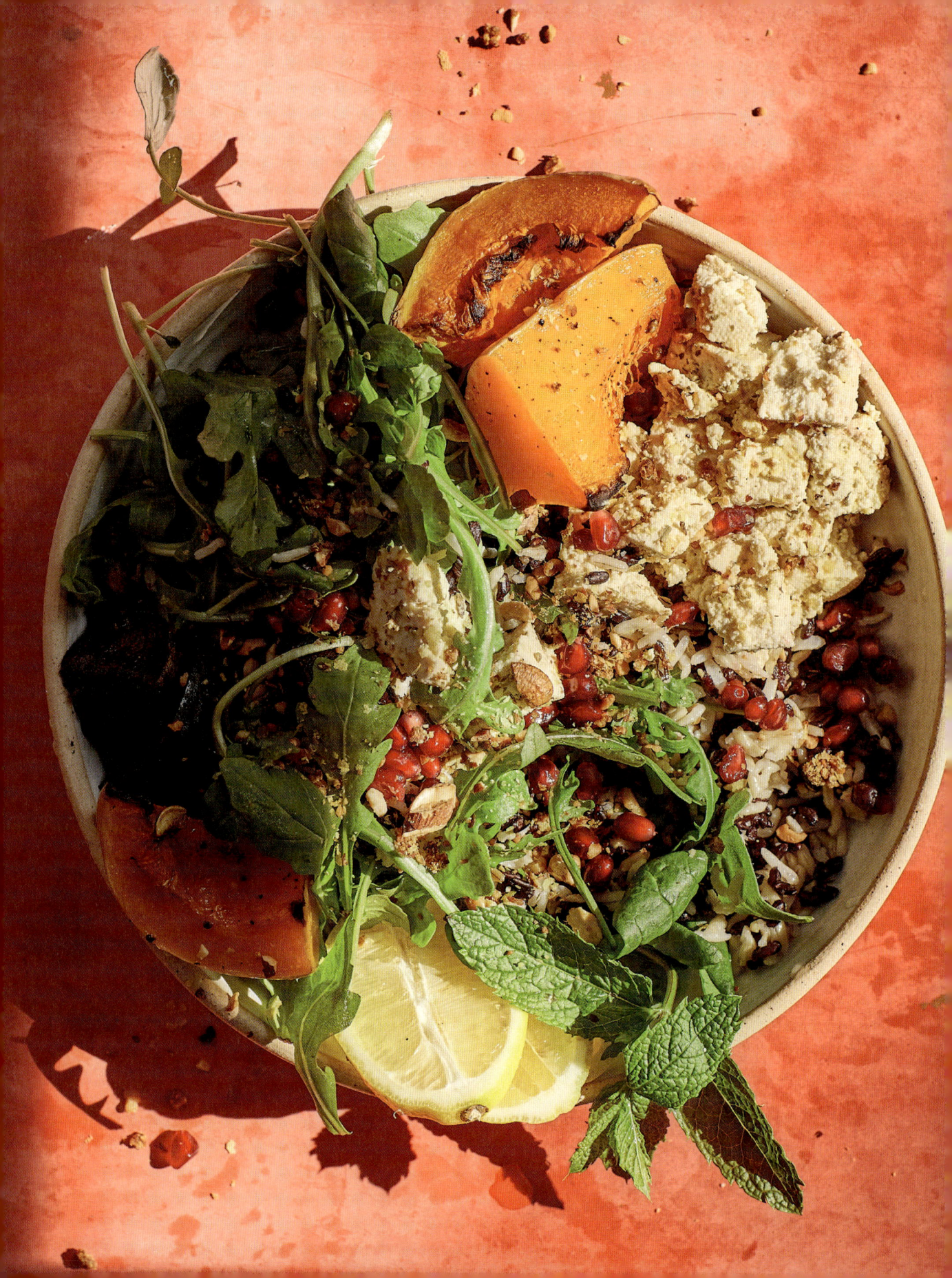

Nourishing Winter
Wild Rice Salad

SERVES 3
TOTAL TIME: 45 MINS
FRIDGE LIFE: 3–4 DAYS

Roasted squash + tofu feta + mint + pomegranate on a bed of black rice with crispy, seedy, noochy crumb. It's everything you want in a winter salad. Hearty goodness with a hint of summer come-soon.

I rarely peel my squash, if organic; I love the nutty flavour of the skin, which is also full of dietary fibre.

200g (7oz/1 cup) wild black rice
½ tsp vegetable bouillon powder
300g (10½oz) butternut squash
2 tbsp extra virgin olive oil
Salt and black pepper

FOR THE TOFU FETA
100g per serving (see page 220)

FOR THE NUTTY, NOOCHY CRUMB
1 tbsp per serving (see page 208)

FOR THE ROCKET AND BEETROOT SALAD
Rocket
Cooked beetroot cubes
1 tbsp extra virgin olive oil
2 tbsp lemon juice
½ tsp sea salt
5–6 twists of fresh black pepper
Sprinkle of pomegranate seeds
Fresh mint

Preheat the oven to 200°C fan/220°C/gas mark 7.

Rinse the rice very well and cook according to the packet instructions, adding the vegetable bouillon powder to the water for extra flavour.

While that's cooking, chop the squash into irregular 1–2cm (½–¾in) shapes and add to a baking dish with the oil and salt and pepper. Pop into the oven to roast for 30–35 minutes, or until the edges are beginning to brown and turn crispy.

Whilst that's roasting, prep the Tofu Feta (page 220) and the Nutty, Nooch Crumb (page 208)

To a large bowl, add the rocket leaves and cubed beetroot. Drizzle over the extra virgin olive oil, sea salt, black pepper and lemon juice, then gently toss together. Season to taste.

Assemble the bowls or containers rice first, then the rocket and beetroot salad, tofu feta, nutty, noochy crumb and top with the pomegranate seeds and fresh mint.

Protein per serving: 22g
Fibre: 8.7g
Plant diversity score: 10

NOTES
Add more tofu feta to up the protein intake

Roasted Cabbage and Bean Salad with Creamy Tahini Dressing

MAKES 3 SERVINGS
TOTAL TIME: 25 MINS
FRIDGE LIFE: 3–4 DAYS

A bowl full of texture. This started life as a shredded cabbage salad, but I felt it wasn't showing the cabbage off in its true star form. Roasted cabbage wedges, although simple, are one of my favourite things to eat. Add a creamy tahini dressing and I'll simply pass away.

200g (7oz/1¼ cups) buckwheat, or other grain of choice
½ vegetable stock cube or ½ tsp vegetable bouillon powder
700g (1lb 9oz) butter beans, from a jar or can, drained and rinsed
100g (3½oz) cooked puy lentils
75g (2½oz) rocket
1 medium sweetheart cabbage
1 medium cucumber, seeds removed and chopped into half-moons
1 fresh red chilli, sliced or chilli flakes, to serve (optional)
50g (1¾oz) Omega-3 Boost (see page 209)
Olive oil
Sea salt

FOR THE GINGER LIME DRESSING
Juice of 2 limes (about 3½ tbsp)
4 tbsp extra virgin olive oil
2cm (¾in) piece of fresh ginger, peeled and minced
1 tsp garlic powder
1 tsp grated shallot (use a Microplane)
1 heaped tbsp brown miso paste
2 tbsp good-quality runny tahini
Pinch of sea salt, more to taste

Preheat your oven to 200°C fan/220°C/gas mark 7.

Chop your sweetheart cabbage into wedges; slice them in half lengthways, then again into quarters. Place them on a baking tray and drizzle with olive oil, sprinkle with sea salt. Cover with foil and bake for 15 minutes, then remove the foil and cook for a further 10-12 minutes, until the cabbage is starting to brown in places and the undersides (if you lift them carefully) are beautifully brown on the edge of each layer.

Now cook your buckwheat or grain of choice. In a small/medium saucepan, dissolve the stock in 400ml (14fl oz/generous 1½ cups) water, pour in the buckwheat and cook according to the packet instructions. Once cooked, allow to cool.

In a small bowl, whisk all the dressing ingredients together. Season to taste.

Add all the beans, rocket, cucumber, lentils and cooked buckwheat to a large mixing bowl and pour over half the dressing. Toss well, divide into bowls or containers, then top with the roasted cabbage wedges, drizzle over the remaining dressing and sprinkle the chilli (if using) and omega-3.

Protein per serving: 25g
Fibre: 17g
Plant diversity score: 12

NOTES
Add Tofu Feta or a Nutty, Noochy Crumb to boost the protein (page 208)

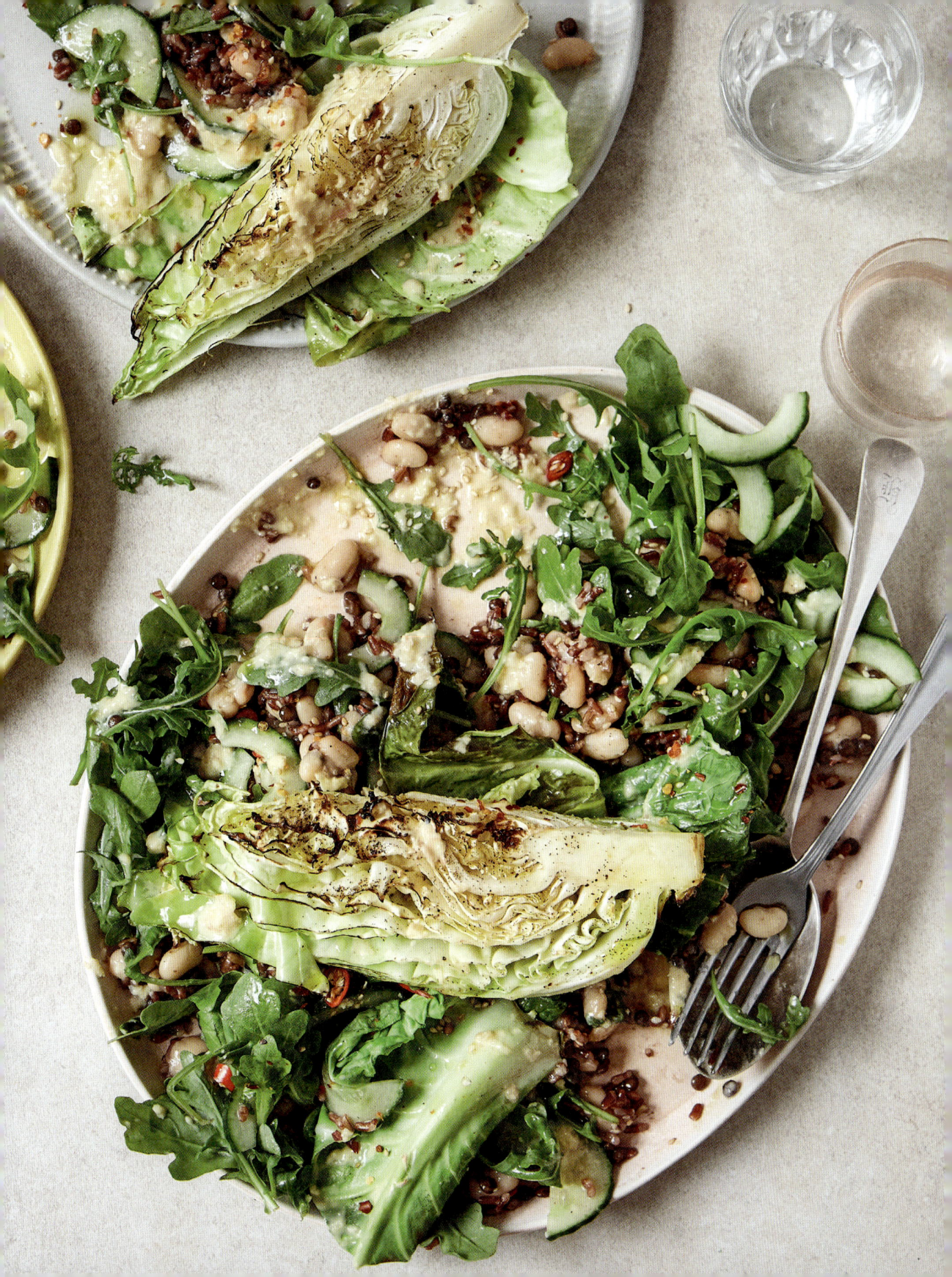

Throw-together Tofu Noodle Salad

MAKES 3 SERVINGS
TOTAL TIME: 30 MINS
FRIDGE LIFE: 4 DAYS

This is my go-to meal prep when I want something light, but still delicious and satisfying, as well as easy to make.

It makes a great stackable salad jar too; just add the dressing in at the bottom and leave the noodles to marinate. If you don't have spelt noodles, buckwheat (soba) or udon work just as well.

250g (9oz) spelt ramen noodles
Toasted sesame oil, for drizzling
300g (10oz) extra-firm smoked tofu
Sesame oil, for frying
2 tsp tamari or soy sauce
90g (3¼oz) edamame beans, fresh or thawed from frozen
90g (3¼oz) cucumber, deseeded and diced
25g (1oz) spring onions (about 3 small), white and green parts finely chopped

FOR THE DRESSING
3 tbsp sesame oil (if you don't have pure sesame, use another neutral oil or olive oil)
5 tbsp tamari
2 tsp maple or agave syrup
3 garlic cloves, minced
Juice of 1½ limes (about 3 tbsp)
1 tbsp toasted sesame oil

TO SERVE
Black sesame seeds
Sprinkle of nori dust (optional)
Lime wedges
Chopped fresh coriander
Thinly sliced red chilli (optional)

Protein per serving: 22g
Fibre: 5.6g
Plant diversity score: 9

Cook the noodles according to the packet instructions, then drain and set aside. Add a little toasted sesame oil to keep them from sticking together.

Wrap the tofu in kitchen paper and give it a good squeeze to remove any excess water. Cut the tofu lengthways into 3 large squares just shy of 1cm (½in) thick, then cut them in half widthways and then in a diagonal line across each half stack to get triangles. In batches, fry the triangles and the white parts of the spring onion in a little sesame oil on a medium heat for 2–3 minutes on each side until nice and golden brown. Add a splash (about 2 teaspoons per batch) of tamari or soy sauce when they are almost done. Remove from the heat when the tamari has been absorbed and coats both sides of the tofu well. Set aside.

If you're using frozen edamame, thaw now. In a bowl, cover the edamame in boiling water and leave for 1 minute, or until thawed. Drain and rinse under cold water.

In another bowl, whisk all the dressing ingredients together.

Divide the dressing between bowls or meal prep containers, then divide the noodles, the tofu, edamame, cucumber and green spring onions and top with sesame seeds, nori dust (if using), coriander, a lime wedge and chilli, if you like. Mix well before eating.

NOTES
Add more tofu or edamame for a more protein dense portion.

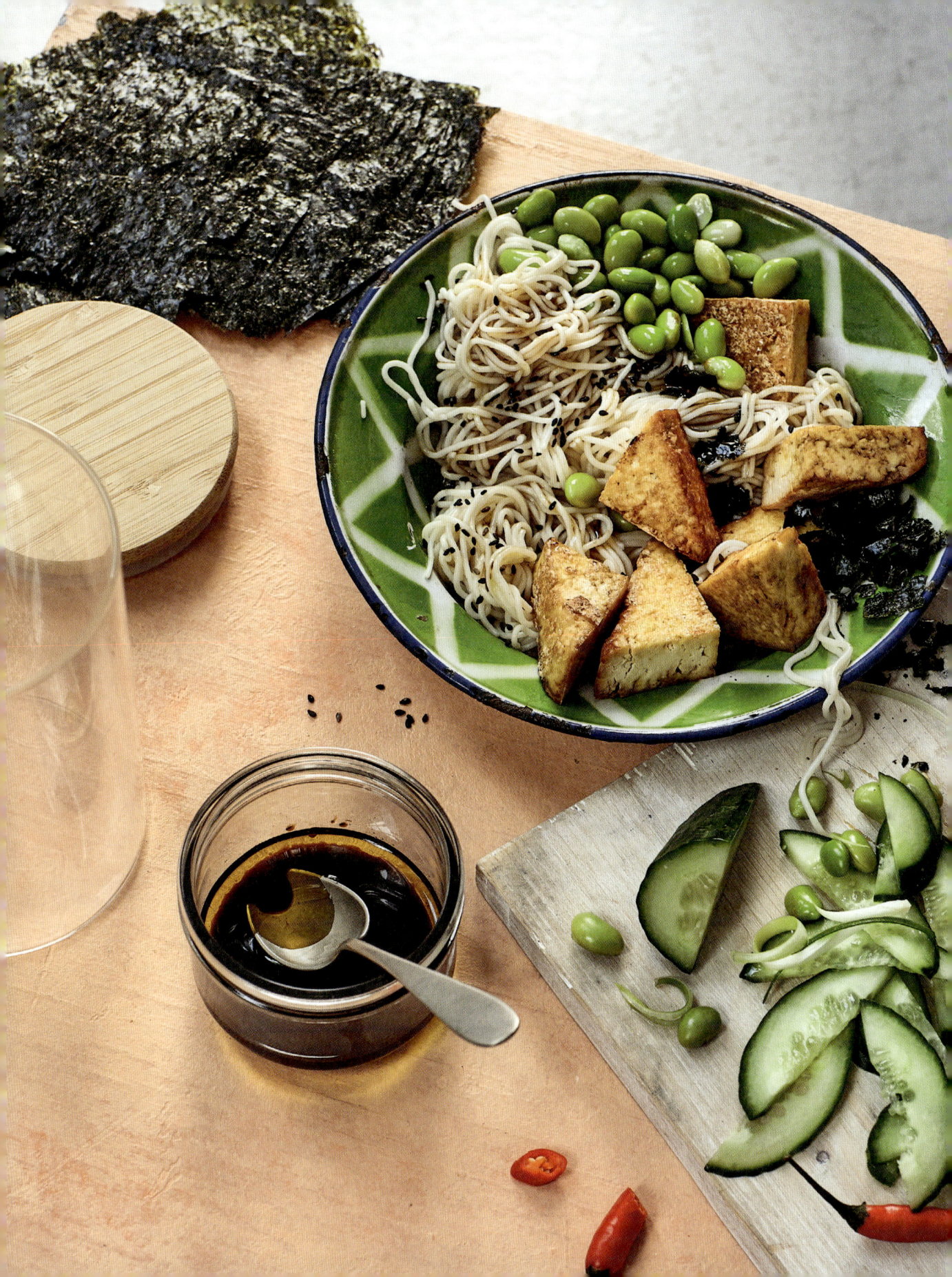

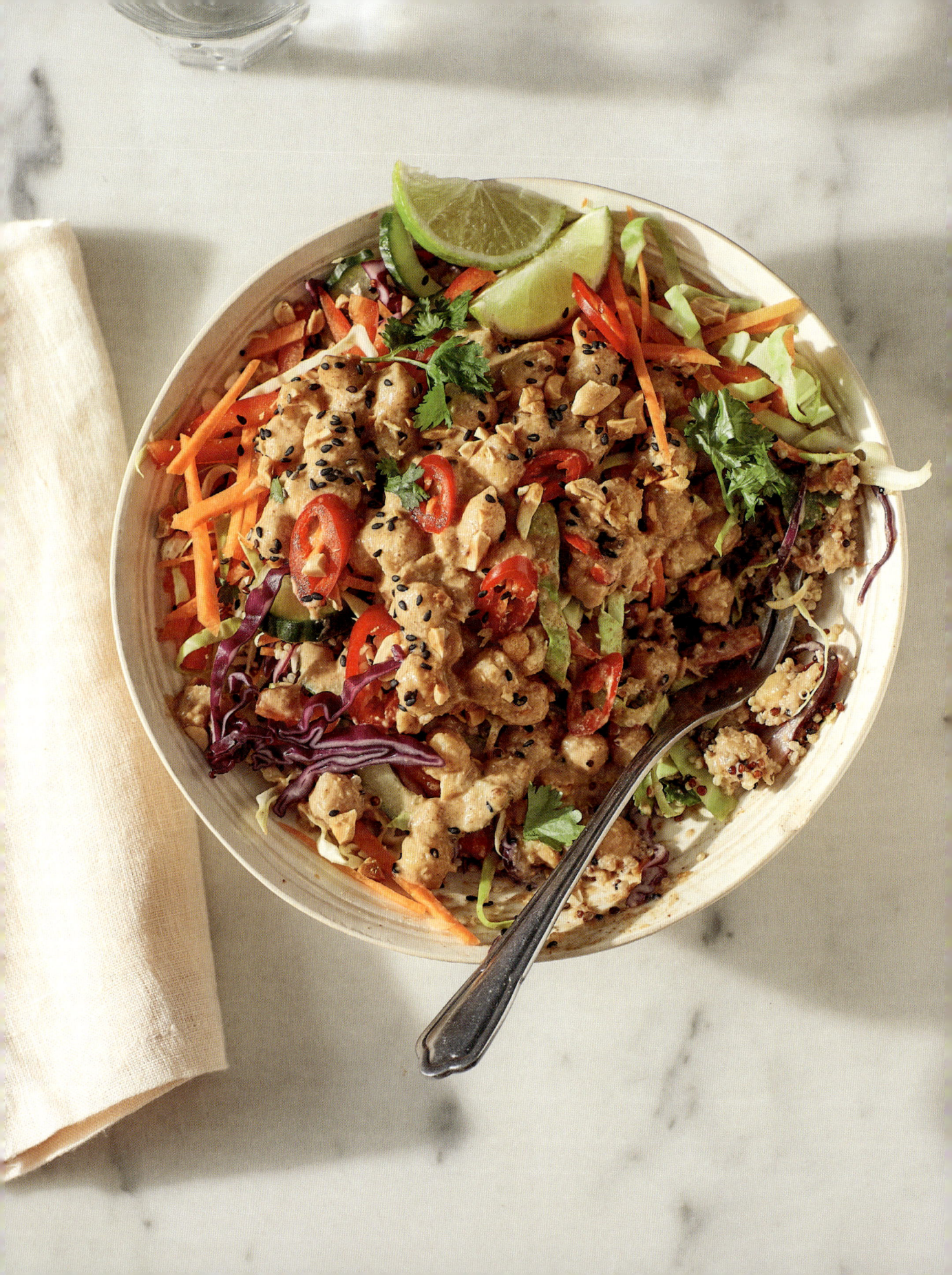

Satay Chickpea and Quinoa Salad

MAKES 3 SERVINGS
TOTAL TIME: 35 MINS
FRIDGE LIFE: 3–4 DAYS

This was a love at first bite. Gorgeous, crunchy rainbow veg with nutrient dense quinoa and grated smoked tofu, topped with a generous helping of unctuous, sweet, salty and creamy chickpeas. It's perfect for dinner, lunch or meal prep, and something I just keep coming back to.

150g (5½oz/¾ cup) tricolour quinoa
1 large or 2 small carrots, peeled and julienned or grated
1 red bell pepper, thinly sliced
¼ red cabbage, thinly sliced
⅓ green sweetheart cabbage, thinly sliced
1 small cucumber, deseeded and cut into 5mm (¼in) half-moons
150g (5½oz) firm smoked tofu, grated or crumbled
700g (1lb 9oz) chickpeas, from a can, drained and rinsed
Salt and black pepper

FOR THE SAUCE
4 heaped tbsp crunchy or smooth peanut butter
Thumb-sized piece of fresh ginger, peeled and grated
3 garlic cloves
2 tbsp soy sauce or tamari
2 tbsp rice vinegar
1 tbsp agave or maple syrup
1 tbsp sesame oil
3–4 tbsp warm water, plus more if needed

TO SERVE
70g (2½oz/½ cup) raw peanuts
Small handful of fresh coriander, leaves picked
Lime wedges
Red chilli, thinly sliced
Sesame seeds

Protein per serving: 31g
Fibre: 14.5g
Plant diversity score: 12

Cook the quinoa according to the packet instructions. You can add some stock powder for extra flavour here!

Add all the sliced veggies to a large bowl, saving one or two bits of each on the side for garnish. Grate the tofu and add this, too, along with the cooked and cooled quinoa.

In a blender cup, blend all the sauce ingredients together. Season to taste. Pour a third into the quinoa tofu mixture, tossing very well with your hands, then combine the rest with the chickpeas in another bowl.

Gently toast the raw peanuts in a dry frying pan for 5–7 minutes, then roughly bash them while warm in a pestle and mortar with a medium pinch of salt. Taste and season to your liking.

Divide into bowls or containers, then generously ladle the peanut butter chickpeas over the salad.

Garnish with coriander, lime wedges, chilli, the roasted and crushed peanuts, sesame seeds and the veggies you kept to the side.

Cheesy, Beany, Broccoli Power Bowl

MAKES 4 PORTIONS
TOTAL TIME: 40 MINS
FRIDGE LIFE: 3–4 DAYS

This one involves a bit of hob time but is well worth it. The cheesy beans work perfectly with the charred broccoli, making this a delicious and super filling lunch – or dinner, if you like.

700g (1lb 9oz) butter beans, from jars or cans, drained and rinsed
1 small/medium head of broccoli, florets sliced through the stems
Olive oil
30g (1oz) sun-dried tomatoes, chopped
Omega-3 Boost (see page 209)
Fresh coriander

FOR THE 'CHEESE' SAUCE WITH BEANS
280g (10oz) silken tofu
3½ tbsp nutritional yeast
2 garlic cloves
1 tsp smoked paprika
½ tsp ground turmeric
½ tsp salt
1 tbsp white wine vinegar
2 tsp Dijon mustard

FOR THE ROASTED CHICKPEAS
480g (1lb 1oz) chickpeas, from a jar or can, drained and rinsed
3 tsp smoked paprika
2 tsp ground cumin
1 tsp salt
5–6 twists of black pepper
1 tbsp olive oil

FOR THE QUINOA/LENTIL BASE
½ onion, diced
3 garlic cloves, minced
200g (7oz/1 cup) quinoa, rinsed and drained
Vegetable stock, to cover
240g (8½oz) cooked brown lentils
Olive oil
Salt and black pepper

Preheat the oven to 180°C fan/200°C/gas mark 6.

Rinse and pat dry the chickpeas. Add the spices, salt and pepper, then roast for 15–20 minutes, or until crispy.

While the chickpeas are roasting, start the quinoa base. In a medium saucepan on a medium heat, sauté the onion in olive oil for 5 minutes with a small pinch of salt until translucent, then add the garlic. Fry for a further 2 minutes, then add the quinoa and cover in the onion and garlic mixture. Add vegetable stock so it covers the mix by at least 1cm (½in). Bring to the boil, then simmer for 10–15 mins, or until the water has evaporated and the quinoa is cooked. If the spiral has not separated from the grain, add a splash more water and cook until it does. Once cooked, add the lentils and stir to combine.

In a blender or bullet blender, blend all the 'cheese' sauce ingredients until smooth and creamy. Season to taste, then add the butter beans and gently heat through – it won't need long, 2 minutes at most.

Lightly fry the broccoli in olive oil and a little salt, cut-side down, for 5–7 minutes until lightly charred. Set aside.

Divide into bowls or meal prep containers, quinoa/lentils first, then the cheesy beans and the broccoli. Add the sun-dried tomatoes, some fresh coriander leaves and sprinkle the chickpeas and Omega-3 seed mix over the top.

Protein per serving: 32g
Fibre: 17g
Plant diversity score: 11

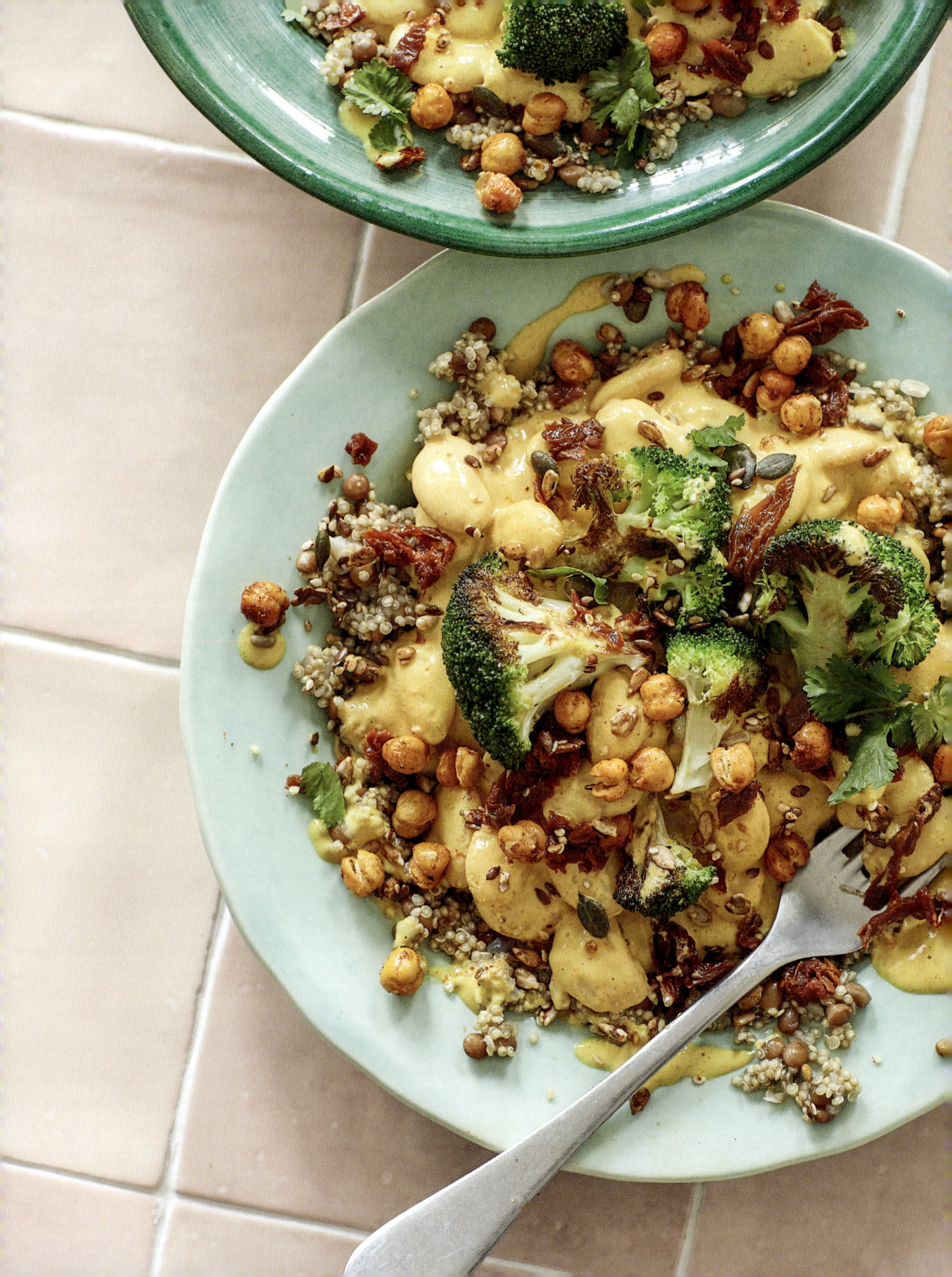

Meal Prep Salad Jars

A selection of my favourite jar recipes from my popular Instagram series. These are perfect for office lunches, just pour them out into a bowl and enjoy. You'll be the envy of everyone. Just go easy on the garlic if you're tight on desk space!

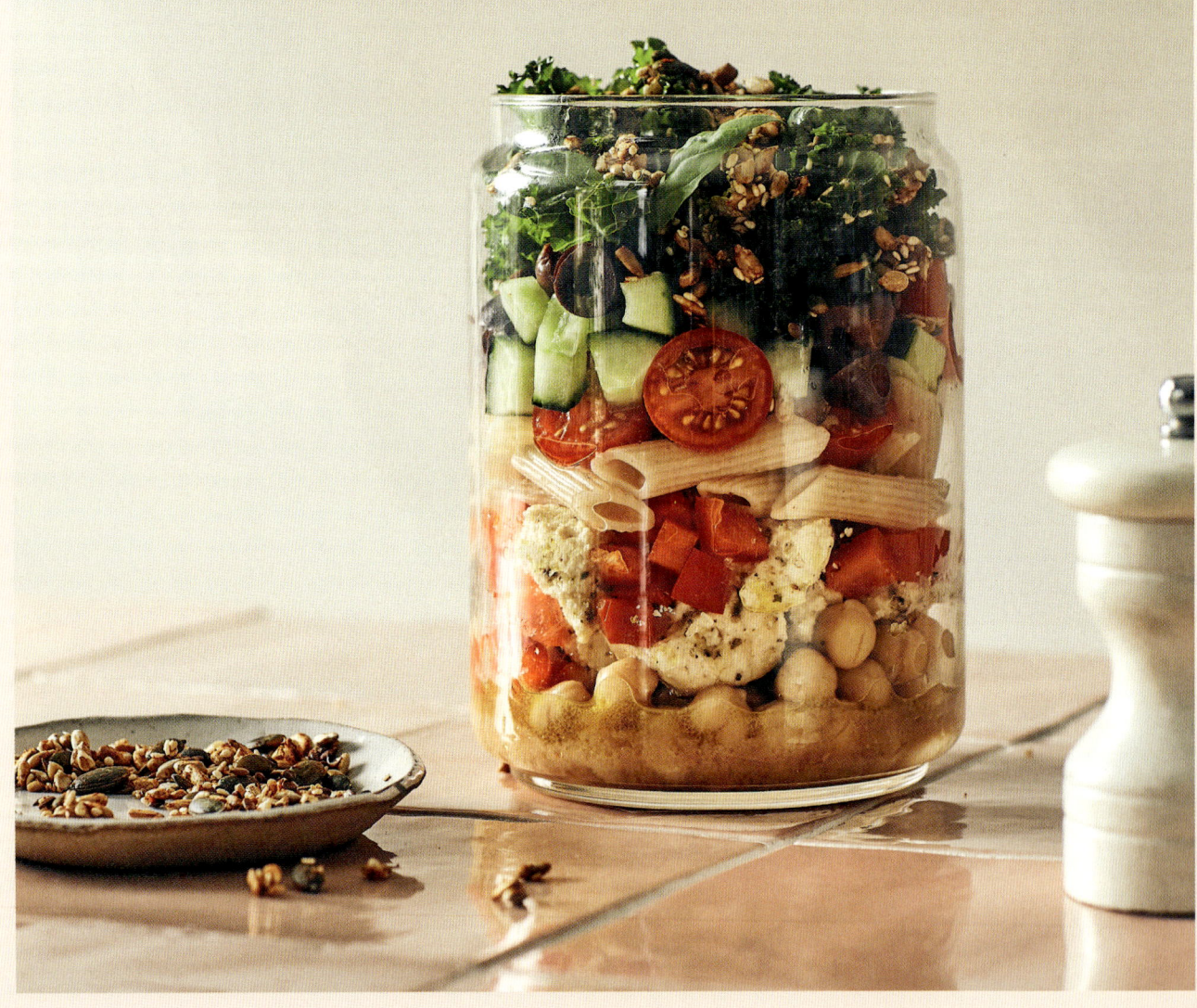

Mediterranean Pasta Salad

MAKES 3 JARS
TOTAL TIME: 30 MINS
FRIDGE LIFE: 4 DAYS

For me, this one embodies Mediterranean flavours. The rich, tangy dressing gives me Greek salad vibes and together with the olives and crunchy veg, all you need to do is shut your eyes and you'll be on the beach.

200g (7oz) cooked pasta of choice
1 red bell pepper, sliced
2 small handfuls of cherry tomatoes, halved
35g (1¼oz) Kalamata olives
Small handful of fresh basil
3 small handfuls of kale
1 tbsp extra virgin olive oil
Squeeze of lemon juice
½ cucumber, deseeded and chopped into small batons
480g (1lb 1oz) chickpeas, from a can or jar, drained and rinsed
250g (9oz) Tofu Feta (see page 220)
2 tbsp Omega-3 Boost (see page 209)

FOR THE VINAIGRETTE
6 tbsp olive oil
2 tbsp red wine vinegar
2 tbsp apple cider vinegar
2 tsp agave syrup
½ tsp salt
½ tsp Dijon mustard
1 fat garlic clove, grated
Black pepper

Start by cooking the pasta in plenty of salty boiling water for one minute less than the packet instructions suggest.

In a small bowl, whisk all the vinaigrette ingredients together.

Chop the red pepper, cherry tomatoes, pitted kalamata olives and roughly tear the basil.

For the kale, de-stem, roughly chop, wash then add to a large bowl and massage with the extra virgin olive oil, until the leaves start to soften. Add a squeeze of lemon and a pinch of salt to taste.

To deseed the cucumber, cut it in half, then swoop the tip of a spoon down the inner layer to remove the fleshy seeds on both sides. Chop into small half-moons.

Layer up the jars: vinaigrette first, then the chickpeas, tofu feta, red pepper, cooked pasta, cherry tomatoes, cucumber, kale, olives, basil and omega-3 seed sprinkle.

Protein per serving: 34g
Fibre: 12g
Plant diversity score: 12

Easy Ginger, Miso and Lime Noodle Salad

MAKES 3 JARS
TOTAL TIME: 20 MINS
FRIDGE LIFE: 3–4 DAYS

Ginger, miso and lime is the holy trinity of dressing ingredients for me. It's the perfect marriage of spice, tang and rich depth. Add any thinly sliced salad veg you have on hand!

60g (2¼oz) red cabbage, shredded
60g (2¼oz) carrot, peeled and grated
3–4 radishes, thinly sliced
150g (5½oz) buckwheat (soba) noodles
100g (3½oz) broccoli, roughly chopped
Splash of sesame oil
250g (9oz) extra-firm smoked tofu, cut into
    small cubes
3 tbsp sauerkraut
80g (2¾oz) edamame beans, fresh or thawed
    from frozen
A few fresh coriander leaves
Sprinkle of sesame seeds

FOR THE LIME, GINGER AND MISO DRESSING
Juice of 3 medium limes
Thumb-sized piece of fresh ginger, peeled and grated
2 garlic cloves, minced
2 tbsp sesame or olive oil
2 tbsp toasted sesame oil
2 tbsp sweet white miso paste
2 tbsp tahini or a nut butter
4–5 tbsp water, to blend to a pourable consistency
Salt and black pepper

Start with the dressing. In a high-speed bullet blender, add all the ingredients and blend until silky smooth. Season to taste.

Slice all your veg: the red cabbage (use a potato peeler to get it extra thin!), the carrots (use a julienne if you have one) and the radishes (use a mandoline if you have one).

Cook the noodles according to the packet instructions, adding the chopped broccoli 4 minutes before the timer ends (this will be not long after the soba goes in). Remove the broccoli with a spider or slotted spoon, set aside, then drain the noodles and give them a good rinse in cold water for about 3 minutes, so they don't clump together. Set them aside in a small bowl with a splash of sesame oil until you're ready to assemble the jars.

Layer up the jars, starting with the dressing, the noodles, the veg, tofu, sauerkraut and edamame, then top with fresh coriander and sesame seeds.

Protein per serving: 25g
Fibre: 10g
Plant diversity score: 12

NOTES
Add more Tofu or swap for Tempeh Crumbles (page 207) for a more protein dense portion

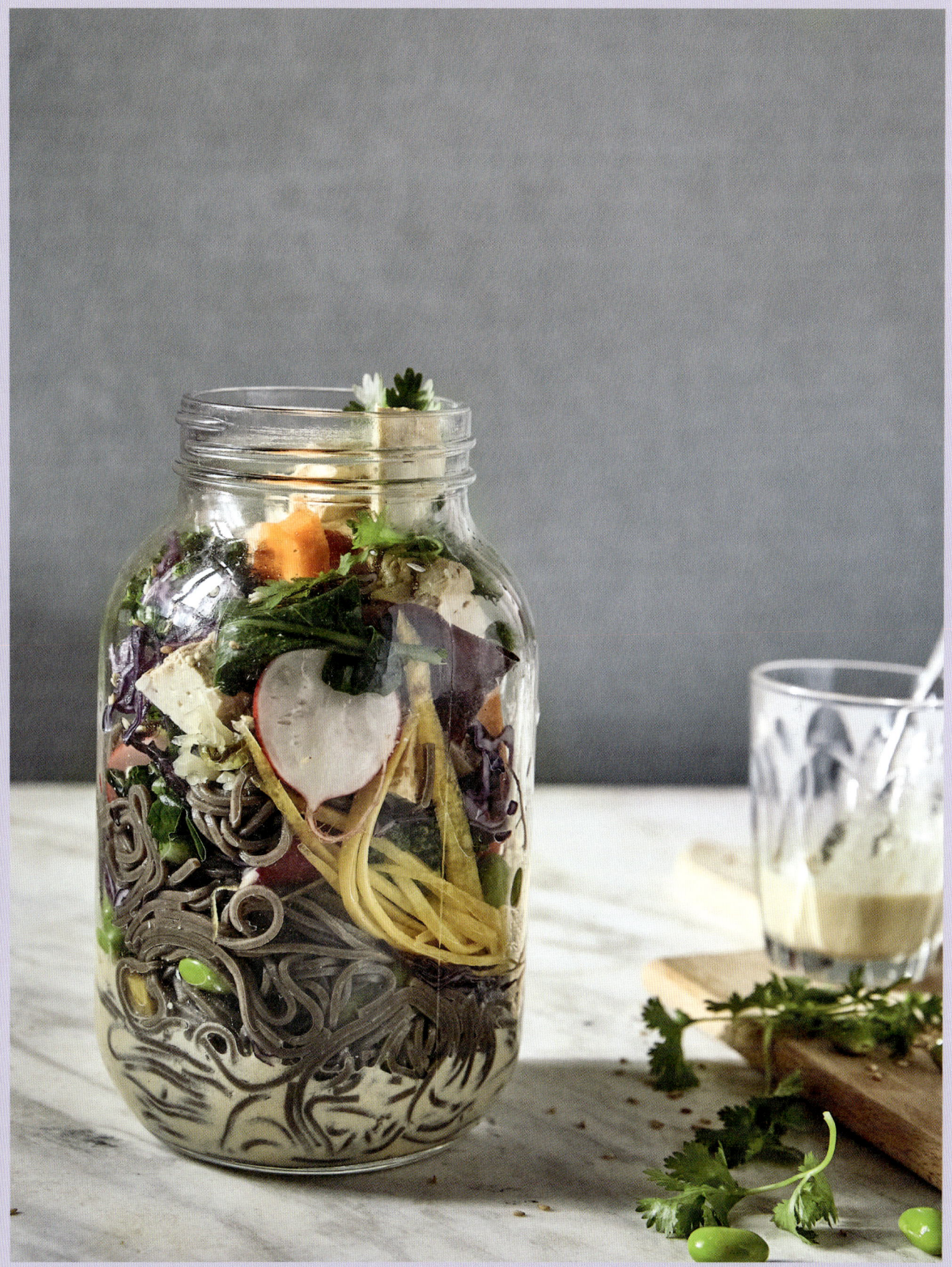

My Favourite Sweet Potato Rainbow Salad

MAKES 3 JARS
TOTAL TIME: 40 MINS
FRIDGE LIFE: 3–4 DAYS

This one brings all the Mexican flavour vibes to the meal-prep jar party. The thick tofu cheese is kind of like queso, the sweet potato dressed in lime brings brightness and vibrancy, and black beans and quinoa back everything up with plenty of protein and fibre.

200g (7oz/1 cup) quinoa
½ vegetable stock cube or 1 tsp vegetable
  bouillon powder
2 medium sweet potatoes
2 tbsp olive oil, plus extra for drizzling
½ small red cabbage
Juice of 2 limes
100g (3½oz) fresh sweetcorn
1 red chilli, finely chopped
½ tsp agave syrup
1 x 400g (14oz) can black beans
1 red bell pepper, sliced
2 handfuls of kale, washed, stems removed, chopped,
  lightly massaged in olive oil
Few fresh coriander leaves
Small handful of pumpkin seeds
Salt and black pepper

FOR THE THICK TOFU CHEESE
250g (9oz) firm smoked tofu
3 tbsp nutritional yeast
2 garlic cloves
1 tsp onion powder
⅓ tsp salt
1 tsp smoked paprika
½ tsp ground turmeric
1 tbsp olive oil
1 tbsp water, plus more to loosen if needed

Preheat the oven to 180°C fan/200°C/gas mark 6.

Cook the quinoa according to the packet instructions, adding the stock to the water for flavour.

Chop the sweet potatoes into 1–2cm (½–¾in) irregular chunks (no need to peel if organic, just give them a good wash), then add to a baking tray with a drizzle of olive oil and salt. Roast for about 20 minutes, or until lightly browned.

To a small, high-powered bullet blender, add all the tofu cheese ingredients and pulse to combine. Season to taste. It will be thick – it's intentional!

Shred the red cabbage into a small bowl with a potato peeler, then add half the lime juice, a pinch of salt and pinch together with your fingers until it turns a pinky-purply shade. Set aside in the fridge.

Heat a dry non-stick frying pan on a medium-high heat and add the sweetcorn. Fry with a pinch of salt, for around 10–12 minutes until lightly charred, then take off the heat and set aside.

Now for the sweet potato marinade. In a small bowl, whisk the 2 tablespoons of olive oil, the remaining lime juice, the red chilli, a pinch of salt and agave syrup together. Pour over the roasted sweet potato and carefully toss to cover.

Time to assemble the jars: put the cooked quinoa in first, then the black beans, sweet potato, tofu cheese, red pepper, kale, red cabbage, charred corn, coriander and pumpkin seeds.

Protein per serving: 33g
Fibre: 18g
Plant diversity score: 12

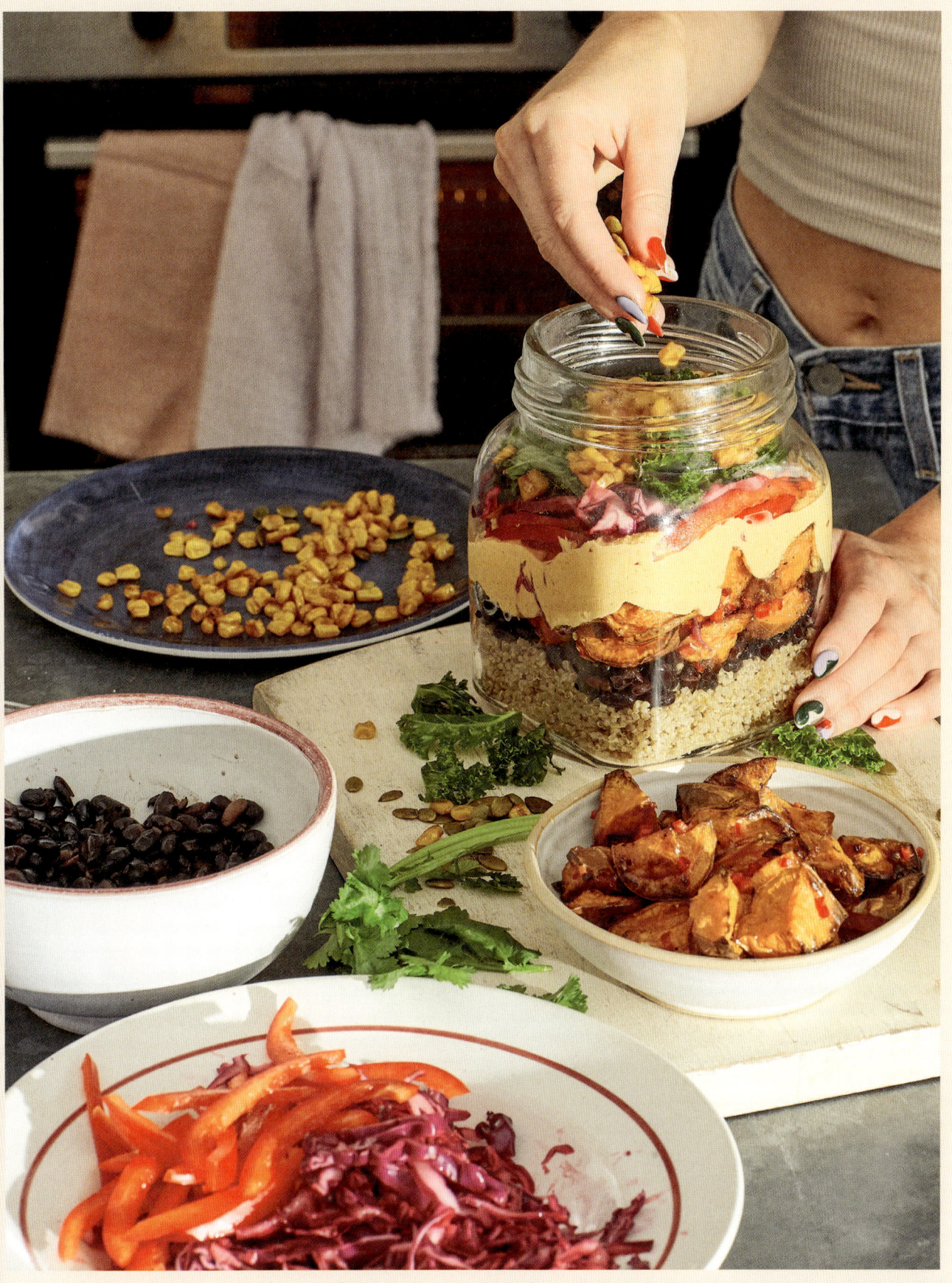

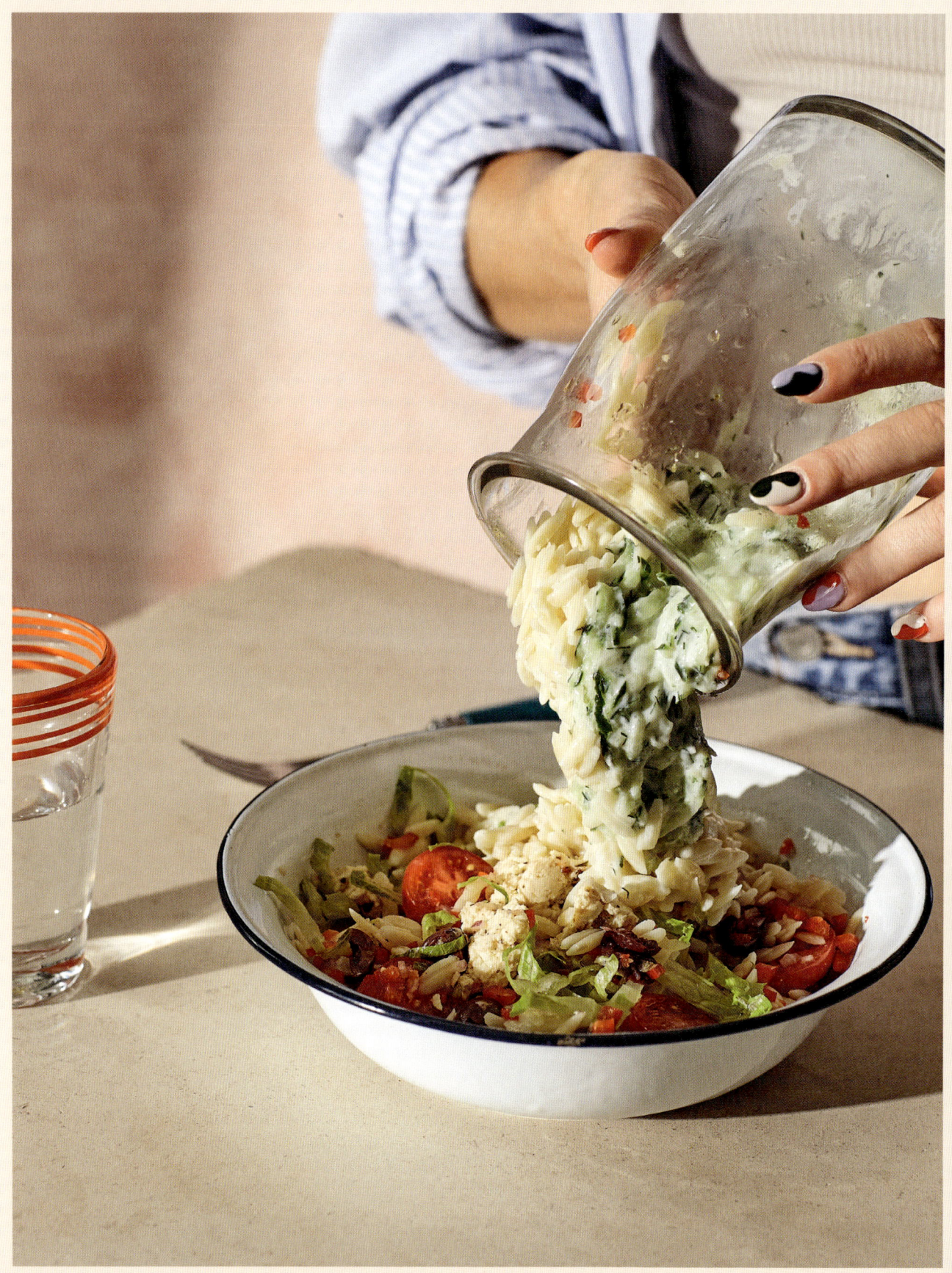

Mezze in a Jar

MAKES 3 JARS
TOTAL TIME: 30 MINS
FRIDGE LIFE: 4 DAYS

Feel free to get creative with this one – replace the orzo for beans, the tofu feta for my savoury meatballs (see page 225) or some falafel. All I ask is you keep the fresh tzatziki sauce at the bottom of the jar, for maximum flavour and so things don't go soggy.

250g (9oz) orzo
2 handfuls cherry tomatoes, halved
70g (2½oz) Kalamata olives, pitted and roughly chopped
1 red bell pepper, finely chopped
300g (10½oz) Tofu Feta (see page 220)
1 medium wedge or about ¼ medium red onion, very finely chopped
3 small handfuls of lettuce leaves, washed and chopped
Pitta breads (optional)
Salt and black pepper

FOR THE TZATZIKI
½ medium cucumber, grated and juice squeezed out
160g (5¾oz/⅔ cup) vegan yoghurt
2 garlic cloves, minced
2 tbsp finely chopped fresh dill
Juice of ½ lemon
½ tsp salt

Cook the orzo in plenty of salty boiling water according to the packet instructions.

In a small bowl, combine all the tzatziki ingredients and mix well. Make sure to squeeze as much water as possible out of the grated cucumber! You can use a muslin cloth or a tea towel. Season to taste.

Assemble the jar: tzatziki first, then the orzo, tomatoes, olives, red pepper, tofu feta, onion and lettuce (to keep it from going soggy!).

If you like, you could toast some pitta and wrap in parchment paper to take alongside the jar.

Protein per serving: 25g
Fibre: 18g
Plant diversity score: 12

NOTES
Add a tablespoon per jar of Nutty, Noochy Crumb to boost the protein (page 208)

Korean Bibimbap-inspired Salad

MAKES 3 JARS
TOTAL TIME: 40 MINS
FRIDGE LIFE: 4 DAYS

Inspired by the Korean dish Bibimbap, this is a celebration of leftovers, so get creative and use whatever you have left over (rice, any grain, roasted veg, crumbled tofu) and quick pickle any slightly sad veg you have laying around. Just keep the sauce the same, and you'll have a delicious meal.

250g (9oz/1¼ cups) quinoa
½ tsp vegetable bouillon powder
2 large or 6 small red, orange or yellow bell peppers, chopped in half and deseeded
1 red onion
2 carrots, julienned
½ cucumber, sliced into thin rounds
Juice of 1 lime
½ small red cabbage, shredded with a peeler
250g (9oz) extra-firm tofu
400g (14oz) shiitake mushrooms
Olive oil
1 tsp smoked paprika
Small handful of fresh coriander
Salt and black pepper

FOR THE PICKLING LIQUID
2 tbsp rice vinegar
½ tsp salt
½ tsp chilli flakes
½ tsp granulated sugar
4 spring onions, finely sliced on the diagonal
2 red chillies, finely sliced

FOR THE GOCHUJANG SAUCE
6 tbsp gochujang paste
3 tbsp mirin or rice vinegar
2 tbsp maple syrup
3 tbsp sesame oil
3 garlic cloves
2 tbsp soy sauce

Preheat the oven to 180°C fan/200°C/gas mark 6.

Cook the quinoa with the vegetable bouillon powder according to the packet instructions.

Slice the peppers and red onion, transfer to a baking tray, add oil, salt and roast for 15–20 minutes until golden.

Mix all the pickling liquid ingredients together in a jar, shake, then add the carrot and cucumber to the jar and shake a little more. Turn up and down every now and then, so the veg gets a good coating. Leave in the fridge.

In a small bowl, pour the lime juice over the red cabbage shreds. Add ½ a teaspoon of salt and gently pinch together with your fingers until it turns a pinky-purply shade. Set aside in the fridge.

In a small blender cup, combine all the gochujang sauce ingredients and blend until smooth.

Grate the tofu and chop or pulse the mushrooms in a food processor a few times. Don't overprocess, you need them a little chunky to get that 'minced beef' texture.

Add the mushrooms and tofu to a hot non-stick pan on a medium-high heat with a little oil and the smoked paprika. Stir in 2 tablespoons of the gochujang sauce. Stir every now and then for about 8 minutes, letting the mixture sit for a bit to get crispy, but being careful not to let it burn. Season to taste.

Layer up the jars: gochujang sauce first, then the quinoa, roasted peppers and onions, crispy tofu and mushrooms, pickled red cabbage and carrot and cucumber pickle. Finish with some fresh coriander.

Protein per serving: 23g
Fibre: 14g
Plant diversity score: 12

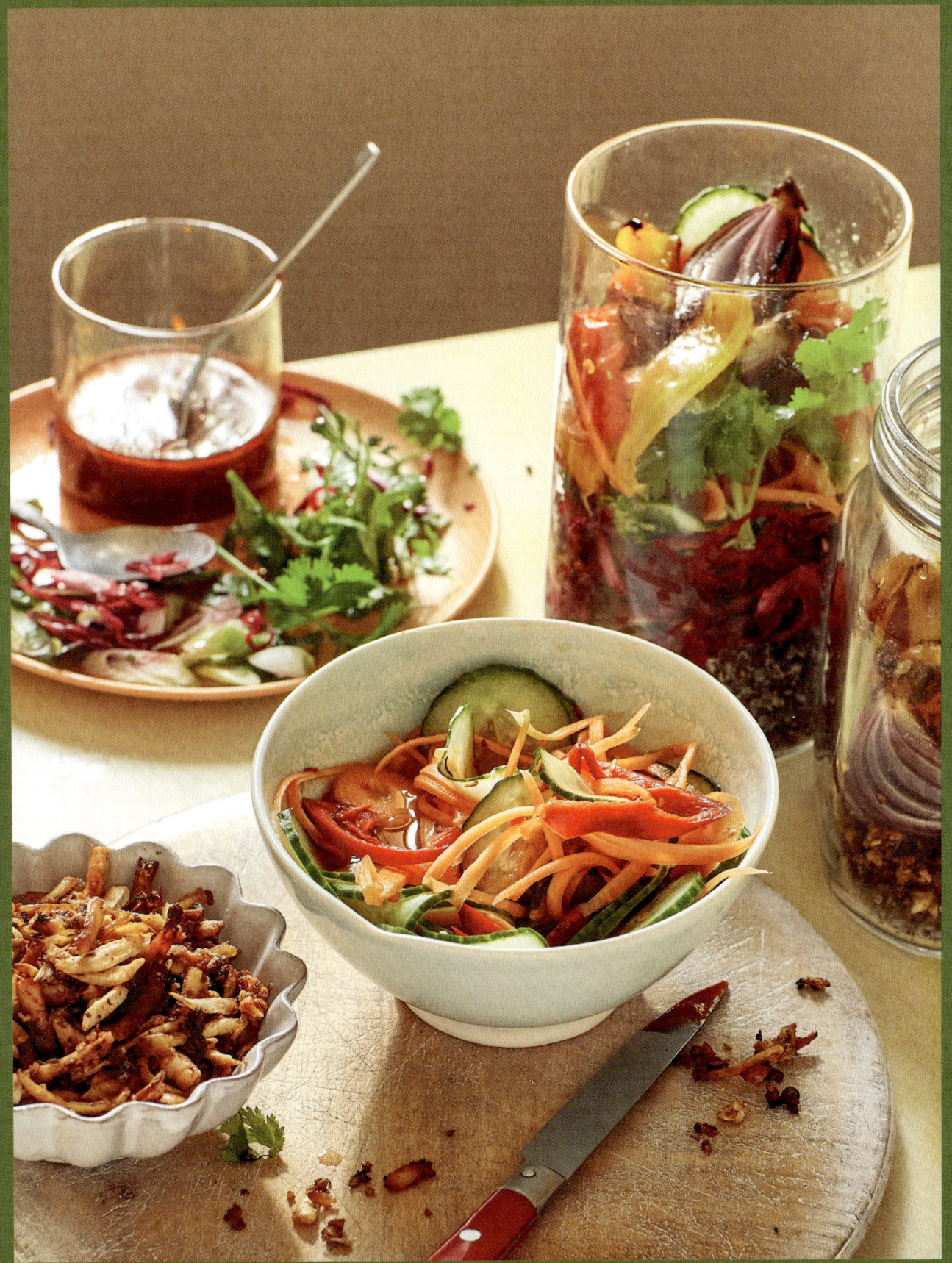

Sandwiches and Soups

I tend to go through obsessions with various sandwich fillings and I've chosen these very carefully as they never, ever fail and are the few filling preps I can't forget. Feel free to shake things up and use wraps or pitas instead of sourdough.

Soups are easy wins for lunch or dinner; I crave them in colder weather or on rest days, but my 20-Minute Ramen (see page 122) is a year-round fave, and always a hit with guests.

Ultimate Chickpea Smash Sandwiches

MAKES 3 SANDWICHES
TOTAL TIME: 20 MINS

OK, all other sandwiches can retire now, this one wins every single award. It's crunchy, tangy, creamy, fresh and, of course, nutrient dense and packed with all the good stuff you need to fuel your workouts effectively.

I used extra firm, deli style tofu when I originally tested this, a brand called Taifun so do get that if you can. The picture shows firm smoked tofu, sliced and marinated in 1 tablespoon of tamari or soy sauce, 1 teaspoon of smoked paprika and 1 tablespoon of olive oil. Grill or fry until a little charred.

200g (7oz) extra-firm smoked tofu
2–3 medium/large tomatoes
1 large ripe avocado
6–8 lettuce leaves
6 slices of wholewheat sourdough bread
6 tbsp Cashew Cream (see page 219)

FOR THE CHICKPEA SMASH MIXTURE
480g (1lb 1oz) chickpeas, from a can or jar, drained and rinsed
4 spring onions, finely chopped
3 tbsp runny tahini
2 tsp Dijon mustard
2 tbsp chopped sun-dried tomatoes, plus 1 tbsp oil from the jar
1 tbsp chopped red chilli (optional)
3 tbsp chopped fresh parsley
Juice of 1 lemon (about 3 tbsp)
½ tsp salt, plus more to taste
Lots of freshly ground black pepper

If you're making the cashew cream, head to page 214 and make this first. You'll likely need to start by soaking cashews in boiling water, which will be your first step.

In a large mixing bowl, combine all the chickpea smash ingredients and mash with a potato masher or fork until they are well mixed. Season to taste. Leave in the fridge whilst you prep the rest.

Thinly slice the tofu, tomatoes and avocado. Separate, wash and dry the lettuce leaves.

Toast the sourdough, then drizzle with a little olive oil and season with a small pinch of sea salt. Layer 3 slices of sourdough with the chickpea smash, then the remaining slices with the cashew cream first, then the lettuce leaves, tomato slices, tofu and avocado slices. Carefully sandwich the two layers together, wrap up, slice down the middle with a serrated knife, and enjoy!

Protein per serving: 29g
Fibre: 19g
Plant diversity score: 13

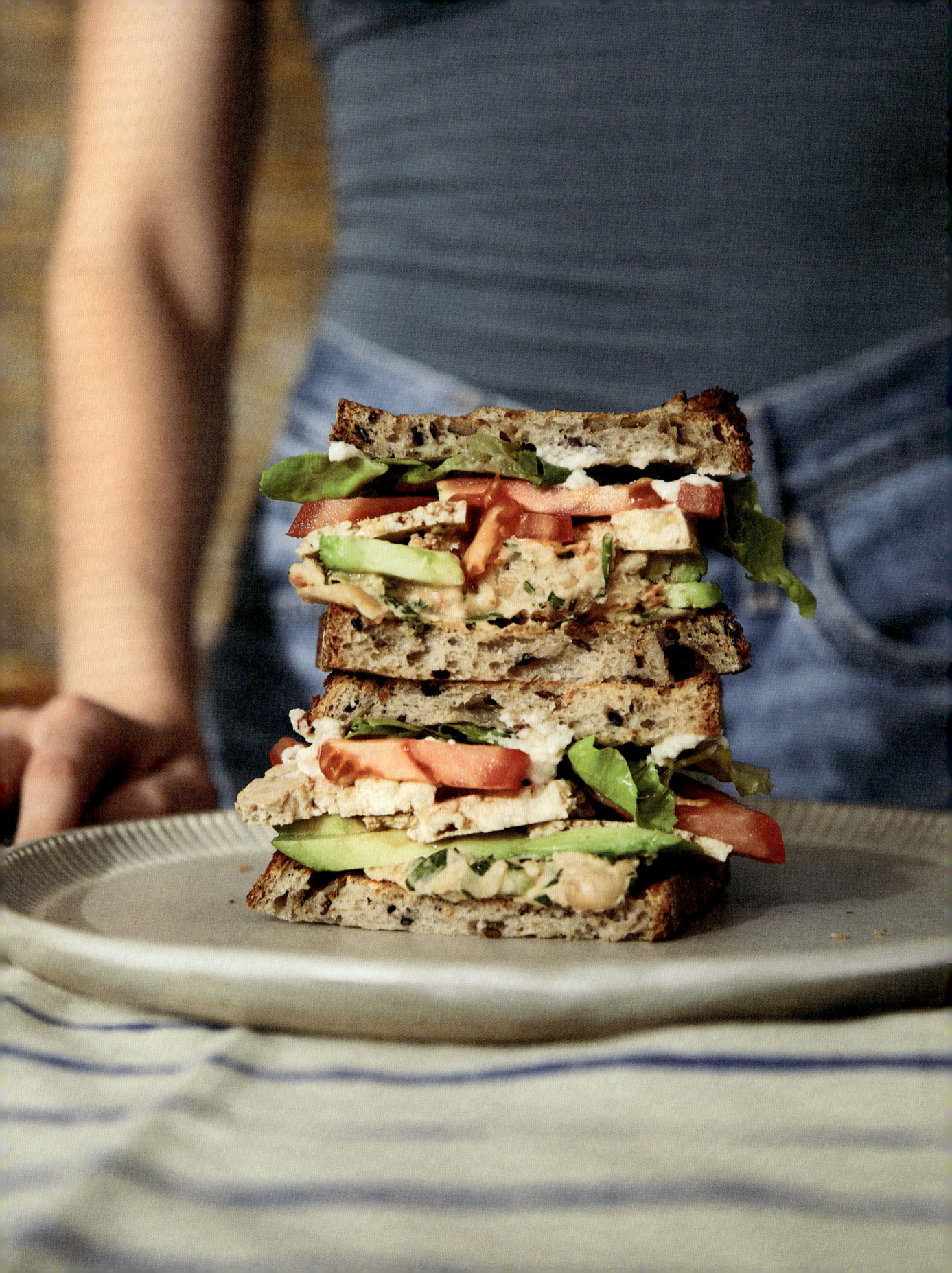

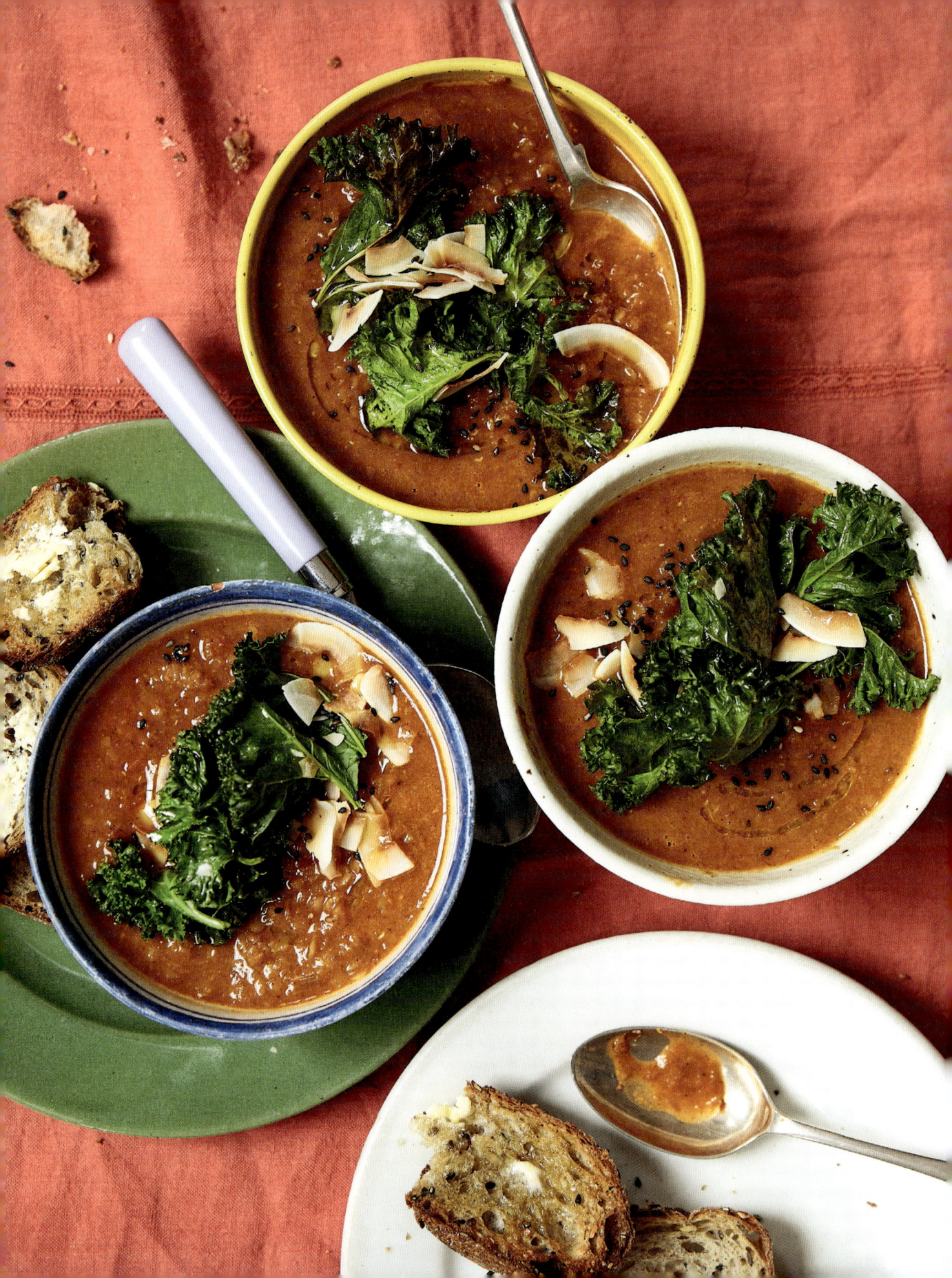

Harissa, Ginger and Coconut Lentils

SERVES 2–3
TOTAL TIME: 35 MINS

The perfect light but nourishing bowl to whip up on a night when you really just can't be bothered but need something healthy and delish. The combination of harissa and toasted coconut results in an earthy, smoky, sweet flavour combination and, served with crispy kale, it's texture heaven.

I tend to crave this when I'm feeling a little under the weather. The warming ginger helps ease any symptoms and the squeeze of lemon helps the body to absorb the plant sources of iron.

1 white onion or shallot, finely chopped
Olive oil
4 garlic cloves, crushed
Thumb-sized piece of fresh ginger, peeled and grated
1 medium carrot, peeled and diced small
1 tsp smoked paprika
1 tsp ground cumin
1 tsp ground coriander
1 tbsp tomato purée
200g (7oz/¾ cup) split red lentils, drained and rinsed
900ml (32fl oz/3⅔ cups) vegetable stock
½ tbsp lemon juice
1 tbsp harissa paste, plus more to drizzle, less if you
    don't like spice
3 tbsp nutritional yeast
Salt and black pepper

TO SERVE
Large handful crispy roasted kale
Toasted coconut flakes
Extra virgin olive oil
Black sesame seeds
Sourdough or other bread of choice

Protein per serving: 15g
Fibre: 11g
Plant diversity score: 9

In a medium saucepan on a medium heat, sauté the onion in plenty of olive oil with a pinch of salt for 8 minutes. Add the garlic, ginger and carrot and fry for a further 3 minutes. Add the spices and a little more oil and continue to fry for 2 minutes.

Add the tomato purée and cook for a further 3 minutes. Add the red lentils and stock, stir well, then cover most of the pot, leaving a slither for steam to escape, and simmer for 15–20 minutes until the lentils are soft, stirring occasionally.

While the lentils cook, dress the kale leaves in olive oil and salt and roast on a baking tray at 180°C fan/200°C/gas mark 6 for 10–15 minutes until crispy. Set aside.

Once the lentils are cooked (taste to test!) take them off the heat, add the lemon juice, harissa paste and nutritional yeast, stir in and season to taste. Scoop out a few ladlefuls, allow to cool, then blend and pour back in, or use a stick blender and pulse a few times to achieve a soup-like consistency.

Serve with the crispy roasted kale, toasted coconut flakes, a drizzle of olive oil, some black pepper, sesame seeds and another squeeze of lemon juice. I like to eat this with toasted sourdough bread!

NOTES
Add 100g Quick Fried Tofu or Tempeh (page 207) or serve with Cheesy Quesadillas (page 126)

Healing Greens and Beans Soup

SERVES 2–3
TOTAL TIME: 25 MINS

A soup as delicious as these rhyming words, fit for any occasion. I eat this at least once a week, sometimes blending the whole mix, sometimes keeping it nice and chunky.

Olive oil
1 medium head of broccoli, chopped (florets, stalk and all)
4 garlic cloves, grated
Finger-sized piece of fresh ginger, peeled and grated
1 tsp ground coriander
1 tsp ground cumin
480g (1lb 1oz) white beans from a can or jar, plus their juices (I used cannellini)
500ml (18fl oz/2 cups) vegetable stock
200g (7oz) fresh spinach
Large handful of fresh basil
150g (5½oz) frozen peas
1 tbsp nutritional yeast
Juice of ½ lemon

TO SERVE (OPTIONAL)
Soy yoghurt or cream
Large handful crispy roasted kale (see page 115 for method)
Pickled radish
Salt and black pepper

Cover the bottom of a medium, heavy-bottomed saucepan with olive oil, then fry the broccoli for 6–7 minutes until bright green. Add the garlic and ginger and fry for a further 2 minutes, then add the spices.

Add the beans, their juices and the stock and stir well. Simmer on a low–medium heat while you blanch the spinach, basil and peas (this helps to keep the bright green colour!). Add them to the broccoli, along with the nutritional yeast and lemon juice. Take it off the heat, allow to cool, then either use a stick blender to blend into a soupy consistency (as much or as little as you like) or transfer to a blender and blend until smooth.

Season to taste, then ladle into bowls and serve with the optional toppings.

Protein per serving: 19g
Fibre: 15g
Plant diversity score: 12

NOTES
Add Quick Fried Tofu or Tempeh (page 207) or serve with Cheesy Quesadillas (page 126)

SANDWICHES AND SOUPS

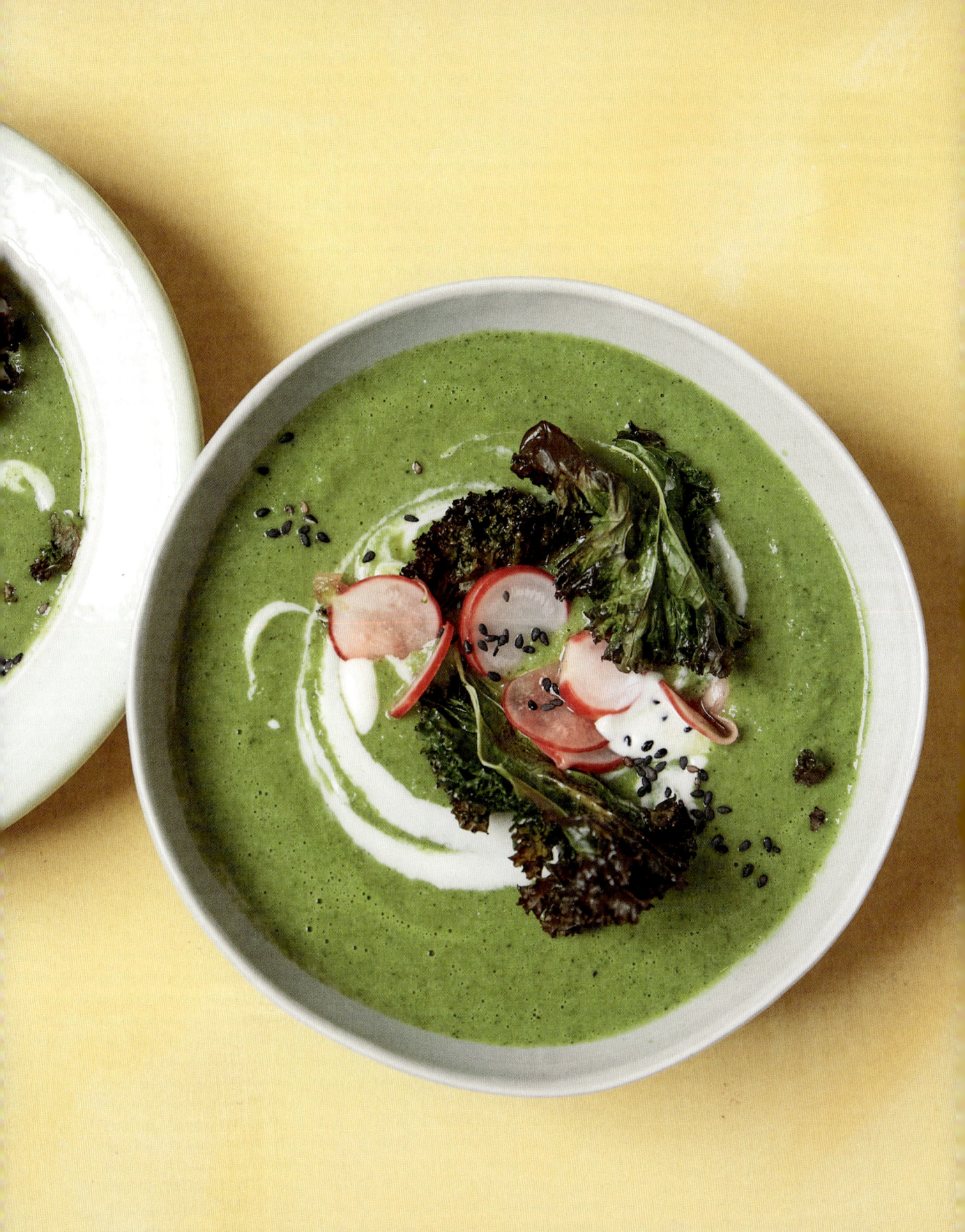

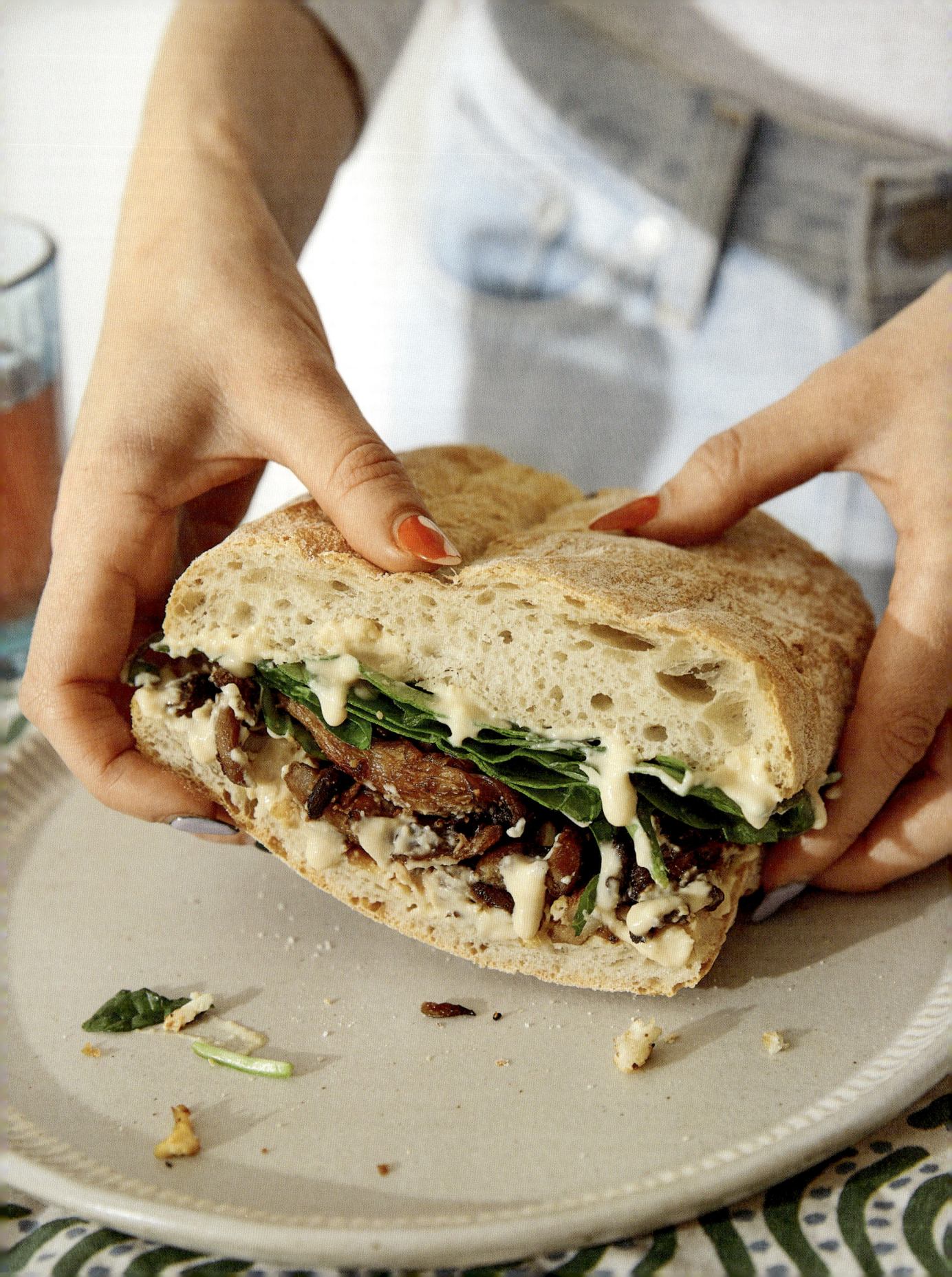

Quick Creamy Miso Mushroom and Crispy Tofu Ciabatta

MAKES 3 SANDWICHES
TOTAL TIME: 30 MINS

Miso cashew cream and mushrooms are a godly combo, which, if you haven't already tried, will blow you away. The bonus is that it's a dump and bake, perfect for a work from home lunch.

400g (14oz) oyster mushrooms
1 tbsp olive oil
1 tbsp tamari
1 tbsp sweet white miso paste
200g (7oz) smoked extra-tofu, grated

FOR THE CASHEW MISO CREAM
80g (3oz/½ cup) cashews
1 tbsp sweet white miso paste
Juice of 1 lemon
1 garlic clove
3 tbsp nutritional yeast
About 3 tbsp water, plus more if needed
Salt and black pepper

TO SERVE
Ciabatta bread, sliced
Rocket or spinach

Preheat the oven to 200°C fan/220°C/gas mark 7.

In a small bowl, soak the cashews in boiling water for 15 minutes. Drain.

Tear the mushrooms into strips with your hands, wiping off any dirt as you go, then add them all to a large bowl with the oil, tamari and miso. Mix to combine well, with your hands, then transfer to a large baking tray and roast for 10–15 minutes.

Remove from the oven, mix, then add the grated tofu and return to the oven for another 10–15 minutes. Once golden and slightly crispy, remove the tray from the oven and leave to cool for 5 minutes (try not to eat it all, it's a challenge!).

Meanwhile, in a small blender, blend all the cream ingredients together and season to taste.

Layer your sandwich with the cashew miso cream on both sides, then the mushroom tofu mix in the middle followed by a handful of rocket or spinach. Make sure you pile it high. Sandwich the slices of bread together firmly, then wrap up and slice down the middle, carefully, with a serrated knife. Enjoy straight away, or take it out for lunch!

Protein per serving: 22g
Fibre: 7g
Plant diversity score: 6

NOTES
Add more Tofu when roasting or swap for Tempeh Crumbles (page 207) for a more protein dense portion

Sweet
Squash Dal

SERVES 4
TOTAL TIME: 50 MINS–1 HR

Indian cuisine is quite possibly my favourite. It can seem intimidating, and there's a fair few internet cooking police out there, but once you've got the base right, and you use enough spice, you'll be in for a tasty meal.

I'm bumping up the protein from the lentils even more here by adding silken tofu to the sauce and giving it a sweeter tang by blending this with roasted squash. It's a bit of a mash-up, but it works, and without a doubt should make it into your weekly rotation during squash season.

250g (9oz/1 cup) split red lentils, drained and rinsed
Olive oil
1 medium pumpkin or squash
1 small white onion, finely diced
4cm (1½in) piece of fresh ginger, peeled and grated
4 garlic cloves, minced
½ red chilli, finely chopped (less if you don't like spice, or omit altogether)
1 tsp ground coriander
1 tsp ground cumin
1 tsp ground turmeric
1 tsp smoked paprika
1 tsp garam masala
Pinch of ground cinnamon
1 tbsp tomato purée
750ml (26fl oz/3 cups) vegetable stock
Sea salt and black pepper

FOR THE SQUASH AND CASHEW CREAM
½ roasted pumpkin or squash (see above), flesh scraped from the skin
200g (7oz) silken tofu
30g (1oz/scant ¼ cup) cashews, soaked in boiling water for 10 minutes then drained
2 tbsp nutritional yeast
1 garlic clove
Juice of 1 lemon
Splash of water, if needed for blending

TO SERVE
Small handful of sage leaves
Sliced red chilli
Soy yoghurt (optional)
Sourdough bread, naan or roti

Preheat the oven to 200°C fan/220°C/gas mark 7.

In a small bowl, soak the lentils in plenty of cold water until ready to use.

Cut the pumpkin or squash in half, de-seed, then cut one of the halves into 4 wedges, leaving the other half intact. Transfer to a roasting tray, drizzle with oil, season with salt and roast for 30–40 minutes until the wedges are browning and the skin on the intact half is starting to collapse when you poke it.

In a medium casserole or other heavy-bottomed saucepan on a medium heat, fry the onion in 2 tablespoons of olive oil with a pinch of salt for 8 minutes. Add the ginger, garlic and chilli and fry for a further 4 minutes. Add another tablespoon of olive oil, heat it up, then add all the spices and fry until fragrant. Add the tomato purée.

Drain the lentils, rinse well and add to the pan. Coat in the spices, then add the stock. Bring to the boil, then simmer on a medium heat, stirring regularly so it doesn't burn. Keep an eye on the consistency. If it's looking too thick, add a splash more water.

In a small blender, whizz up all the creamy sauce ingredients, then season to taste.

In a small frying pan on a medium-high heat, fry the sage leaves in oil until crispy, rest them on kitchen paper and sprinkle with a little sea salt.

Once the lentils have been cooking for 25–30 minutes, taste to see if they're ready. When they're

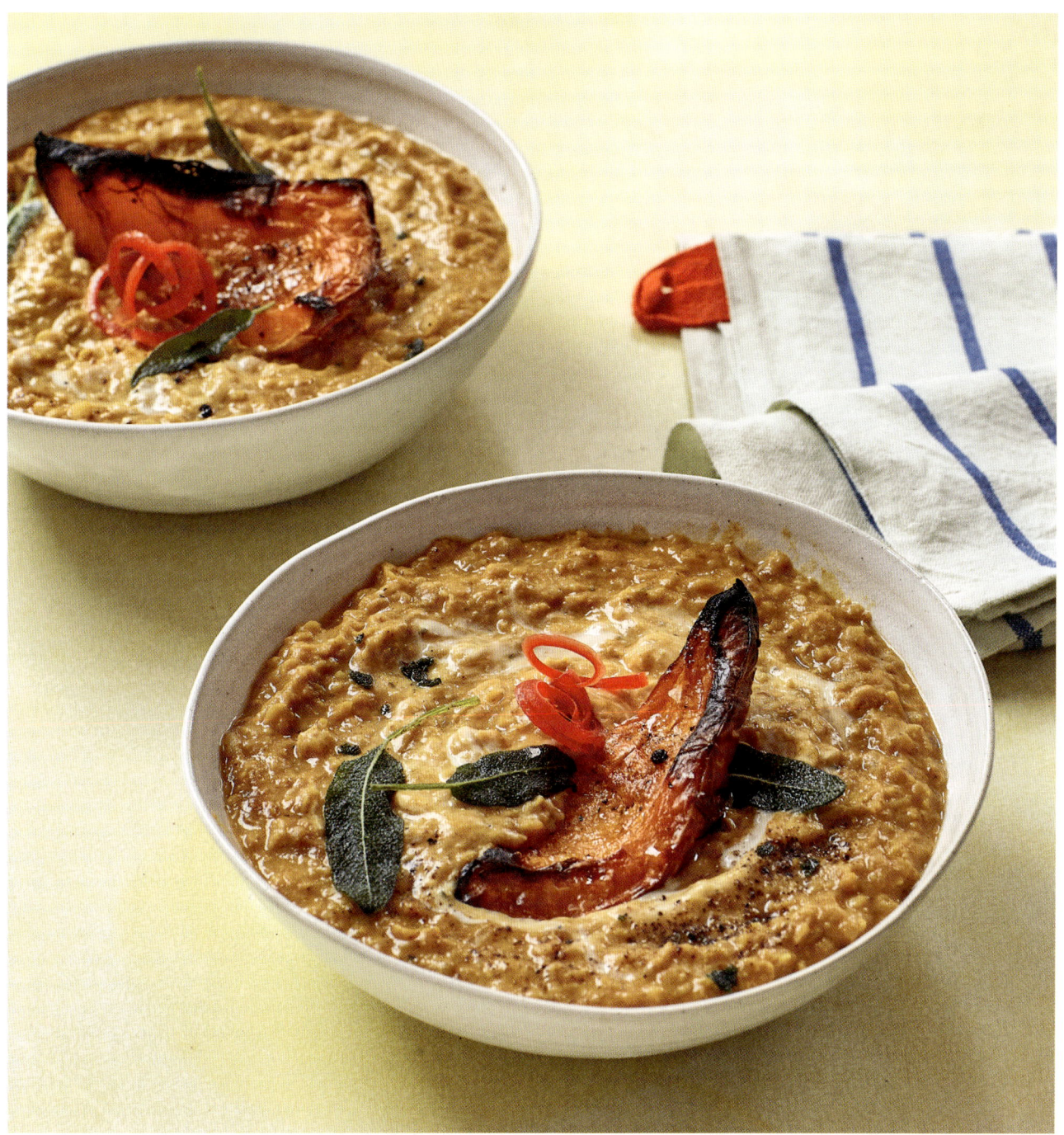

soft, add the squash and cashew cream and stir through.

Divide the dal between bowls and decorate with the roasted pumpkin wedges, crispy sage, chilli and yoghurt. Serve with sourdough bread, naan or roti.

Protein per serving: 23g
Fibre: 11g
Plant diversity score: 11

20-minute Ramen

SERVES 3
TOTAL: 20 MINS

Another easy win weeknight meal to whip out on a cold evening. A true bowl of comfort, absolutely bursting with flavour. Adjust the chilli quantities to your liking!

3 tbsp sesame oil
3 spring onions, white parts finely chopped, green parts finely chopped for the topping
1 tbsp chopped red chilli
Large thumb-sized piece of fresh ginger, peeled and grated
3 garlic cloves, grated
200ml (7fl oz/¾ cup) soy milk
200ml (7fl oz/¾ cup) vegetable stock
1 tsp brown miso paste
2 tbsp rice wine vinegar
2 tbsp tamari
200g (7oz) buckwheat (soba) noodles
Sesame oil, for drizzling

FOR THE TOPPINGS
Olive oil
300g (10oz) extra-firm smoked tofu, crumbed into small pieces
Splash of tamari or pinch of sea salt
Large handful of cooked chickpeas (optional)
Sliced red chilli
A sprinkle of black and white sesame seeds
Crispy chilli oil (optional)

Start with the broth. Heat the sesame oil in a heavy-bottomed saucepan on a medium heat and add the white spring onion, chilli, ginger and garlic. Fry for 2–3 minutes until fragrant.

Add the veg stock and soy milk, mix everything together and bubble on a medium heat. Add the miso, rice vinegar and tamari. Stir well and keep on a low heat while you prep the toppings.

Heat up some olive oil in a non-stick pan on a medium-high heat and add the tofu. Cook off with the tamari until golden and crisping at the edges. Season to taste.

Cook the noodles according to the packet instructions. Drain and wash well in cold water, then set aside. Drizzle a little sesame oil over to stop them from sticking together.

Divide the elements into bowls, starting with a large ladle of broth, then a large handful of noodles, the crispy smoked tofu, green parts of the spring onions, chickpeas (if using), fresh chilli, sesame seeds and crispy chilli oil.

Protein per serving: 27g
Fibre: 14g
Plant diversity score: 11

NOTES
Get creative with the toppings! Add fried beans, crispy lentils or a crumbled veg sausage or Homemade Meatballs (see page 225).

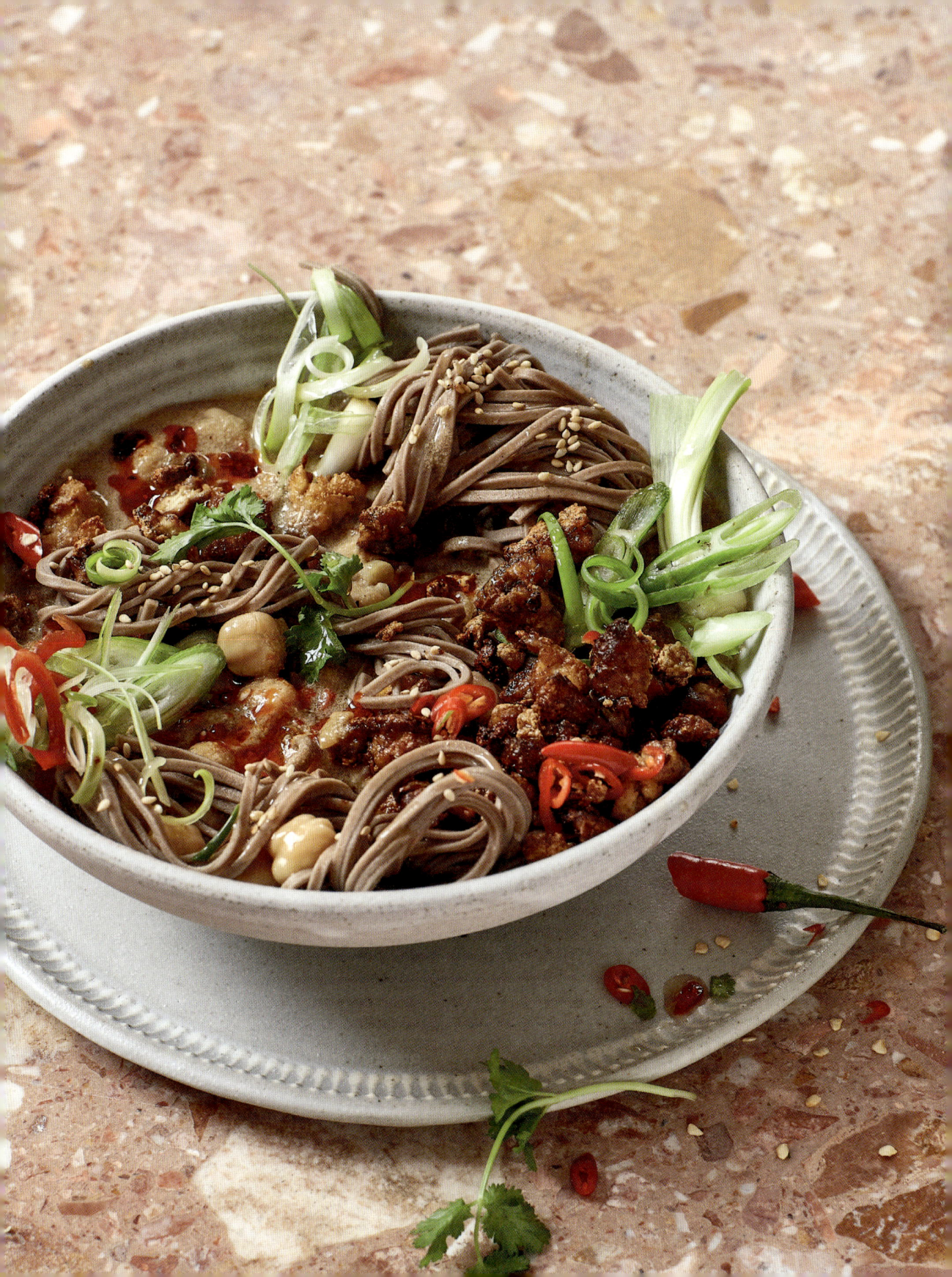

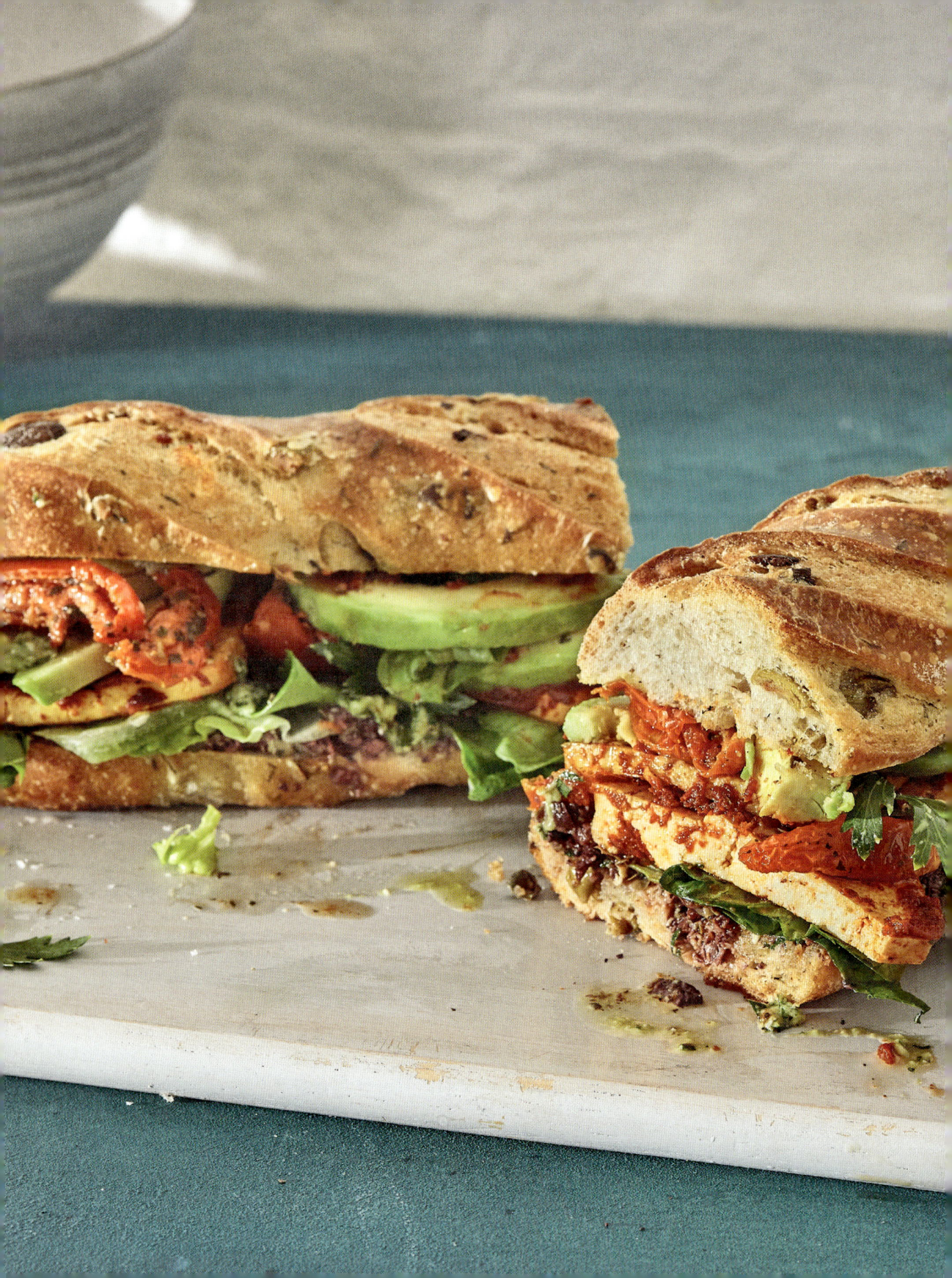

Avo, Olives, Toms and Tofu Baguette

SERVES 2
TOTAL TIME: 30 MINS

A remake of one of my favourite sandwiches from a popular sandwich chain in the UK. I've added tofu for extra protein!

200g (7oz) extra-firm smoked tofu
40g (1½oz) Kalamata olives, pitted
1 tbsp red wine vinegar
1 tbsp olive oil
1 tbsp capers
½ avocado
Small handful of rocket
1 sourdough baguette
5 sun-dried tomatoes
2 tbsp Hemp Seed Pesto (see page 216)

FOR THE TOFU MARINADE
1 tbsp tomato purée
3 tbsp olive oil
2 tbsp lemon juice
½ tsp smoked paprika
½ tsp dried oregano
½ tsp ground cumin
Pinch of ground cinnamon
Pinch of ground turmeric
Pinch of cayenne pepper
½ tsp onion powder
½ tsp garlic powder

Preheat the oven to 160°C fan/180°C/gas mark 4.

In a small bowl, mix all the marinade ingredients together.

Give the tofu a good squeeze, wrapped in kitchen paper, to drain off any excess water. Slice it into 5mm (¼in) slices, then lay on a baking tray and coat both sides with the marinade using a pastry brush. Bake for 20 minutes, turning over halfway through cooking.

In a small bullet blender, add the olives, vinegar, olive oil and capers. Blend to a thick paste.

Slice the avocado and toast the baguette in the oven on a low temperature for 2–4 minutes at most. Cut the baguette almost in half and scoop out a little of the fluffy white bread, to make way for the fillings. Spread the bottom with the olive paste, and the top with hemp pesto. Then add the rocket, tofu, avocado and sun-dried tomatoes.

Sandwich together, wrap in baking parchment, slice in half and enjoy!

Protein per serving: 21g
Fibre: 6.3g
Plant diversity score: 8

Cheesy Quesadillas

SERVES 2–3
TOTAL: 30 MINS

A quick, savoury, moreish snack. Fun to make, great to do with kids, too.

6 wholemeal tortillas
7–8 tbsp Cashew Queso (see page 219)

FOR THE CHICKPEA MIXTURE
1 x 400g (14oz) can chickpeas, drained and rinsed
2 tbsp roughly chopped sun-dried tomatoes
2 spring onions, white parts finely sliced
1 tsp Dijon mustard
3 tbsp vegan mayonnaise (sub soy yoghurt)
2 tbsp olive oil
2 garlic cloves, crushed
1 tsp smoked paprika
½ tsp salt, plus more to taste
6–8 twists of black pepper
Small handful of finely chopped fresh coriander

FOR THE GUACAMOLE
1 ripe avocado, deseeded and diced
5 cherry tomatoes, quartered
Small wedge of red onion, finely chopped
1 garlic clove, minced
Small handful of finely chopped fresh coriander
Juice of 1 lime
1 tbsp olive oil
½ tsp sea salt

In a large mixing bowl, roughly mash all the chickpea mixture ingredients. It should resemble a chunky breadcrumb texture. Season to taste.

In a medium-sized mixing bowl, combine/mash all the ingredients for the guacamole. Season to taste.

Add one tortilla to a dry frying pan (don't turn the heat on yet) and spread half of the chickpea mixture on half of the tortilla. You want about 1cm (½in) in thickness, about 3–5 tablespoons of the mixture, depending on the size of your tortilla. Drizzle a generous layer of the cashew queso on top and smooth out to the edges with the back of a spoon. Then fold the other half of the tortilla on top neatly and press down with a spatula.

Put the heat on high. After a few minutes, carefully check to see if the tortilla is browning underneath by lifting the edge. If it is, carefully flip the tortilla over to cook the other side.

Repeat the above process with the rest of the tortillas and filling.

When cool enough to touch, cut each tortilla into 3 segments with a sharp knife, quickly, so the filling doesn't splat everywhere.

Serve with the guacamole.

Protein per serving: 20g
Fibre: 23g
Plant diversity score: 10

NOTES
Serve with my Harissa, Ginger and Coconut Lentils (page 115) or Healing Greens and Beans Soup (page 116) for a more filling meal

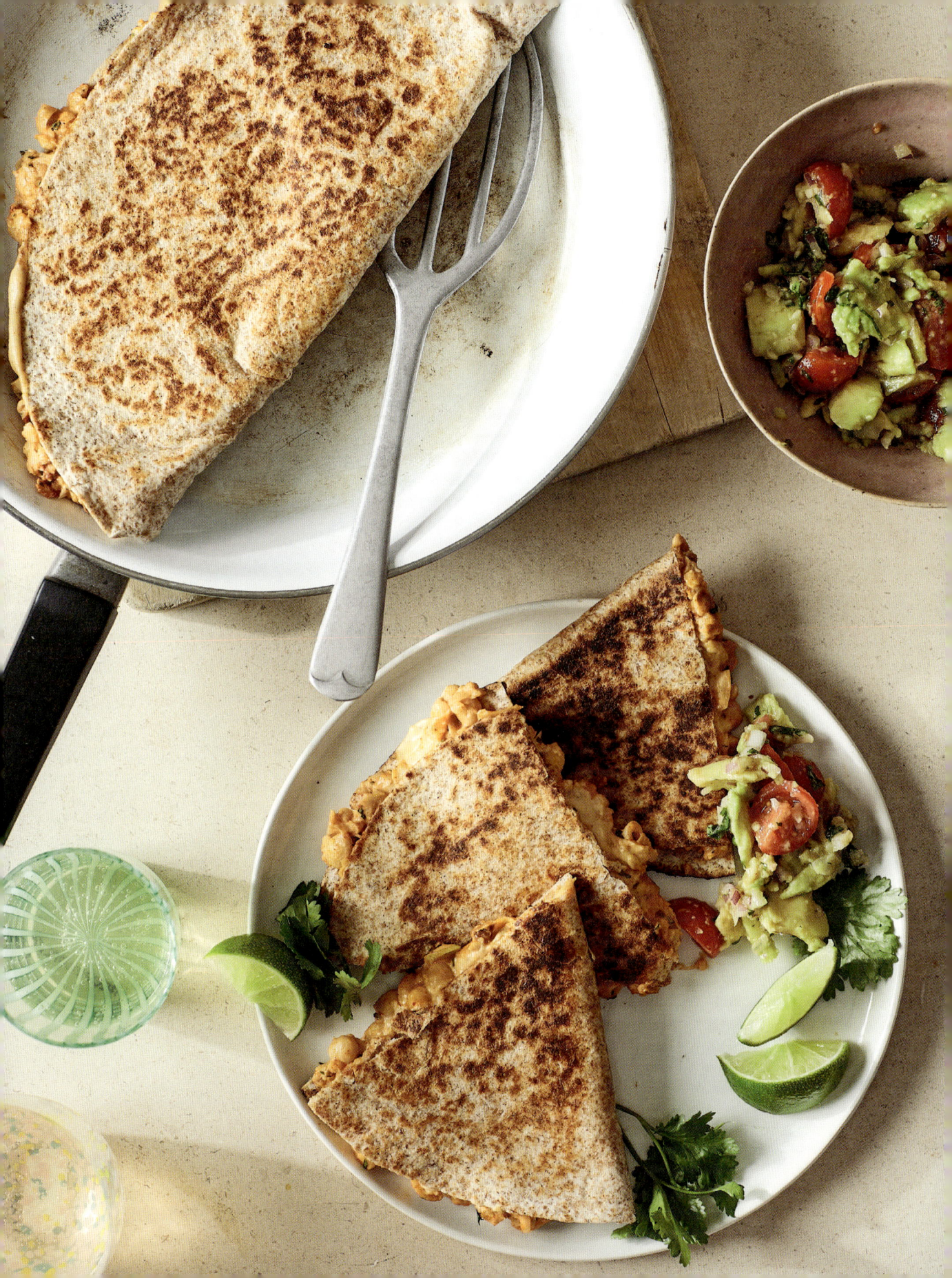

30/30

Each of these recipes should take less than 30 minutes, and contains over 30g of protein. You'll *probably* be able to make these in under 30 minutes, but it will depend on the speed of your chopping. I recommend investing in a mini chopper for ease and speed if you find chopping boring and laborious.

There's a bit of everything in here, from my Ultimate Bean Bowl (see page 132) to Loaded Caesar Pasta Plates (see page 138) and Tantalising Tempeh Fried Rice (see page 145), so you'll be able to keep things interesting on weeknights without spending the whole evening in the kitchen.

Teriyaki Tofu with Mango Edamame Salsa

I've never been organised enough to marinate my tofu for hours, so my shortcut is to go for the smoked variety, make sure to crisp it up, then add the sauce and fry lightly until it's nice and glazed – not for too long, as this can dull the flavour of the sauce. Paired with the zingy mango and crunchy Tenderstem broccoli, this one really hits the spot!

200g (7oz/1 cup) brown rice
½–1 tsp vegetable bouillon powder (optional)
150g (5½oz) Tenderstem broccoli, washed and ends chopped off
Flaky sea salt

FOR THE QUICK TERIYAKI-STYLE TOFU
250g (9oz) extra-firm smoked tofu
2 tsp cornflour
2 tbsp sesame oil
2½ tbsp tamari
1 tbsp maple syrup or agave
½ tbsp rice wine vinegar
3 garlic cloves, minced
1 tbsp grated fresh ginger

FOR THE MANGO SALSA
100g (3½oz) fresh mango, finely diced
6–8 cherry tomatoes, quartered
4 spring onions, white parts finely chopped, green parts finely chopped and saved for garnish
Handful of fresh coriander, leaves finely chopped
1 tsp apple cider vinegar
Pinch of sea salt

TO SERVE
Cucumber slices
Edamame beans, fresh or thawed from frozen
Black sesame seeds
Chilli flakes
Lime wedges

Cook the rice according to the packet instructions, adding the vegetable bouillon powder if you wish for extra flavour!

Get the tofu out of the packet, drain well and give it a good squeeze, wrapped in kitchen paper or a tea towel. Tear it into medium/large irregular chunks and add to a bowl. Sprinkle over the cornflour and a little flaky salt. In a non-stick pan on a medium heat, fry the tofu in the sesame oil for 8–10 minutes until the edges start to firm up and the tofu turns a shade darker. While it's frying, prep the teriyaki tofu sauce by whisking all the remaining tofu ingredients together in a small bowl. Pour this over the tofu and fry until sticky and unctuous.

Set the tofu aside, then, in the same pan, lightly fry the broccoli. The residual water from the wash will lightly steam the broccoli, and the leftover sauce in the pan will give it some bite. When the broccoli starts to turn a bright shade of green, remove from the pan and set aside.

In a small bowl, combine all the mango salsa ingredients and season to taste.

Divide all the elements between bowls, starting with the rice, then the broccoli, tofu, mango salsa, cucumber, edamame beans, sesame seeds, chilli flakes and a lime wedge on the side. Squeeze over the lime before you eat!

Protein per serving: 32.5g
Fibre: 13
Plant diversity score: 10

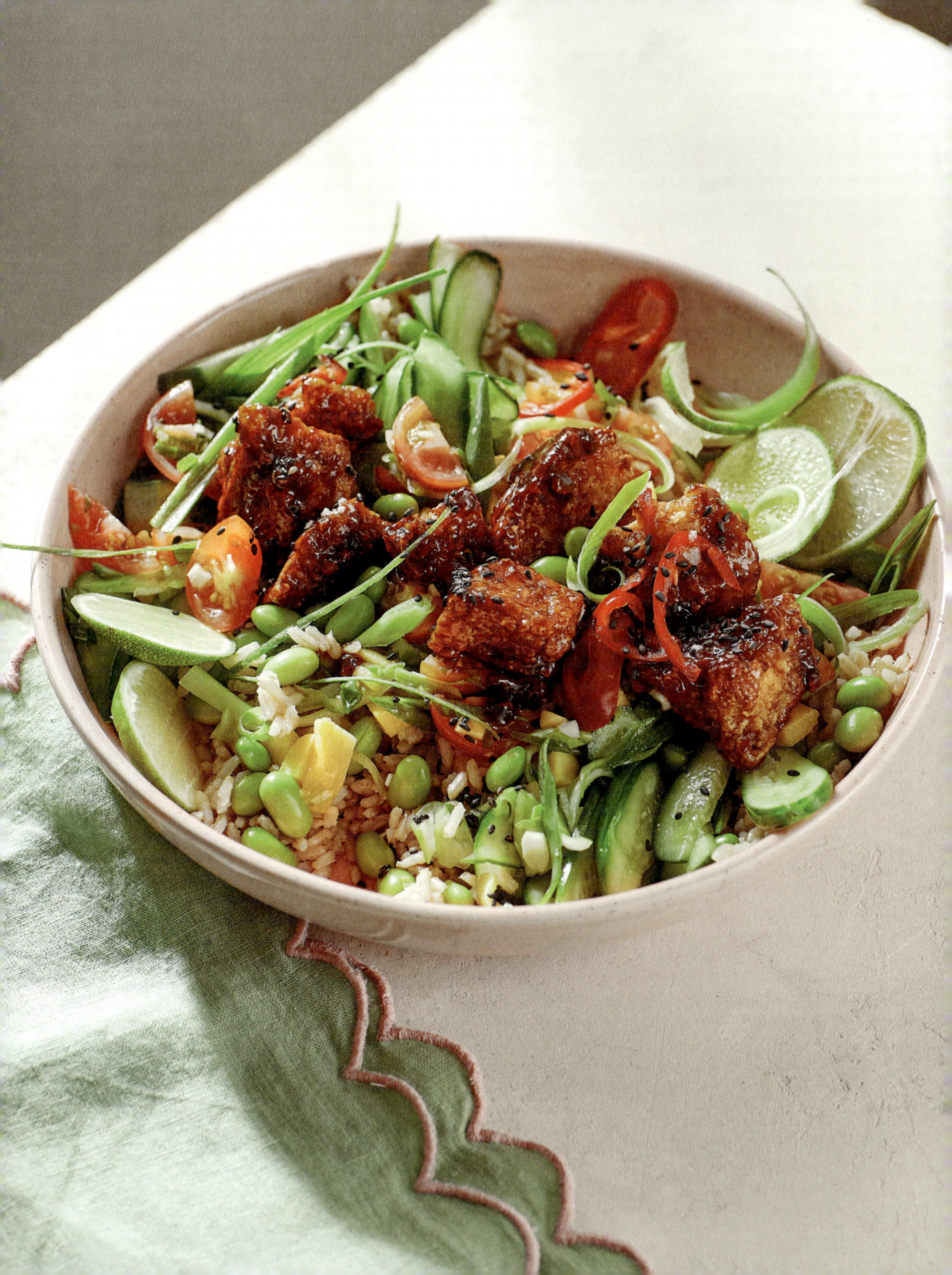

The Ultimate
Bean Bowl Method

SERVES 2–3
AVERAGE TOTAL TIME: 15–30 MINS

If you follow me on socials, you'll know I'm a huge advocate for a simple, seasonal bean bowl. If you don't know what to cook, and you'd rather not spend hours in the kitchen, but want something easy, tasty and healthy, this is your ultimate guide.

It's the epitome of my 'protein layering' method. Start with a legume, add a nutty cream, tofu cubes or a crunchy seed topping and enjoy with bread or a wholegrain.

I highly recommend the ritual of going to a local market at the weekend, and picking up whatever is in season to add to the bean bowls. Not only will it be tastier and more sustainable, but it's also a way to get more in tune with mother nature, as well as being a great way to meet like-minded people.

The Formula

FOR THE BASE (per person, multiply for the number you're cooking for)

1 small shallot or ½ white onion, finely chopped (sub a leek!)
Olive oil
2 garlic cloves, grated
Any fresh herbs you like! Think sage, thyme, rosemary, coriander etc.
About 1 x 400g (14oz) can beans, plus their juices if the can is organic and BPA free, or you can use 160ml (5½fl oz/⅔ cup) water per person, plus ¼ vegetable stock cube or ½ tsp vegetable bouillon powder
About 1–2 tbsp nutritional yeast
Extra virgin olive oil, for drizzling
Salt and black pepper

FOR THE VEG

Seasonal veg you can find easily in the local supermarket, or even better, a local farmer's market A few ideas:

Spring: Peas, Asparagus, Radish, Spinach

Summer: Tomatoes, Courgettes, Aubergines

Autumn: Squash, Jerusalem artichokes, Pak choi, Parsnips, Mushrooms

Winter: Cavolo nero, Kale, Cabbage, Carrots, Cauliflower, Broccoli

Of course, you can buy these all year round in the supermarket, but buying locally and seasonally will ensure you're getting the best-tasting meal, and the most environmentally friendly one.

You can choose to pan-fry this veg with the onion, chopping stems finely (broccoli/asparagus) and leaving more water-dense veg (courgettes) diced or sliced, or you can roast it and add in later, steam on top of the pan, or boil in with the liquidy beans. All are delicious methods and will depend on the texture, size and shape of your veg.

Leaves and thinner, more water-dense veg like leeks, spinach and kale will cook a lot quicker, whereas thicker, starchier winter veg like squash and potatoes will probably need either par-boiling or roasting. Roasting is a great way to add additional spices and plant points, too.

132

FOR THE ADD-INS

Cashew Cream (see page 219)
Coconut, soy or oat cream
Miso paste
Chilli oil
Harissa

FOR THE TOPPINGS

Garlicky Sourdough Breadcrumbs (see page 207)
Nutty, Noochy Crumb (see page 208)
Cashew Parmesan (see page 221)
Tofu feta (page 220)
Crumbled tofu or tempeh (page 207)
Red Lentil or Chickpea Tofu (see pages 210–211)
Tofu Cream Cheese (see page 220)
Other legumes, such as cooked lentils
Crispy roasted legumes (see page 78)

Basic method

In a wide casserole pan or frying pan on a medium heat, start by cooking down the onion in plenty of olive oil and a pinch of salt. If you're pan-frying larger veg, such as courgette or carrot, chop and pop this in, too. You want the veg to be a little tender and the onion translucent before you move on to the next step.

Add the garlic and any fresh herbs, ground spices or other aromatics like ginger to layer those flavours in. For some hardier, woodier herbs like rosemary, you would throw the whole stem in and remove it later, before eating. For a more delicate leaf like coriander or parsley, wait until the end to put the leaves in, but chop the stems up finely and use those – they're full of flavour. Basil I like to layer in, some torn in halfway and some on top or stirred in when the pan comes off the heat.

Ground spices I love using in bean bowls are usually coriander, cumin, smoked paprika, cayenne chilli pepper, curry powder and garam masala.

Pour in the beans and their juices. If you'd prefer to not add the bean water, that's fine, just add water plus a little bit of crumbled vegetable stock cube or bouillon powder, being mindful of the salt level and only adding as much stock cube as you prefer (bear in mind - some of the toppings might also have salt in them).

Next up, the add-ins. Choose from cashew cream to make it creamier, or you could add coconut cream, soy or oat cream if desired, silken tofu for extra protein, then anything else you fancy. For a bit more umami, add nutritional yeast or miso paste, for something spicier, maybe chilli oil or harissa. Endless possibilities!

Once you are happy with the flavour and level of seasoning, it's time to choose your toppings. You'll want to add some crunch, so maybe crispy, garlicky breadcrumbs, tamari roasted seeds, nutty, noochy crumb, or maybe you're looking for a 'cheesy' boost – add cashew parm in this instance.

I always squeeze over some lemon juice (if the dish isn't loaded with acidity – like tomato flavours) just before serving, to add brightness, some more extra virgin olive oil, plenty of cracked black pepper and fresh herbs.

For an extra protein boost, fry up some tofu cubes, tempeh crumble, or you can use chickpea tofu or red lentil tofu (page 210).

The bottom line is: cooking is all about experimentation. Have fun with the process of cooking seasonal, healthy and high-protein plant-based whole foods. You now have all the tools to effectively layer your protein, in an easy and straightforward way.

Up next is an example to get you started.

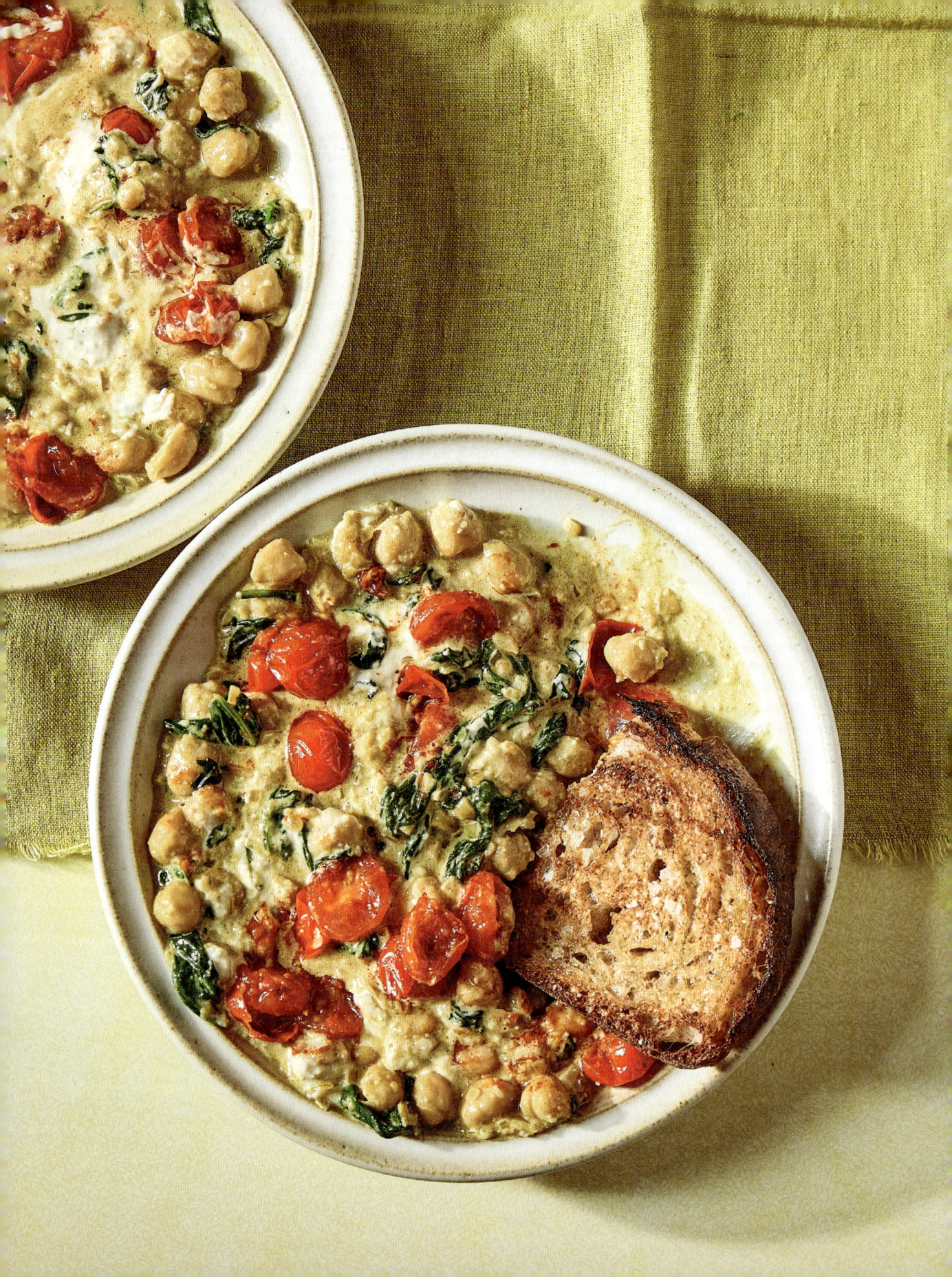

Healing Creamy Bean Bowl

SERVES 2
TOTAL TIME: 30 MINS

1 small/medium white onion, finely chopped
4 garlic cloves, minced
3cm (1¼in) piece of fresh ginger, peeled and grated
1 tsp ground cumin
1 tsp ground coriander
1 tsp ground turmeric
½ tsp cayenne chilli pepper (less if you don't like spice)
2 x 400g (14oz) tins cooked chickpeas
200ml (7fl oz/ ¾oz)coconut milk, from a can
2 large handfuls (about 120g/4oz) chopped spinach
200g (7oz) cherry tomatoes, cut in half
1 tsp smoked paprika
Salt and black pepper

FOR THE SAUCE
290g (10¼oz) silken tofu
Juice of 1 lemon
3 tbsp nutritional yeast
50g (1¾oz/⅓ cup) cashew nuts, soaked in boiling water for 10 minutes then drained
1½ tbsp sweet white miso paste

TO SERVE:
Fresh basil leaves
Chilli flakes
Nigella seeds (optional)

Begin by soaking your cashew nuts in a small bowl. If you have a nut allergy, swap these for sunflower seeds.

In a medium pan on a medium heat, fry off the onion in plenty of olive oil for 8 minutes with a pinch of salt until lightly caramelised, then add ¾ of the garlic and all of the ginger, frying for a further 3 minutes. Add the spices and toast for 1 minute more, until fragrant. Add the chickpeas, coconut milk, spinach, and a splash of water to loosen the dish, then turn the heat down whilst you blend the sauce ingredients together.

In a small blender cup, blend up the all white creamy sauce ingredients and season to taste, adding salt if you need to. Pour into the pan, mix well. Turn the heat up to a bubble, then down to a simmer and cook, stirring occasionally for 5 minutes, whilst you prepare the tomatoes.

In a medium frying pan on a medium/high heat, fry the tomatoes in olive oil and a pinch of salt for 5–6 mins, until they start to visibly break down. Add the smoked paprika and remaining garlic, fry for a further 3–4 minutes. Season to taste.

Divide into bowls, place the fried tomatoes on top and garnish with the chilli flakes, fresh basil and nigella seeds.

Enjoy with a cooked grain of choice or a slice of toasted sourdough bread.

Protein per serving: 41g
Fibre: 22g
Plant diversity score: 12

Hot 'Honey'
Tofu Bowls

Hot honey is what all the cool kids eat these days, so I thought why not see what all the fuss is about? Turns out, it's really quite good. Paired with a quinoa, lentil and veg base and a tangy dressing to bring everything together, this is an instant winner.

150g (5¼oz/ ¾ cup) quinoa
½ tsp vegetable bouillon powder (optional)
200g (7oz) cooked Puy lentils, from a can or jar, drained and rinsed
½ small red cabbage, thinly sliced
3 spring onions, white and green parts finely chopped
250g (9oz) extra-firm tofu
Olive oil
2 tsp cornflour
1 tbsp agave syrup
2 tbsp tamari
1 tsp chilli flakes (adjust the heat to your liking)

FOR THE DRESSING
1 tbsp lemon juice
1 tbsp olive oil
Pinch of sea salt
Pinch of black pepper
½ tsp Dijon mustard
½ agave syrup

TO SERVE
½ cucumber, roughly sliced at an angle
4 radishes, finely sliced
Sesame seeds
Fresh coriander leaves

Start by cooking the quinoa according to the packet instructions. I usually cook mine with vegetable bouillon powder.

Once cooked and cooled, mix the quinoa with the lentils, red cabbage and spring onions. Mix all the dressing ingredients in a small bowl and pour over. Gently combine and season to taste.

Give the tofu a good squeeze, wrapped in kitchen paper or a tea towel, to remove any excess water, then tear it apart with your hands into irregular sized chunks, ranging from 1–4cm (½ –1½in). Add the chunks to a mixing bowl and sprinkle over the cornflour. Toss the chunks around in the bowl so they're well covered.

Heat the oil in a non-stick pan on a medium heat and fry the tofu on all sides for a few minutes each, until golden. Drizzle over the agave, tamari and chilli flakes, adding more if you need so all the tofu chunks are generously coated and starting to char and go golden. Taste one of the chunks, add a little more tamari if you think it needs more salt. Remove from the heat.

Divide into bowls, plating the quinoa lentil salad first, followed by the hot honey tofu chunks, the cucumber and radishes. Garnish with sesame seeds and fresh coriander leaves.

Protein per serving: 33g
Fibre: 14g
Plant diversity score: 12

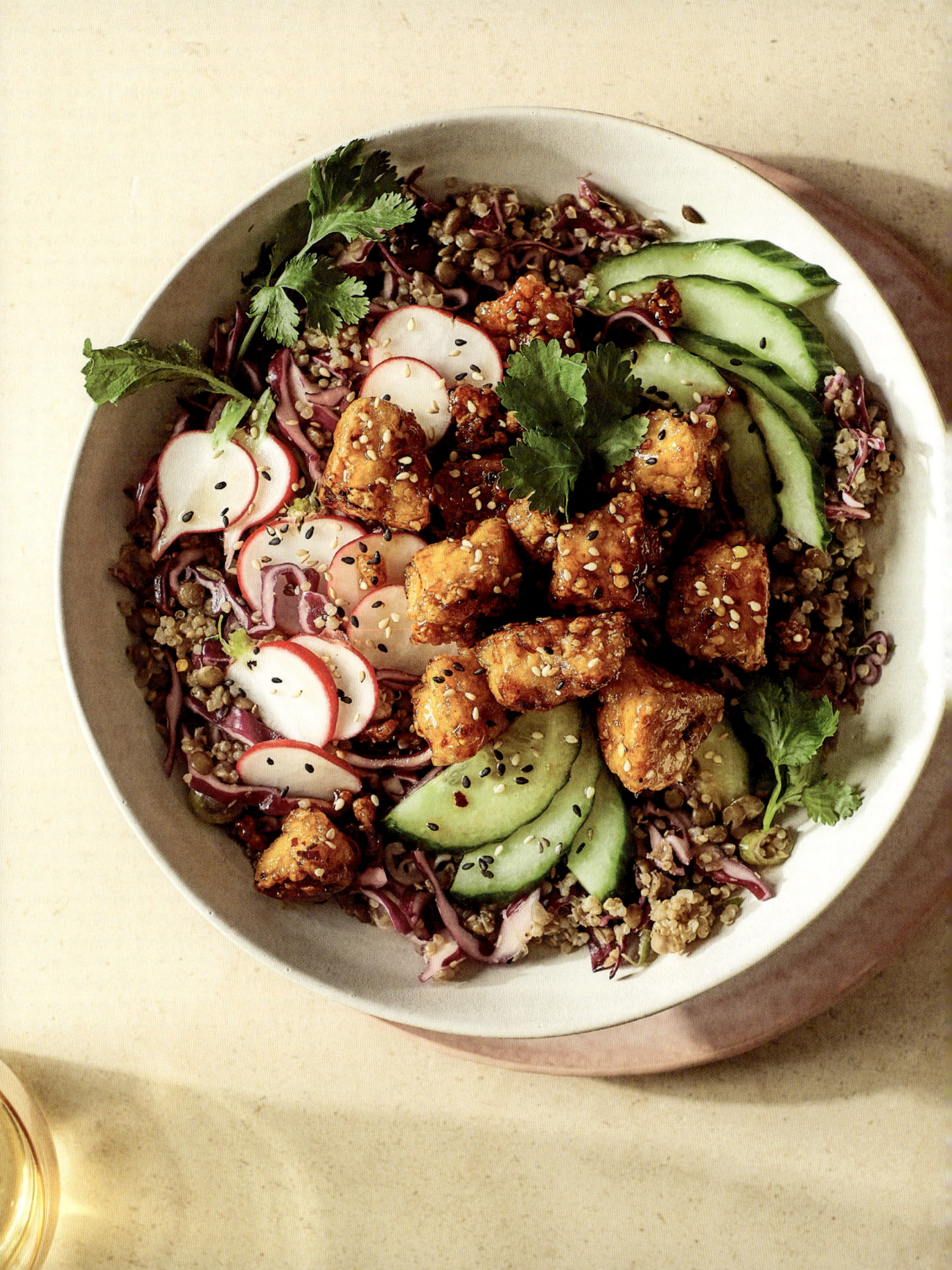

Loaded Caesar Pasta Plates

This dressing is so good I could drink it straight from a cup. It's slightly weaker than a typical Caesar dressing, and a little creamier. I've swapped the traditional cos lettuce for kale, as the kale holds the dressing very well and keeps better in the fridge, so you can enjoy the leftovers for lunch the next day.

Feel free to customise it with whatever you have on hand – add new potatoes or roasted sweet potato instead of pasta, swap the tofu for tempeh or seitan, add garlicky croutons, etc. It's an easy winner and a great recipe to have on hand!

1 x 400g (14oz) can chickpeas, rinsed, drained and dried
1 tbsp olive oil
250g (9oz) spelt pasta
200g (7oz) kale, washed, stems removed, leaves roughly chopped
50g (1¾oz) rocket
200g (7oz) extra-firm smoked tofu
1 tbsp tamari (optional)
Salt and black pepper

FOR THE CAESAR SAUCE
80g (3oz/½ cup) cashews, soaked in boiling water for 15 minutes then drained
½ tbsp Dijon mustard
1 tbsp capers, plus 1 tsp of their brine
100g (3½oz) silken tofu
4 tbsp nutritional yeast
Juice of 1 large lemon, plus more to taste
6–7 twists of black pepper
1 tsp maple or agave syrup
1 tbsp olive oil, plus more if needed
3 fat garlic cloves, minced

TO SERVE
Cashew Parm (see page 221) or your favourite vegan parm, shaved (optional)

Omega-3 Boost (see page 209)
Lemon wedges

Preheat the oven to 180°C fan/200°C/gas mark 6.

On a roasting tray, toss the dried chickpeas in the olive oil, ½ teaspoon of salt and a few twists of black pepper. Bake for 15–20 minutes or until golden and crispy.

Meanwhile, cook the pasta in plenty of salted water for 1 minute less than the packet instructions, reserving a large mugful of the water before draining.

While that's cooking, prep the dressing. In a bullet or blender cup, blend all the dressing ingredients until smooth. Season to taste.

In a large bowl, combine one-third of the dressing with the washed kale leaves, massaging briefly with your hands until it starts to soften. Add a little more olive oil, if you need to. Add the pasta and a little more dressing, combine well, then add the rocket and toss again, lightly.

Chop the smoked tofu into 1cm (½in) cubes. If you're using a brand that tastes good without cooking, skip straight to the next step. If not, fry the tofu in a little olive oil for a few minutes each side until it starts to brown, then add 1 tablespoon of tamari and fry until all the sauce has been absorbed.

Divide the cooked pasta between bowls or plates, topping with the roasted chickpeas, smoked tofu, cashew parm, Omega-3 seeds, more of the gorgeous dressing, and the lemon wedges for squeezing over before you eat it.

Protein per serving: 33g
Fibre: 25g
Plant diversity score: 9

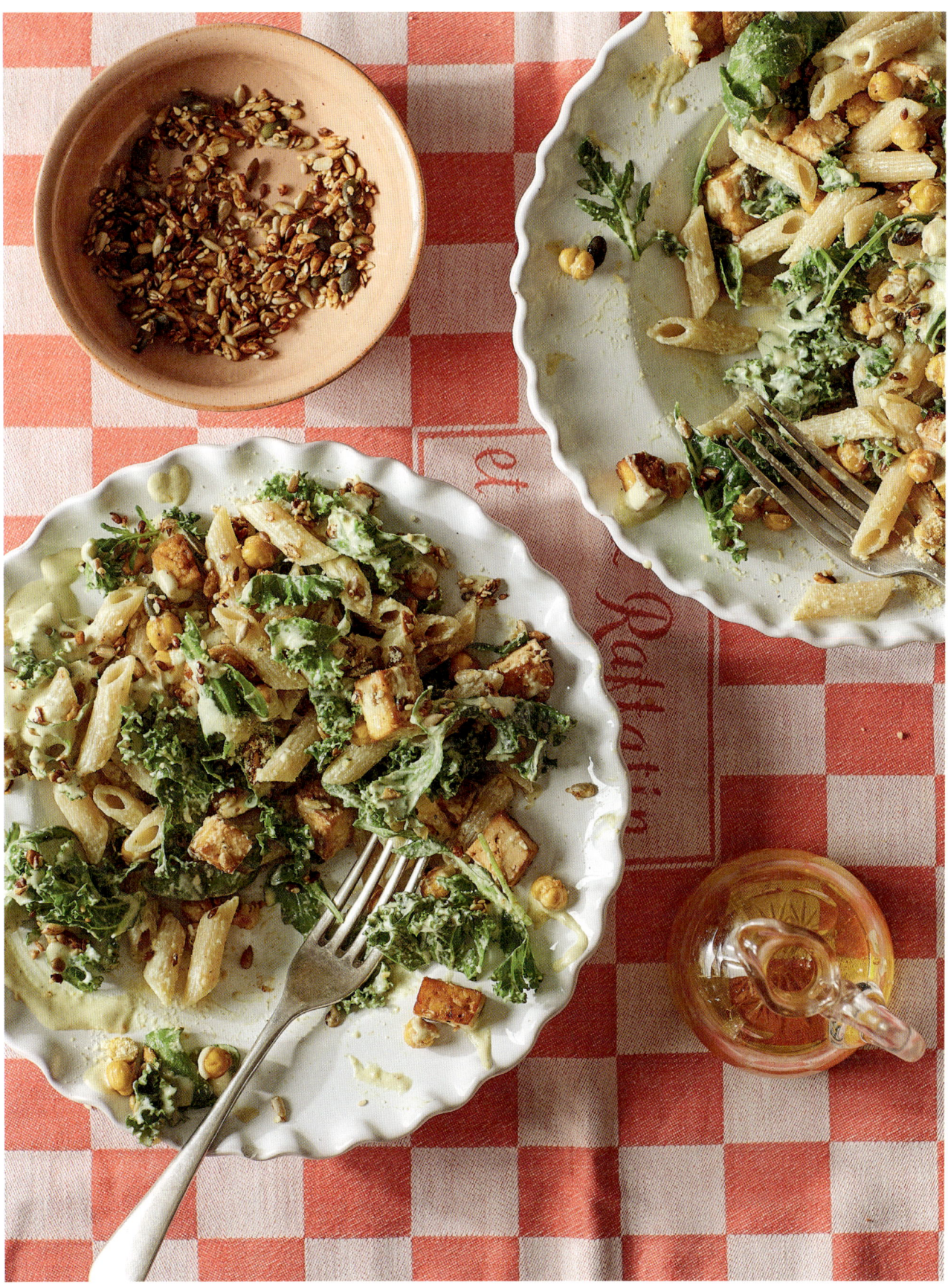

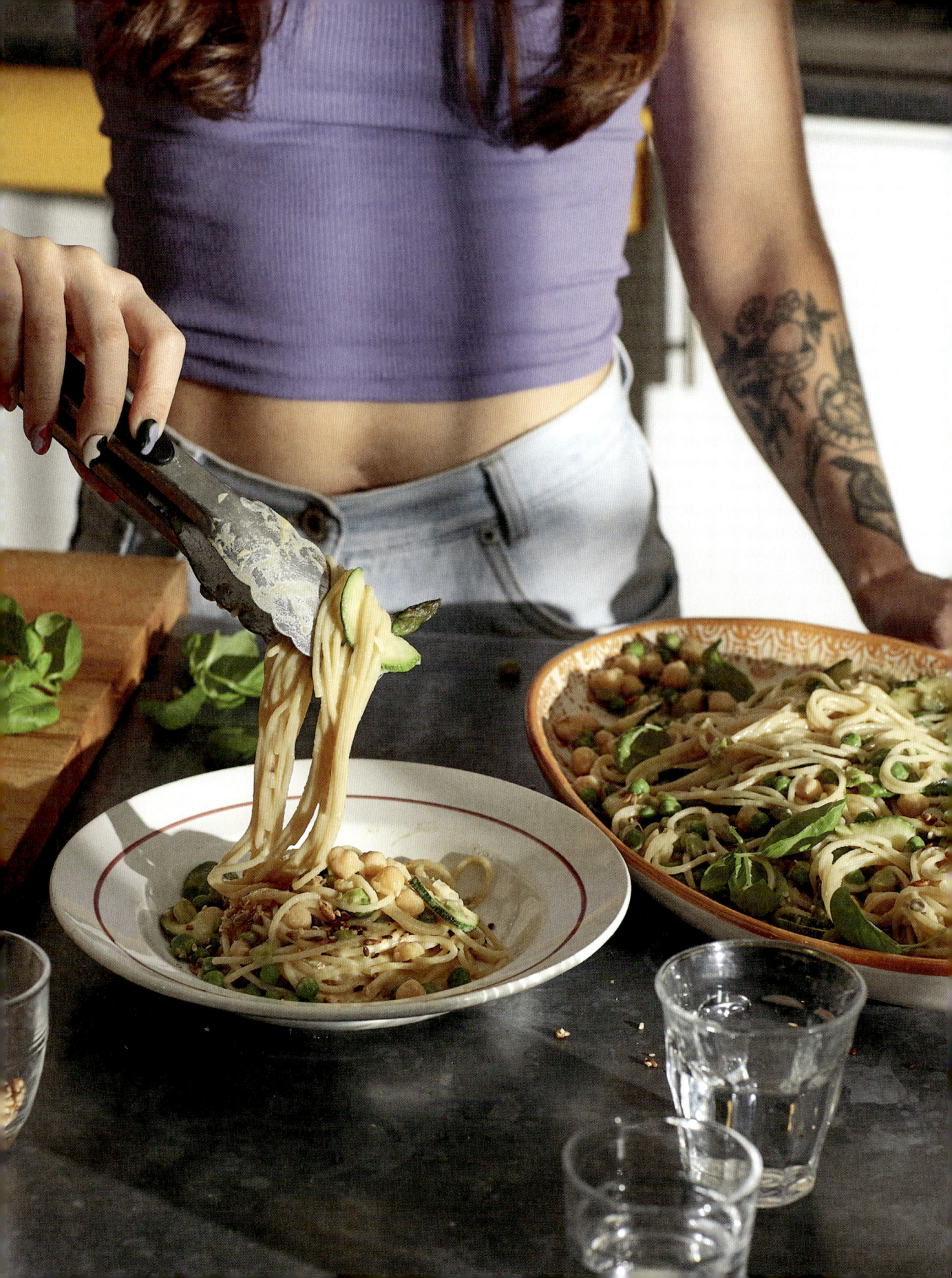

Creamy Springtime Spaghetti

SERVES 3
TOTAL TIME: 30 MINS

Fresh, crunchy veg, juicy peas, cheesy sauce, soft-cooked chickpeas and starchy pasta. It's filling, quick and super healthy!

If asparagus is not in season, feel free to substitute with any seasonal veg – cauliflower, broccoli, tomato, fennel, cabbage would all work.

1 large shallot or ½ white onion, finely diced
1 bunch (about 200g/7oz) of asparagus, woody stems snapped off, stalks finely chopped, tops halved
4 garlic cloves, minced
1 large courgette, cut into half-moons
Olive oil, for frying
200g (7oz) spelt spaghetti
150g (5½oz) frozen garden peas
480g (1lb 1oz) chickpeas, from a can or jar, drained and rinsed
3 tbsp sweet white miso paste
Juice of 1 lemon
3 tbsp nutritional yeast
Sea salt and black pepper

TO SERVE
Fresh basil
Lightly dressed rocket
Omega-3 Boost (see page 209, optional)

In a medium frying pan on a low–medium heat, cook the shallow or onion in plenty of olive oil with a small pinch of sea salt for 5 minutes. Add the finely chopped asparagus stems and cook for a further 6–7 minutes. Add the garlic, the courgette, asparagus tops and another pinch of sea salt to help it all caramelise. Add more olive oil if you need to.

Cook the spaghetti for 1 minute less than the packet instructions. Add the frozen peas 1 minute before the pasta is done. Drain the pasta and peas. Save one large mug (about 80ml/3fl oz) of pasta water.

Add half the chickpeas to the pan and blend the other half with the miso paste, lemon juice, nutritional yeast and the pasta water.

Add the pasta and the creamy chickpea sauce to the pan of veg, combine very well and add more pasta water if you think it needs it.

Divide into bowls, top with black pepper, fresh basil, lightly dressed rocket (washed rocket tossed with a little olive oil, lemon and salt) and roasted seeds (if using for an extra protein boost).

Protein per serving: 33g
Fibre: 22g
Plant diversity score: 10

TIP
Don't wash the pasta in cold water when it's ready, as it'll wash off some of the starch that makes the glossy sauce stick to it. Try to time the sauce for when the pasta will be ready, so you can take it directly out of the pan and add it straight into the sauce.

Bang Bang Bowls with a Quick Pickled Salad

SERVES 2
TOTAL TIME: 30 MINS

Punchy, zingy, fresh bowls of tofu goodness. I'm obsessed with lightly dressed pickled salads (if you can't already tell) as they add a delightful crunch to an otherwise yummy, spicy bowl of slop. Did I sell it?

100g (3½oz/½ cup) brown rice
½ vegetable stock cube or ½ tsp vegetable bouillon powder (optional)
1 x 400g (14oz) can or jar chickpeas, drained and rinsed
250g (9oz) extra-firm tofu
1 tsp ground coriander
½ tsp cayenne pepper
1 tsp garlic granules
¼ tsp ground cinnamon
3 tsp cornflour
2 tbsp sesame oil, plus extra for frying
1 onion, finely diced
3 garlic cloves, minced
Thumb-sized piece of fresh ginger, minced
2 tbsp gochujang paste
2 tbsp sriracha
1 tbsp agave syrup
Pinch of sesame seeds
Salt and black pepper
Lime wedges, to serve

FOR THE QUICK-PICKLED CUCUMBER
1 medium cucumber
Small handful of fresh coriander
2 tsp apple cider vinegar
Pinch of sea salt

Protein per serving: 31g
Fibre: 12g
Plant diversity score: 10

Preheat the oven to 200°C fan/220°C/gas mark 7.

Put the rice on to cook according to the packet instructions, in some seasoned water (with the crumbled stock cube/powder, if you like).

Unwrap the tofu, drain the water out, then wrap it up in a kitchen towel and give it a good squeeze. Repeat with another piece of kitchen towel until it's quite dry.

Break the tofu apart into irregular 2cm (¾in) chunks, then add them to a mixing bowl along with the chickpeas, spices, cornflour and sesame oil. Combine well, then add them to a baking dish and bake for about 20 minutes.

Meanwhile, prepare the sauce. In a small frying pan on a medium heat, fry the onion, garlic and ginger in some sesame oil with a little salt for 5–8 minutes until fragrant. Take off the heat and stir in the gochujang, sriracha and agave syrup.

Tip the baked tofu and chickpeas into the sauce and mix well until most of the sauce has been absorbed or covering the tofu and chickpeas.

Cut the cucumber into ribbons, using a potato peeler with a bowl underneath to catch them. Do this on 3 sides of the cucumber until you have a skinless triangular middle shape. Finely slice half of this, add to the bowl and save the rest for another salad.

Wash the coriander leaves, then roughly chop them (including the stalks) and add them to the bowl. Pour over the vinegar and add the sea salt. Delicately toss everything together with your hands.

Divide the components into bowls, then sprinkle over some sesame seeds, serve with a lime wedge and dig in.

30/30

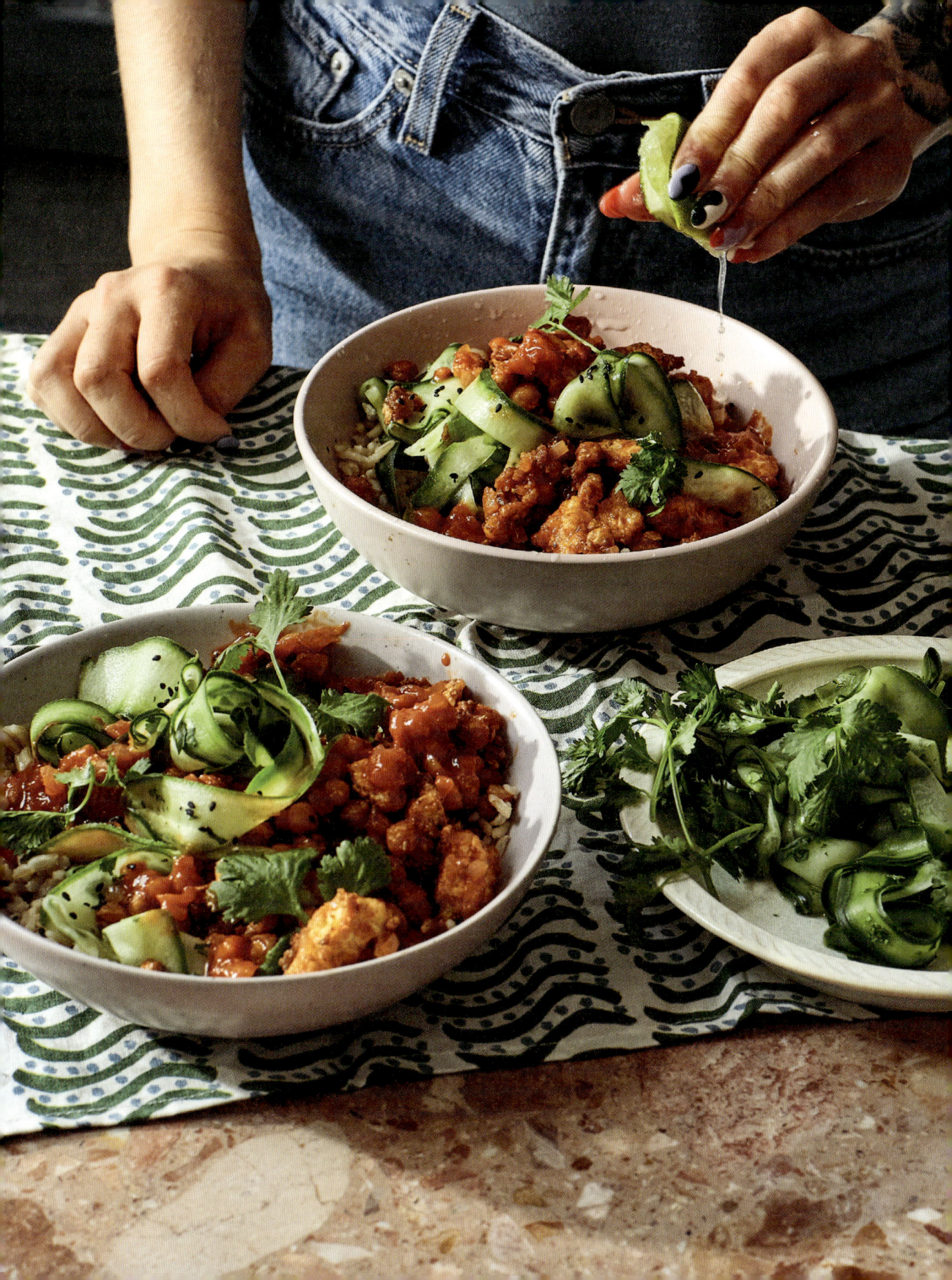

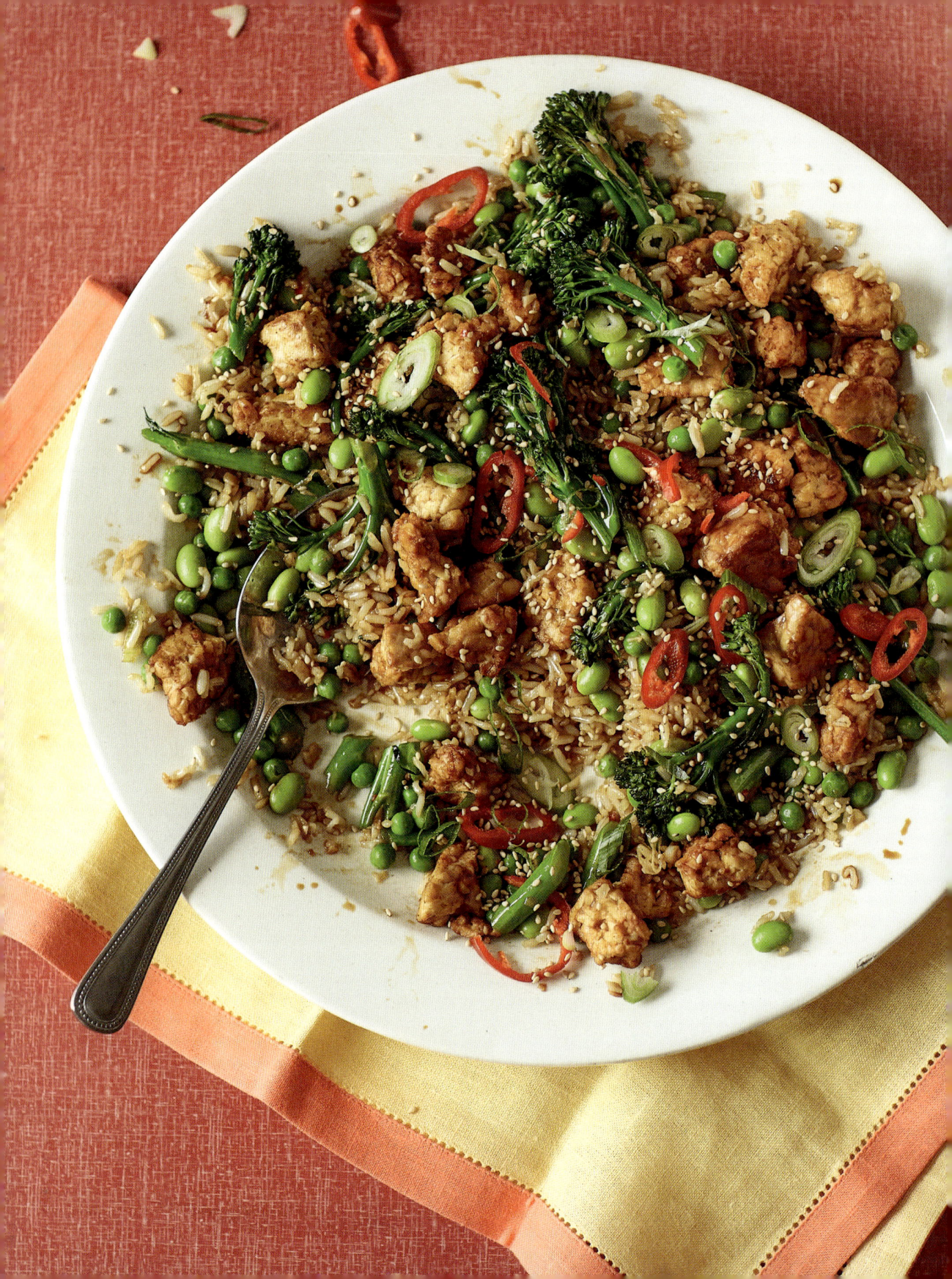

Tantalising Tempeh Fried Rice

Whatever you do, don't skip past this one. It's one of my favourite recipes in this book. Bookmark it! Tempeh and edamame beans do the heavy lifting here, in terms of protein count, so feel free to get creative with any other veg you've got lying around to avoid food waste.

300g (10½oz/1½ cups) brown rice
½ vegetable stock cube
300g (10½oz) block of tempeh
2 tbsp sesame oil
1 tbsp tamari
1 bunch of spring onions, white and green parts finely chopped
Thumb-sized piece of fresh ginger, peeled and minced
4 garlic cloves, minced
½–1 mild red chilli, finely chopped, depending on your spice preference, plus more to serve
150g (5½oz) Tenderstem broccoli, stems roughly chopped into 2cm (¾in) pieces
80g (3oz) frozen edamame beans
80g (3oz) frozen peas
Sesame seeds, to serve

FOR THE QUICK TERIYAKI-STYLE SAUCE
1 tbsp sesame oil
2½ tbsp tamari
1 tbsp maple or agave syrup
1 tbsp mirin
1 tsp toasted sesame oil

Cook the rice according to the packet instructions, with the vegetable stock cube if you like for extra flavour.

In a small bowl, mix together all the quick teriyaki sauce ingredients. Set aside.

Over a small bowl, crumble the tempeh into small chunks with your hands. Heat 1 tablespoon of the sesame oil in a non-stick frying pan on a medium–high heat and, once hot, add the tempeh. Fry for 5 minutes until browning. Add the tamari and mix well. Taste and add a little more tamari if you think it needs more salt.

In a wok or frying pan, add the remaining sesame oil and fry the spring onion whites, ginger, garlic and chilli for 3–4 minutes until fragrant. Add the broccoli and stir-fry for 3–4 minutes until it turns bright green. Add the cooked rice, edamame and peas (straight from frozen is fine, they will thaw in the pan), then tip in the sauce. Mix well, then add the cooked tempeh and heat through.

Divide into bowls and serve topped with chilli, the spring onion greens and sesame seeds.

Protein per serving: 30g
Fibre: 16g
Plant diversity score: 8

Crispy Pulled Mushroom, Kale and Chickpea Bowls

SERVES 3
TOTAL TIME: 25 MINS

The answer to: I want something that tastes naughty but is actually very healthy!

These chickpeas and mushrooms are full of texture and bite, the kale bright and healthy, the sauce creamy and moreish.

1 shallot or ½ white onion, finely chopped
3 garlic cloves, minced
700g (1lb 9oz) chickpeas, plus their juices, from a jar or can(s)
8 large kale leaves, stems removed, leaves chopped
Olive oil
Salt

FOR THE MUSHROOMS
300g (10½oz) oyster mushrooms, roughly torn
1 tbsp tamari
1 tbsp olive oil
1 tbsp red miso paste

CHEESY MISO CASHEW CREAM
80g (3oz/½ cup) cashews
4 tbsp nutritional yeast
1 tsp Dijon mustard
Juice of 1 lemon
1½ tbsp sweet white miso
3½ tbsp water, plus more if needed to blend to a thick but pourable consistency

TO SERVE
Fresh flat-leaf parsley leaves
Sesame seeds
Grain of your choice or toasted sourdough bread

Preheat the oven to 180°C fan/200°C/gas mark 6 and line a large baking tray with baking parchment. Soak the cashews in boiling water for 15 minutes.

Tear up the mushrooms with your hands over a bowl. Add the remaining mushroom ingredients to another small bowl and whisk to combine. Pour the marinade over the torn mushrooms and work it into them with your hands. Spread the mushrooms on a lined baking tray in an even layer. Bake for 18–20 minutes, or until crisping up and golden.

In a wide frying pan on a medium heat, sauté the shallot or onion in plenty of olive oil with a pinch of salt for 8 minutes. Add the garlic, fry for a further 2 minutes, then add the chickpeas and their juices. Alternatively, drain and add the equivalent in filtered water plus some stock powder if you prefer to rinse. Add the kale leaves, mix and bubble on a low heat while you make the cheesy miso cashew cream.

In a small blender cup, add all the cheesy miso cashew cream ingredients and blend until silky smooth. Add more water if you think you need to. Season to taste, adding lemon for brightness or more miso for umami and salt. Pour at least half the cream into the chickpeas, saving the rest for drizzling on top.

Divide into bowls, assemble the mushrooms on top, garnish with parsley, sesame seeds, the remaining miso cashew cream and serve with your grain of choice or slices of toasted sourdough bread.

Protein per serving: 30g
Fibre: 18g
Plant diversity score: 9

30/30

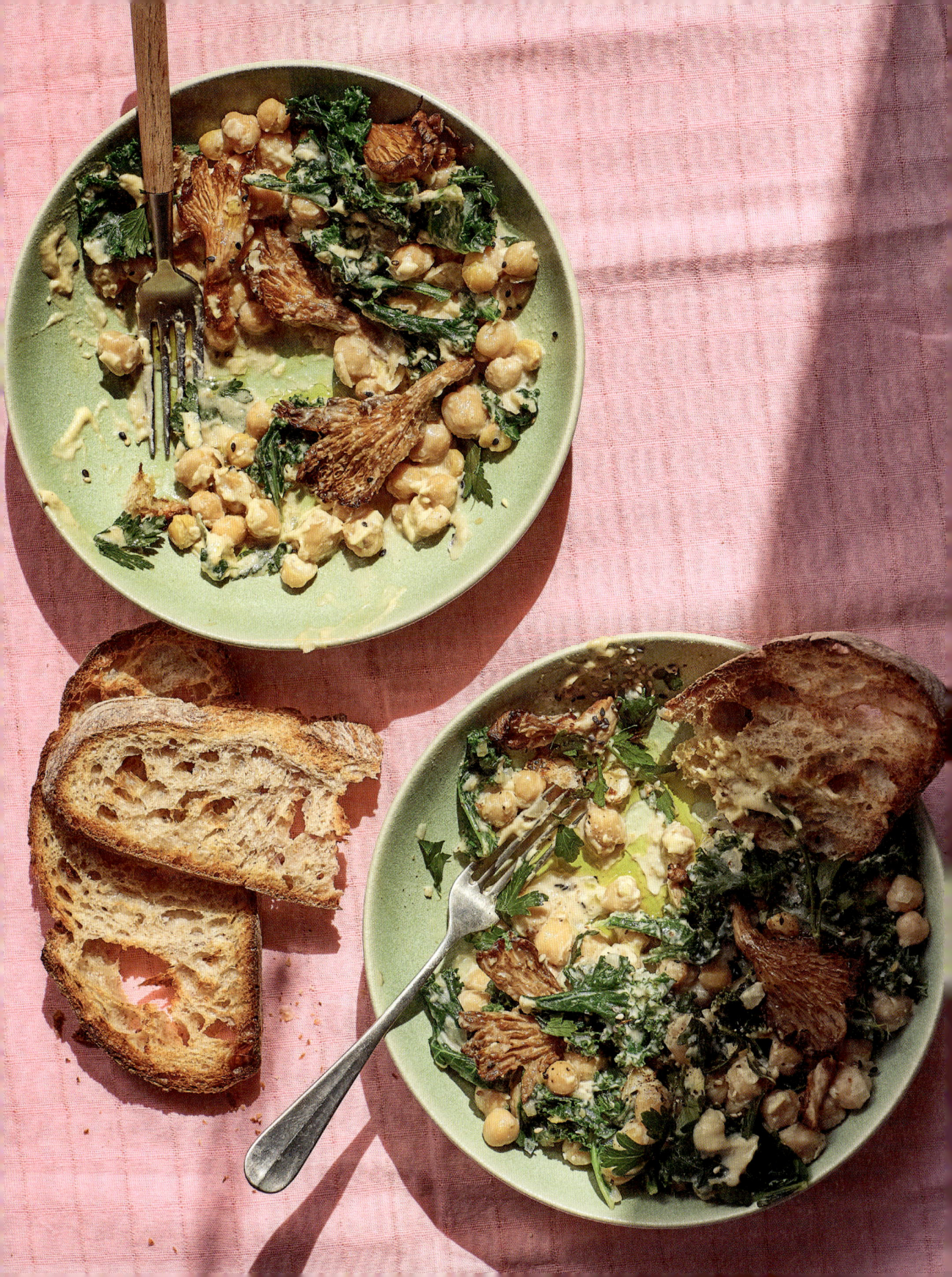

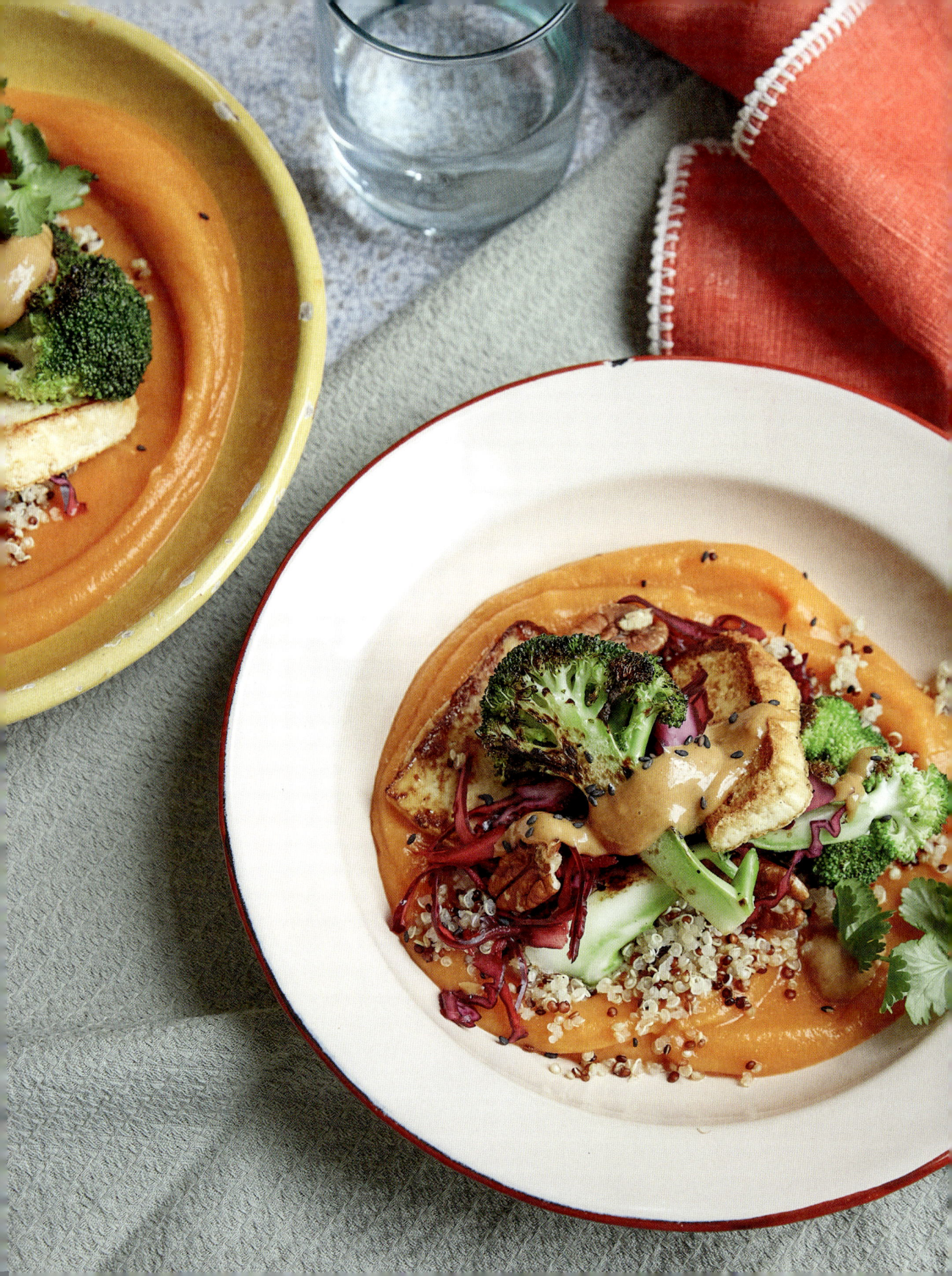

Miso Sweet Potato Protein Bowl

SERVES 3
TOTAL TIME: 30 MINS

I called this a salad on social media and got a fair bit of push back and fair enough, I guess it's more of a warm bowl than your typical salad! It's inspired by a dish I had at a plant-forward restaurant in Porto, Portugal, which consisted of grilled veg and tofu on a bed of delightful miso sweet potato mash. I added peanut sauce for extra depth, and the result is quite wonderful.

4 medium sweet potatoes
1½ tbsp brown miso paste
1 small head of broccoli
Olive oil
½ small red cabbage
1 tbsp lime juice
300g (10½oz) firm smoked tofu
Small handful of pecans
2 tbsp coconut or brown sugar
200g (7oz/1 cup) cooked tricolour quinoa
Salt and black pepper

FOR THE PEANUT SAUCE
3 tbsp natural peanut butter
1 tbsp sesame oil
1 garlic clove, crushed
1 tbsp maple or agave syrup
1 tbsp soy sauce
Water, to loosen

TO SERVE
Black sesame seeds
Fresh coriander leaves

Protein per serving: 30g
Fibre: 15g
Plant diversity score: 10

Peel the sweet potatoes, cut into chunks and boil for 5–7 minutes, or until soft (so a knife easily penetrates). Drain and blend in a food processor with the miso paste, and season to taste.

Cut the broccoli into wedges through the stem and add to a frying pan on a medium-high heat with a pinch of salt. Pan-fry in olive oil for 6-8 minutes, or until browning/charring at the edges.

In a medium bowl, shred the cabbage with a potato peeler, or simply chop finely. Add the lime juice and a pinch of salt. Pinch together with your fingers until the cabbage turns a little pink in colour. Set aside in the fridge whilst you prep the rest.

Cut the smoked tofu into strips and pan-fry on a medium heat with a splash of soy sauce (you can use the same pan as you used for the broccoli) for 3–4 minutes each side, until lightly browning. Remove the tofu and add the pecans, sugar and a splash of water. Heat, stirring regularly, until lightly caramelised (they will be quite sticky, that's intentional!).

In a small blender cup, blend all the peanut sauce ingredients together. Season to taste.

Layer on plates – the sweet potato miso mash first, then the quinoa, veg, tofu, candied pecans, peanut sauce, sesame seeds and coriander. Garnish with the fresh coriander leaves and sesame seeds.

TIP
If you have leftover peanut sauce, use it in stir-frys, or as a sauce for roasted veg!

Warm Noodles, Charred Broccoli and Peanut Sauce

SERVES 2
TOTAL TIME: 30 MINS

Soba noodles are a firm favourite of mine. I prefer the 100% buckwheat variety, as they're really high in protein and fibre. I always have a few packets in the cupboard so I can whip up one of these dishes during the week, using any leftover veggies I have. Please feel free to sub any veg you like – this is another great recipe for avoiding food waste.

200g (7oz) buckwheat (soba) noodles
Sesame oil
1 head of broccoli, sliced through the stems
200g (7oz) firm smoked tofu, sliced
1 tbsp tamari
100g (3½oz) edamame beans, fresh or thawed
   from frozen

FOR THE SAUCE
3 heaped tbsp natural peanut butter
Thumb-sized piece of fresh ginger, grated
2 garlic cloves
1½ tbsp tamari
2 tbsp rice vinegar
1 tbsp agave
1 tbsp sesame oil
2–3 tbsp warm water, plus more if needed to blend to
   a smooth pourable consistency

TO SERVE
Red chilli
Sesame seeds
Fresh coriander leaves

In a small blender cup, blend all the sauce ingredients together until you have a smooth, pourable consistency, adding more water if you need it.

Cook the noodles according to the packet instructions. Rinse in cold water, then set aside in a bowl with a little sesame oil to stop the noodles from sticking together.

Cut the broccoli down the stem and add it to a non-stick or griddle pan on a medium-high heat with a little oil and salt. Sear for 5–7 minutes until golden and charring around the edges. Remove and set aside. In the same pan, fry the tofu with a little sesame oil and the tamari for 3–4 minutes each side, until golden and sizzling.

If using frozen edamame, add them to a sieve and pour over boiling water for 10 seconds, or until thawed. Rinse off in cold water.

Divide between bowls or plates. I like pouring most of the sauce on the bottom, then adding half the noodles, some broccoli, tofu, more noodles, broccoli and tofu, then drizzling the rest of the sauce on top and finishing with sliced red chilli, sesame seeds and coriander leaves.

Protein per serving: 38g
Fibre: 14g
Plant diversity score: 10

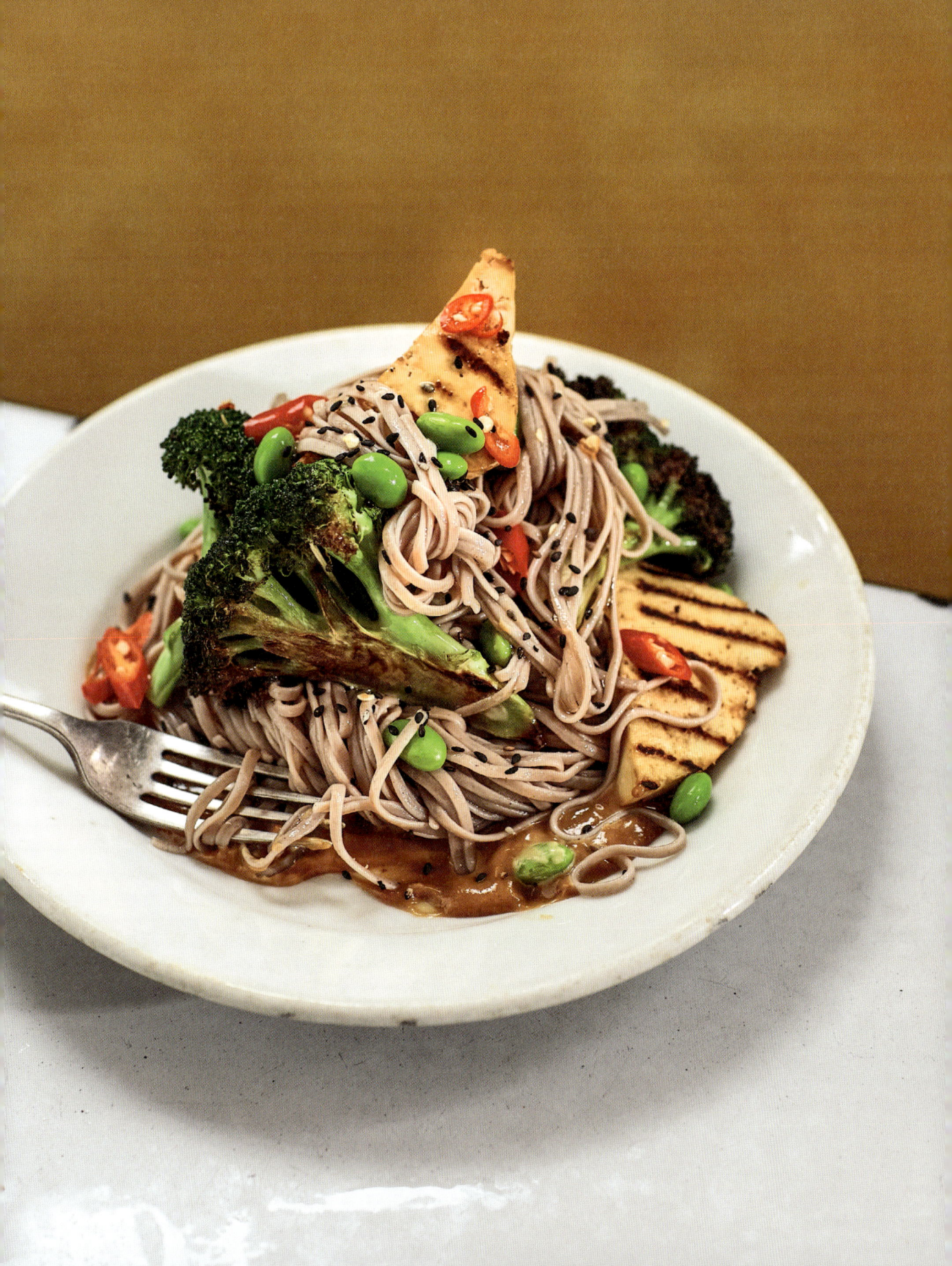

Dinners

Comforting
Classics

Think bangers and mash and meatballs, given a high-protein, plant-based, wholefood makeover. These recipes take up to an hour, or ever-so-slightly over, but that includes oven time. The taste is defined by patience, cooking off aromatics and spices in olive oil. You'll get a much tastier bowl of food by doing this, trust me. If you're spending more time cooking, it's a good idea to make a large portion so you'll have leftovers for lunch or dinner the next day.

Double Tofu Katsu

The Vegatsu is one of my favourite orders from Wagamama. This is my take, heavier on the fresh, crunchy veg with more of that gorgeous katsu sauce.

200g (7oz/1 cup) wild rice
½ vegetable stock cube or ½ tsp vegetable bouillon powder

FOR THE KATSU SAUCE
½ large or 1 small white onion, finely diced
2 medium carrots, peeled and finely diced
Olive oil
3 garlic cloves
Thumb-sized piece of fresh ginger, peeled and grated
1 tsp garam masala
2 tsp medium curry powder
1 tsp ground turmeric
1 tsp ground coriander
1 tsp ground cumin
1 tsp smoked paprika
Pinch of cayenne pepper
250ml (9fl oz/1 cup) vegetable stock
4 tbsp nutritional yeast
280g (10oz) silken tofu
1 tbsp tamari
1 tbsp coconut sugar
Salt and black pepper

FOR THE CRISPY TOFU
250g (9oz) extra-firm tofu
100g (3½oz/¾ cup) plain flour

½ tsp sea salt
Few twists of black pepper
½ tsp smoked paprika
½ tsp ground cumin
½ tsp ground coriander
100ml (3½fl oz/scant ½ cup) soy milk
150g (5½oz/3 cups) plain, sugar-free cornflakes, whizzed into crumbs, or panko breadcrumbs
Sesame oil

FOR THE EASY ZINGY SLAW
Handful of cucumber ribbons
Small handful of fresh coriander leaves
½ tbsp apple cider vinegar
Pinch of salt

TO SERVE
3–4 large radishes, cut into strips
White and black sesame seeds
Lime wedges
Red chilli, finely chopped

Cook the rice according to the packet instructions, tossing the vegetable stock cube into the water and stirring well to dissolve, before adding the rice.

In a medium pan on a medium heat, sauté the onion and carrots in plenty of olive oil with a pinch of salt for 10 minutes. Add the garlic and ginger and fry for another 2–3 minutes until the raw aroma of the aromatics has subsided. Add the spices and a few twists of black pepper. Fry for a further 1–2 minutes, then add the stock.

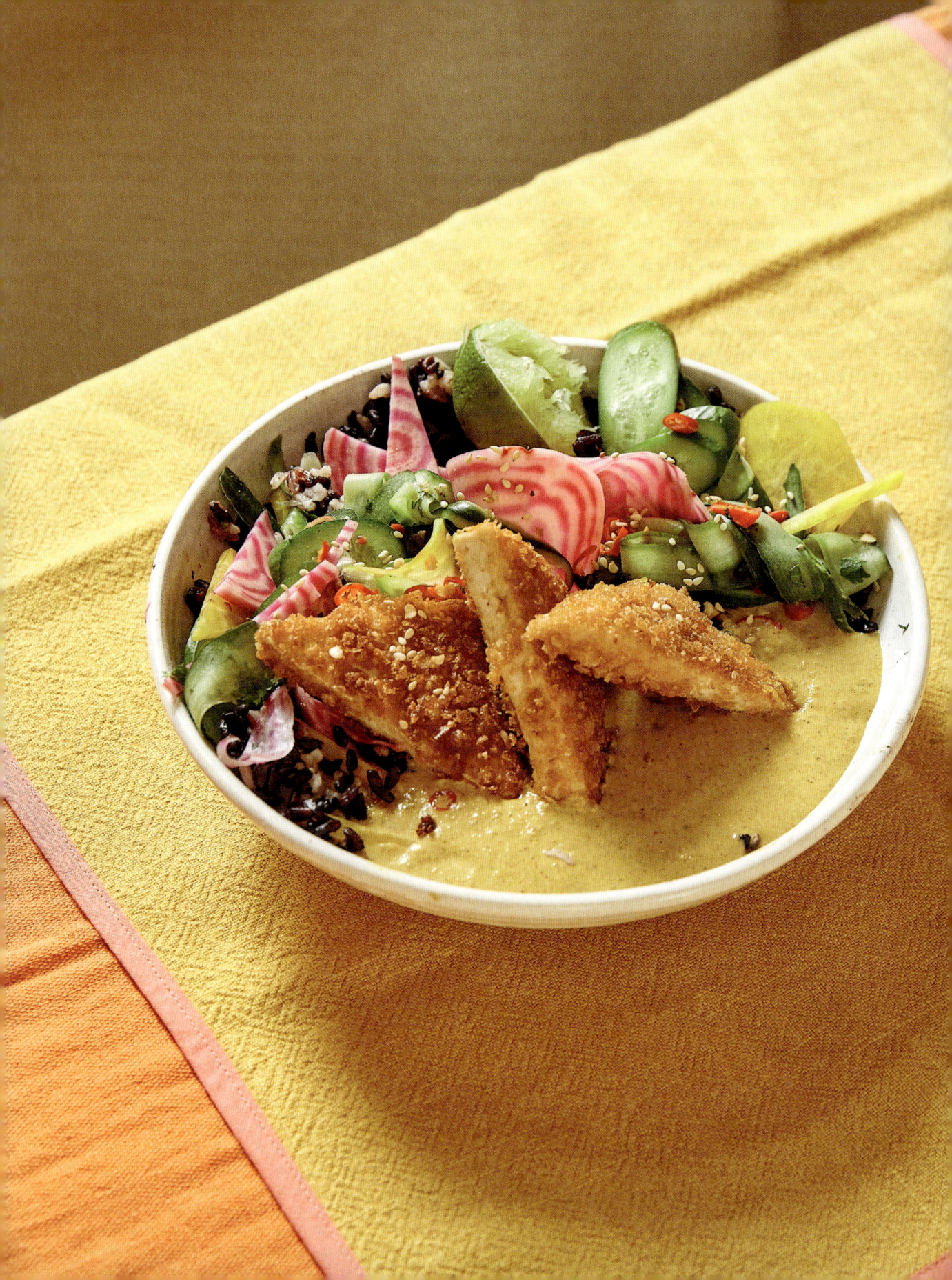

In a small blender, blend the nutritional yeast and silken tofu together. Add the creamy mixture to the pan, along with the tamari and coconut sugar. Mix well and season to taste. Allow to cool, then blend the mixture with a stick blender, or transfer to the same blender you used to blend the silken tofu. Purée the mixture, then pour back into the saucepan and keep on a low heat while you prep the crispy tofu.

Give the tofu a good squeeze, wrapped in kitchen roll or tea towel, to drain off any excess water. Cut into 1cm (½in) strips, then diagonally into triangles.

Grab 3 small bowls. In the first, add the flour, salt, pepper and spices. In the second, the soy milk. In the third, the cornflake crumbs.

Dip the tofu in the spiced flour first, then the soy milk, then the cornflake crumbs. Make sure each triangle is well covered. Lay them on a baking tray or large plate, while you heat sesame oil (you want enough to cover the bottom of the pan entirely) in a nonstick frying pan on a medium-high heat. Fry the coated tofu for 2–3 minutes on each side, or until golden. Place on a plate lined with kitchen paper when done.

Add the cucumber ribbons to a mixing bowl with the coriander leaves, vinegar and salt. Gently toss to combine.

Divide into bowls and serve the rice first, then the katsu sauce, the salad over the rice/sauce line, the radishes, sesame seeds and, finally, the crispy tofu triangles, nestled into the sauce. Finish with a lime wedge and sliced fresh red chilli.

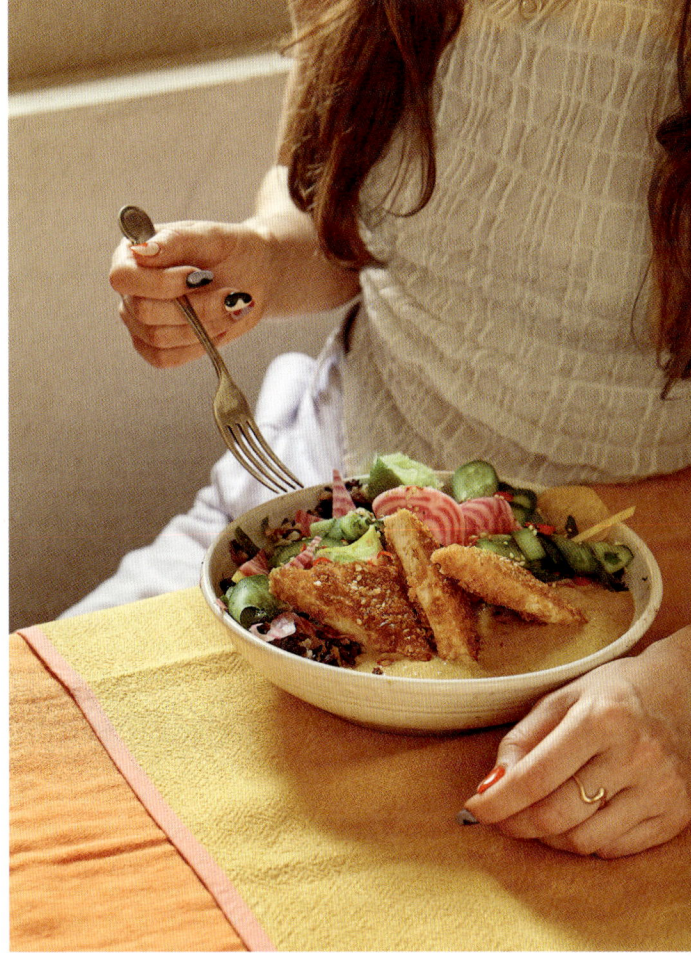

Protein per serving: 37g
Fibre: 13g
Plant diversity score: 10

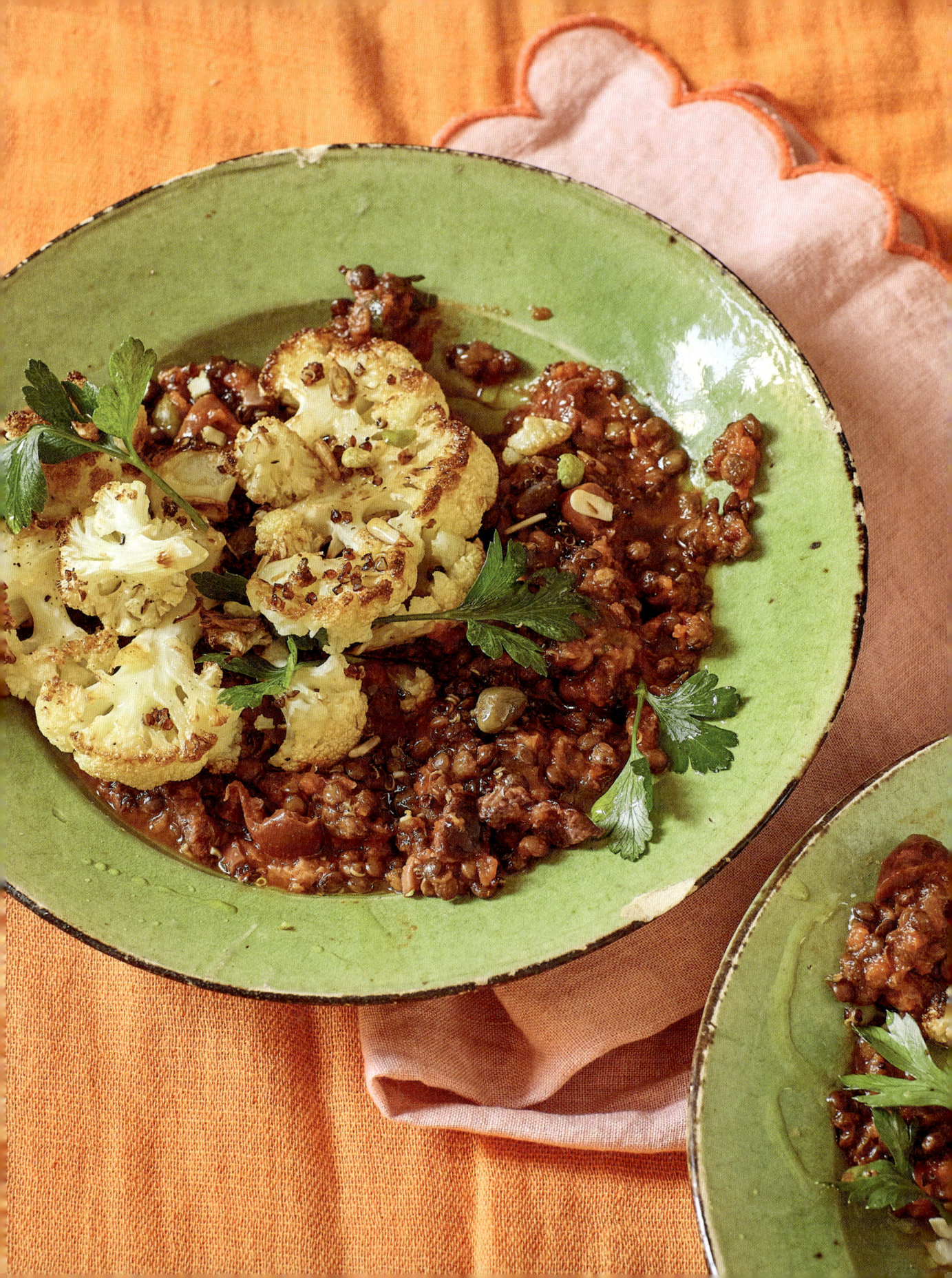

Puttanesca Lentils with Buttery Roasted Cauliflower

SERVES: 3
TOTAL TIME: 45 MINS

This one is a perfect example of what I call 'protein layering'. You have a base legume, a grain and a crispy, crunchy seed topping. All pack protein and flavour. This puttanesca lentil dish was a revelation – the salty, tomato-y, earthy goodness paired with the buttery cauli is really quite sensational.

1 small–medium head of cauliflower, cut into 1.5cm (⅝in) thick steaks, the rest of the florets broken off the stem and chopped or broken in half
Olive oil
80g (3oz/⅓ cup) quinoa
1 tsp smoked paprika
3 garlic cloves, minced
2 x 400g (14oz) cans chopped tomatoes
60g (2oz) Kalamata olives, pitted and chopped, plus 1 tbsp of their brine
2 tbsp capers, plus 1 tbsp of their brine
15g (½oz) fresh parsley, chopped, plus a few leaves for garnish
400g (14oz) cooked Puy lentils
Salt and black pepper
Omega-3 Boost (see page 209), to serve (optional)

Preheat the oven to 200°C fan/220°C/gas mark 7.

Add the cauliflower steaks and chopped cauliflower to a roasting tray and cover liberally in olive oil, salt and pepper. Get into all the crevices. (You can reserve some of the baby cauliflower leaves and roast these too; just be mindful that they take less time to cook, so add them 5–6 minutes before your cauliflower is done.) Roast for 30–35 minutes until turning golden brown and charring in a few places, flipping the steaks halfway through.

While that's roasting, cook the quinoa according to the packet instructions. I often cook it with half a stock cube, to add flavour.

Heat the olive oil in a pan on a low heat and fry the garlic for 30 seconds, then add in the smoked paprika and stir until fragrant. Be careful to not let the garlic take on any colour or burn, as this will make the final result taste bitter! Now pour in the tomatoes, olives and capers, plus the brine from both their jars and a big pinch of salt. Cook for another 10 minutes, then add the chopped parsley.

Season to taste, then pour in the lentils and cooked quinoa. Combine, then ladle into bowls, adding the roasted cauliflower and garnishing with fresh parsley and roasted Omega-3 seeds, if you like.

Protein per serving: 25g
Fibre: 14g
Plant diversity score: 7

NOTES
Add 100g Tofu Feta (page 220) on top to add another 16g protein to this meal

Red Lentil Ragù with Homemade 'Meatballs'

SERVES: 3
TOTAL TIME: 35–40 MINS

Meatballs will forever conjure up a picture of The Lady and the Tramp in my head. I also can't decide if they're horrendously unsightly or actually kind of cool looking?

This recipe uses my wholefood 'meatballs' (see page 225) but you can always buy some for ease. The sauce is a mix of tangy, cheesy notes buried in a rich and earthy red lentil and soffritto base. Comfort food at its finest!

½ white onion, very finely chopped
1 small carrot, peeled and very finely chopped
1 celery stalk, very finely chopped
Olive oil
5 garlic cloves, crushed
1 tbsp fresh thyme leaves
2 tbsp tomato purée
150g (5½oz/⅔ cup) red lentils, rinsed
1 x 400g (14oz) can good quality plum tomatoes
350ml (12fl oz/scant 1½ cups) vegetable stock
1½ tbsp red wine vinegar
2 tbsp nutritional yeast
6 Homemade 'Meatballs' (see page 225) or other plant based meatballs
6–7 nests of tagliatelle
Salt and black pepper

TO SERVE
Cashew Parmesan (see page 221)
Extra virgin olive oil
Fresh parsley leaves

In a heavy-bottomed pan covered with olive oil on a low–medium heat, cook the onion, carrot and celery with a pinch of salt for about 10 minutes. Add the garlic and thyme and cook for another 4 minutes.

Add the tomato purée, cook for 5 minutes, then add the red lentils and can of tomatoes. Then fill the can up halfway with water, swill it around to get all those juices and tip that in, too. Add the stock, give it a good stir, then bring to the boil, lower the heat and simmer for 20 minutes until the lentils are cooked and the water greatly reduced. It should be a thick-ish soup consistency. Add the red wine vinegar, nutritional yeast, mix and season to taste.

Preheat the oven to 160°C fan/180°C/gas mark 4 Warm up the 'meatballs' in the oven for 5–8 mins, making sure to brush them with olive oil first.

Meanwhile, cook the pasta in plenty of salty boiling water for 1½ minutes less than the packet instructions. Once cooked, ladle it straight into the soupy sauce and stir gently.

Divide between bowls, top with the 'meatballs', cashew parm, olive oil, freshly cracked black pepper and parsley.

Protein per serving: 23g
Fibre: 16g
Plant diversity score: 15

NOTES
Change the pasta to a legume pasta to up the protein content if desired

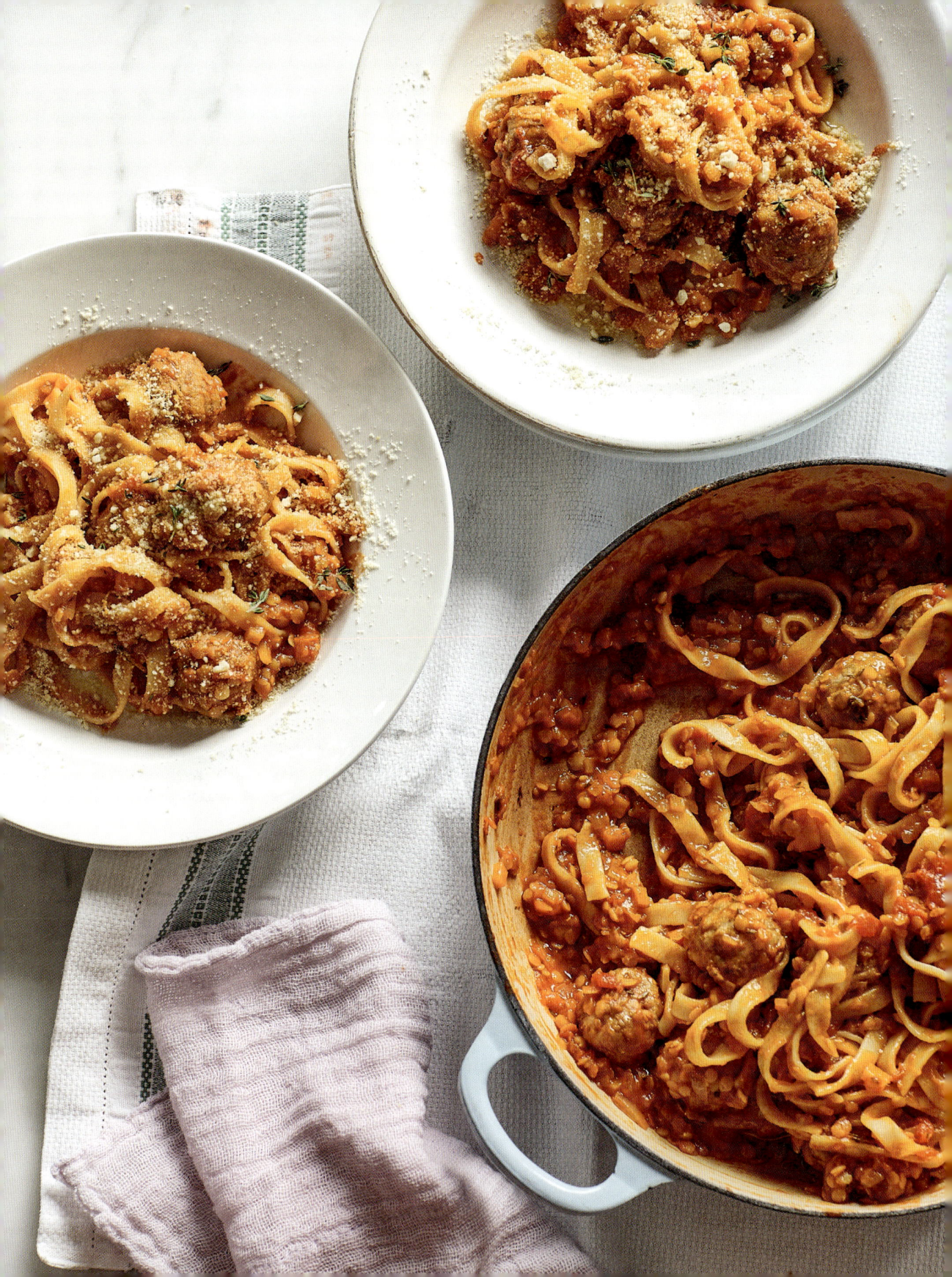

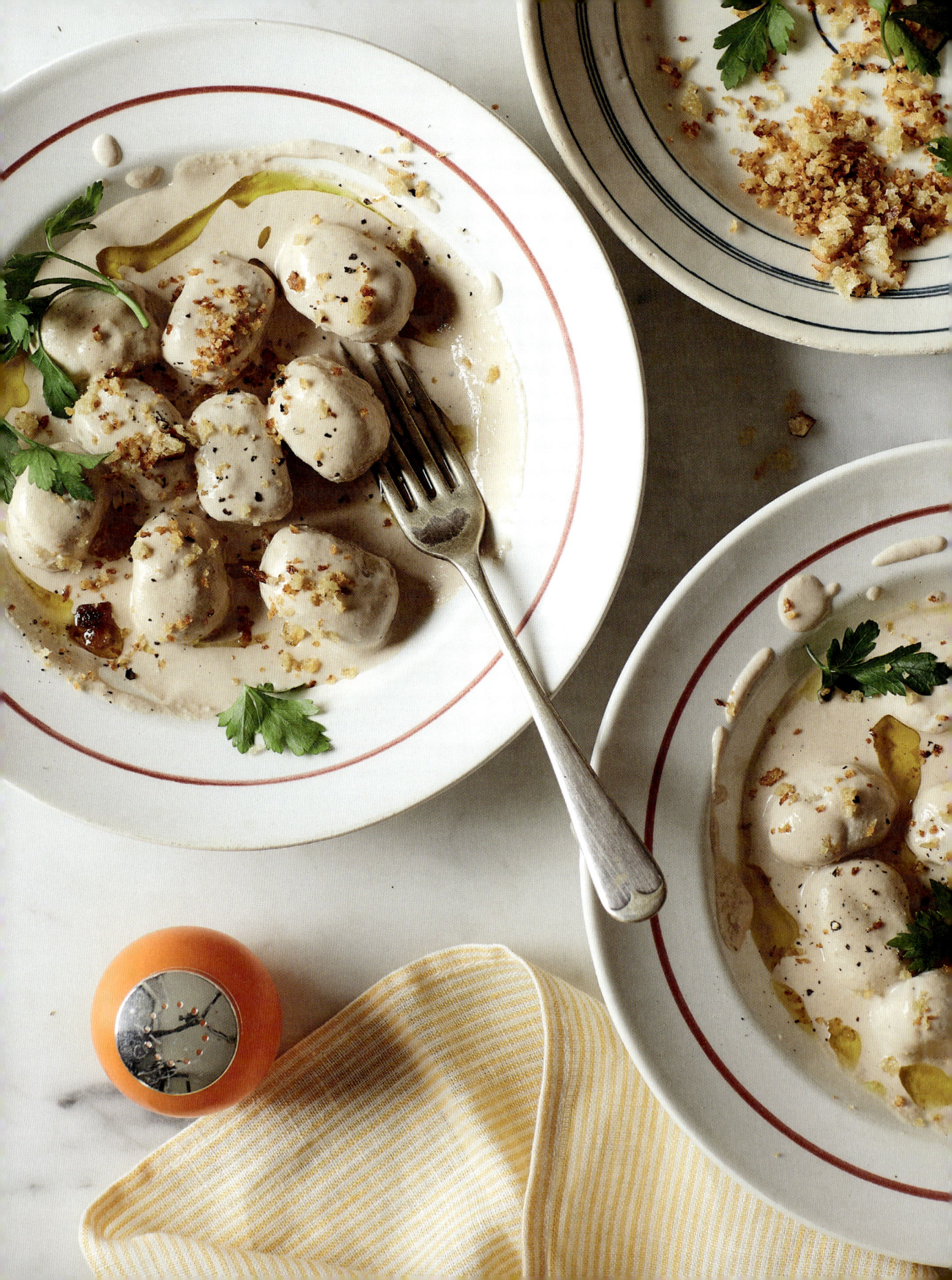

Giant Tofu Gnocchi with Creamy Walnut Sauce

SERVES 3
TOTAL TIME: 25 MINS

Making gnocchi seems like an arduous task, but rest assured, all you need for this one is a food processor, rolling pin (or wine bottle) and about 15 minutes.

The creamy walnut sauce is an interpretation of the Italian Salsa di Noci, traditionally made with milk, white bread, walnuts and Parmesan. Instead, I've used soy milk, silken tofu, cashews, plus some other ingredients to achieve the depth of umami here. Although it may look unassuming, it's certainly not one to skip past!

FOR THE TOFU GNOCCHI
250g (9oz) firm tofu
70g (2½oz/½ cup) spelt flour, plus more for dusting
2 tbsp nutritional yeast
½ tsp salt
2 tbsp olive oil

FOR THE CREAMY WALNUT SAUCE
100g (3½oz/1¼ cups) walnuts, soaked in boiling water for 15 minutes
50g (1¾oz) silken tofu
2 garlic cloves
20g (¾oz/1½ tbsp) cashews
3 tbsp nutritional yeast
150ml (5fl oz/⅔ cup) soy milk
1 tbsp sweet white miso paste
1 tbsp olive oil
½ tbsp apple cider vinegar
Salt and black pepper

TO SERVE
Garlicky Sourdough Breadcrumbs (see page 207)
Fresh parsley leaves
Extra virgin olive oil

Start by making the gnocchi. In a food processor, pulse the tofu a few times until it reaches a crumb-like consistency. Add the flour, nutritional yeast, salt and olive oil, then pulse a few more times until it resembles fine-ish breadcrumbs. Lightly flour a work surface, then tip out the mixture and press/knead into a ball for about 3 minutes. Add a little more flour to your hands if it's sticking.

Once it resembles a smooth ball, divide the tofu gnocchi dough into 4 pieces and roll each one into a long sausage. Using a knife or a dough scraper, cut the dough into small pillows, about 1.5–2cm (⅝–¾in) in length. Cover with a damp tea towel. At this point, you can either leave them as they are or use a gnocchi board or fork to make grooves in the little pillows.

Creamy walnut sauce time! Add all the ingredients to a high-speed blender and blend until you get a silky smooth texture. Season to taste. Pour into a small non-stick frying pan or saucepan and very gently heat up while you cook the gnocchi. Make sure to stir it, otherwise the sauce will stick to the pan. It should be creamy, but runny. If it starts to look too thick, add a splash of water.

Bring a large saucepan of salted water to the boil and add the tofu gnocchi. When the gnocchi floats to the top, fish it out using a slotted spoon and add it directly to the sauce with a little cooking water. Gently toss to combine, then serve straight away with the optional garnishes.

Protein per serving: 29g
Fibre: 10g
Plant diversity score: 8

My 'Bangers and Mash'

SERVES: 2
TOTAL TIME: 40 MINS

I'm obsessed with turning quintessential British dishes into collages of colour, as I'm sure we can all agree, they're almost a bit too beige sometimes.

Don't sleep on my wholefood 'sausage' recipe. I suggest making a double batch and whipping them out on a rainy day.

6 of my Homemade 'Sausages' (see page 224, or another plant-based sausage)
Salt and black pepper

FOR THE BUTTER BEAN AND HEMP PESTO MASH
1 large shallot, diced
3 garlic cloves, minced
480g (1lb 1oz) butter beans, from a jar or can, most of the canned liquid drained off the top
2 tbsp Hemp Pesto (optional) (see page 216)
Olive oil
Salt and black pepper

FOR THE JAMMY SPICED PEPPERS AND TOMATOES
1 large red bell pepper, thinly sliced lengthways
150g (5½oz) cherry tomatoes
2 tsp crushed garlic
1 tsp smoked paprika
1 tsp ground cumin
1 tsp ground coriander
¼ tsp cayenne pepper (adjust spice to your own preferences)

TO SERVE
Avocado chunks, dressed with a little apple cider vinegar, olive oil and salt
Fresh coriander
Extra virgin olive oil
Black sesame seeds (optional)

Start with the mash. In a medium pan on a medium heat, fry the shallot in olive oil with a small pinch of salt for 5 minutes, then add the garlic and cook for another 3 minutes. Add the butter beans and most of their canned juices (pour a little out the top of the can first) and cook down for another 5 minutes until the liquid has reduced. Season to taste. Leave to cool while you start the jammy peppers and tomatoes.

In a small saucepan on a medium heat, sauté the red pepper and tomatoes with a pinch of salt for 8 minutes until they start to become soft and you can almost squish the cherry tomatoes with your spatula. Add the garlic, spices, some salt, pepper and a little more oil. Keep on a low heat, stirring regularly, until it starts to melt into the pan and become super soft and jammy.

Transfer the cooled beans to a food processor and pulse until a chunky, mashy texture is achieved. Season to taste.

Fry or grill the sausages until cooked through, about 5 minutes (170°C fan/190°C/gas mark 5 or in a frying pan on medium heat).

Assemble the plates! Mash first, then swirl through the hemp pesto with a spoon or edge of a knife. Place the jammy tomatoes and peppers on next, followed by the cooked 'sausages' and avocado. Dress with coriander, a little extra virgin olive oil and lots of cracked black pepper.

Garnish with sesame seeds, if you wish.

Protein per serving: 33.4g
Fibre: 27g
Plant diversity score: 12

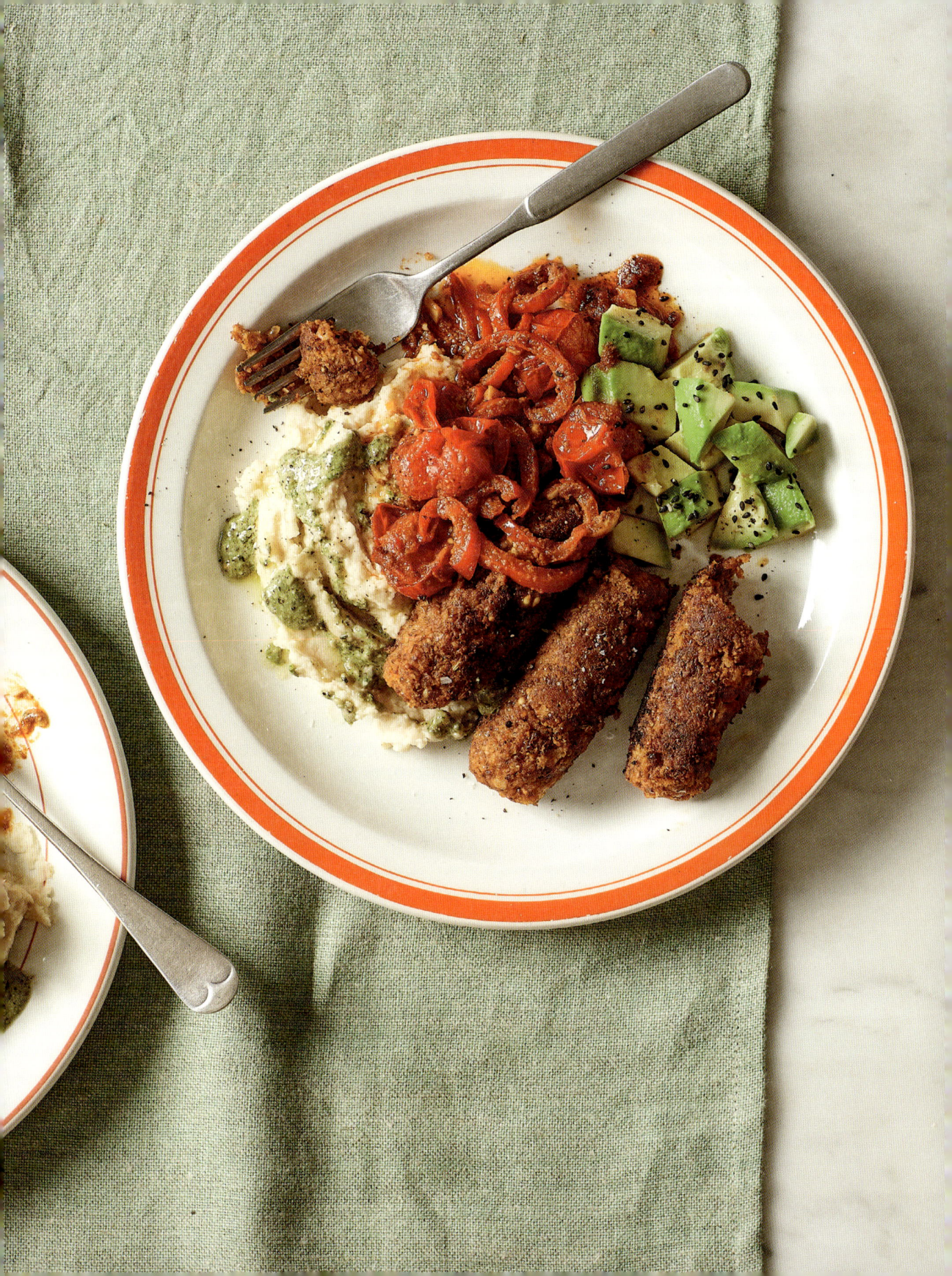

Smoky Lentil, Walnut and Sun-dried Tomato Pasta

SERVES: 3
TOTAL TIME: 40 MINS

The amount of flavour in these ingredients astounds me, let alone the fact that this dish takes just 40 minutes from start to finish. It was a huge hit on social media, too, which made me enormously happy as this is truly one of the best dishes I have ever made. Enjoy!

½ red onion, finely chopped
300g (10½oz) chestnut mushrooms, chopped
Olive oil
4 garlic cloves, minced
7 large sun-dried tomatoes, finely chopped
2 tsp smoked paprika
1 tbsp tomato purée
2 x 400g (14oz) can of plum tomatoes
300g (10½oz) cooked Puy lentils
40g (1½oz/⅓ cup) walnut pieces, soaked in boiling water for 15 minutes
250g (9oz) durum semolina pasta
Salt and black pepper

TO SERVE
Cashew Parmesan (see page 221)
Extra virgin olive oil

In a medium pan on a medium heat, fry the onion and mushrooms in olive oil and salt for about 10 minutes until all the steam has subsided (this means the water has evaporated!). Add the garlic, sun-dried tomatoes and smoked paprika. Fry for another 3 minutes, then add the tomato purée and cook for a further 3 minutes.

Add the plum tomatoes, lentils, walnuts and a large pinch of salt and pepper. Break the tomatoes up with your spatula or a fork. Don't add too much salt here as you'll be adding some salty pasta water.

Simmer the sauce on a low heat while you cook the pasta for 1–2 minutes less than the packet instructions suggest. Drain, then add the pasta directly into the sauce with a ladle, so you get lots of lovely salty pasta cooking water. Season to taste, you shouldn't need much. Reserve an additional mug of pasta water to stir in later if you're not eating straight away.

Serve with cashew parm, extra virgin olive oil and cracked black pepper.

Protein per serving: 31.5g
Fibre: 14g
Plant diversity score: 9

NOTES
Look for Durum Semolina pasta to get the protein amount listed. Find it in larger supermarkets or your local Italian deli.

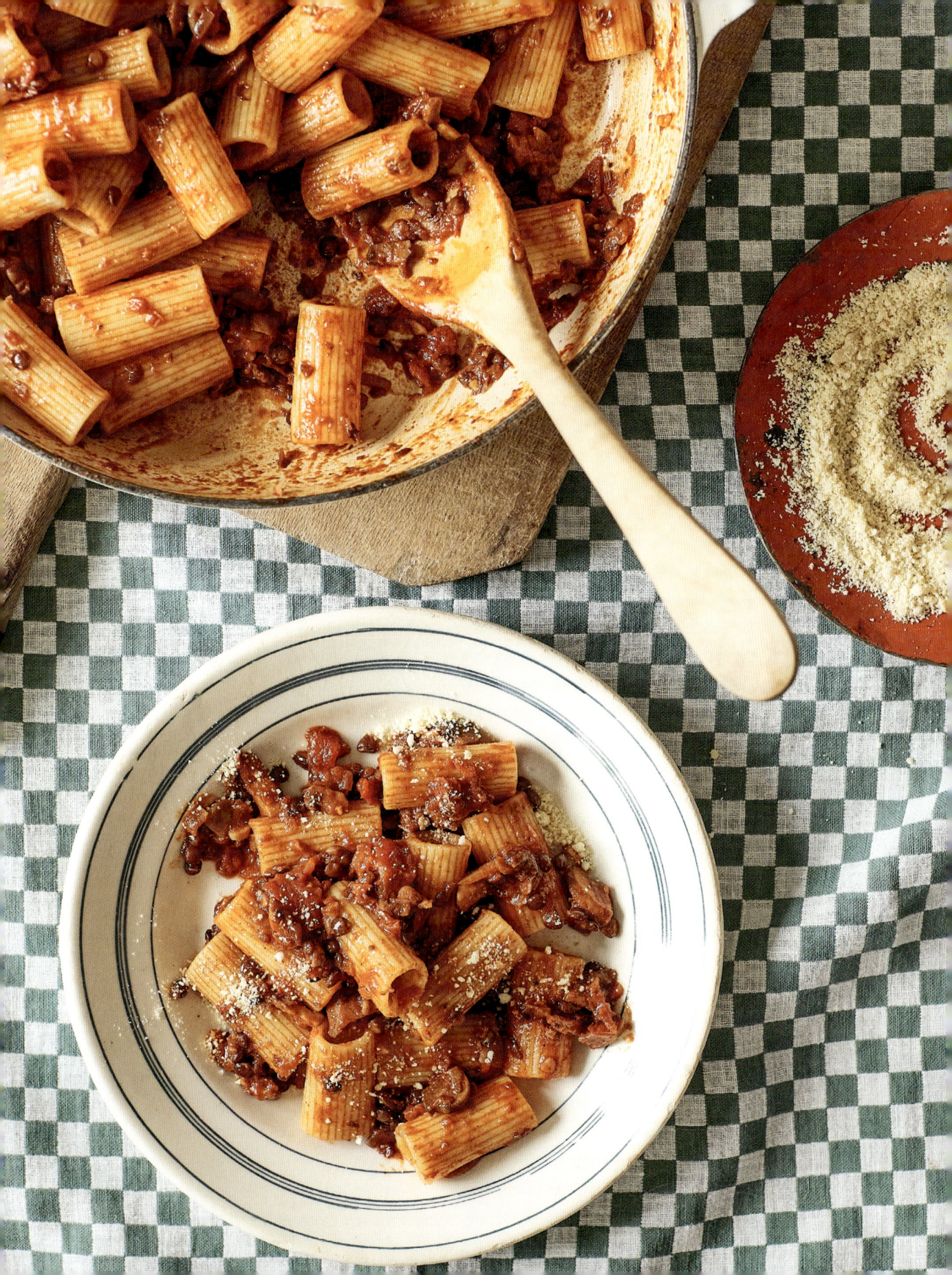

Kimchi Burgers

SERVES 2
TOTAL TIME: 50 MINS

This is based on my favourite burger on the menu at Miranda cafe in Crouch End, where I worked for a short time as an assistant chef. Find the burger recipe in the Protein Layering chapter!

2 medium sweet potatoes
240g (8½oz) chickpeas, from a jar or can
Olive oil, for drizzling
1 tsp smoked paprika
1 tsp ground cumin
2 x 90s Baby Beanburgers (see page 217)
2 heaped tsp gochujang paste
1 tsp tomato purée
6 tbsp Cashew Cream (see page 219)
½ small red cabbage, shaved with a potato peeler
Juice of 1 lime
2 burger buns (I use wholemeal)
Small handful of lettuce leaves
3 heaped tbsp kimchi
1 small cucumber, sliced into ribbons with a potato peeler
Black sesame seeds
Sea salt and black pepper

FOR THE SIDE SALAD
A handful of lettuce leaves
3–4 cherry tomatoes, quartered
Splash of apple cider vinegar
Sea salt

Preheat the oven to 180°C fan/200°C/gas mark 6.

Wash the sweet potatoes thoroughly, then prick with a fork a few times and microwave on high for 2 minutes. Rinse and dry the chickpeas well.

Once the potatoes are softened, cut into chunky home-style wedges and place on a large baking tray with the chickpeas. Drizzle over some olive oil and season with sea salt and black pepper, the smoked paprika and cumin. Toss to combine, then bake for 30–35 minutes until crisping at the edges. Once they are 20 minutes into the cooking time, add the cooked burger patties to another small baking tray and place on the bottom rack to warm through.

Add the gochujang and tomato purée to the cashew cream to make the burger sauce.

To a small bowl, add the shredded red cabbage, lime juice and a pinch of salt. Stir to combine.

Slice and toast the burger buns in a frying pan, grill or toaster. Once ready, layer up the burgers. Gochujang cashew sauce first, a few lettuce leaves, then the burger patties, 1½ tablespoons of kimchi on top of each burger, the lightly pickled red cabbage, the cucumber ribbons and black sesame seeds. Add more sauce, then complete your burger!

Serve with the sweet potato wedges and crunchy chickpeas, and a small side salad of lettuce and cherry tomatoes, dressed with a splash of apple cider vinegar and a small pinch of sea salt.

Protein per burger: 25g
Fibre: 21g
Plant diversity score: 14

NOTES
You can also crumble these cooked burgers over salads to add taste, nutrients and crunch!
Add an extra burger patty to up the protein content

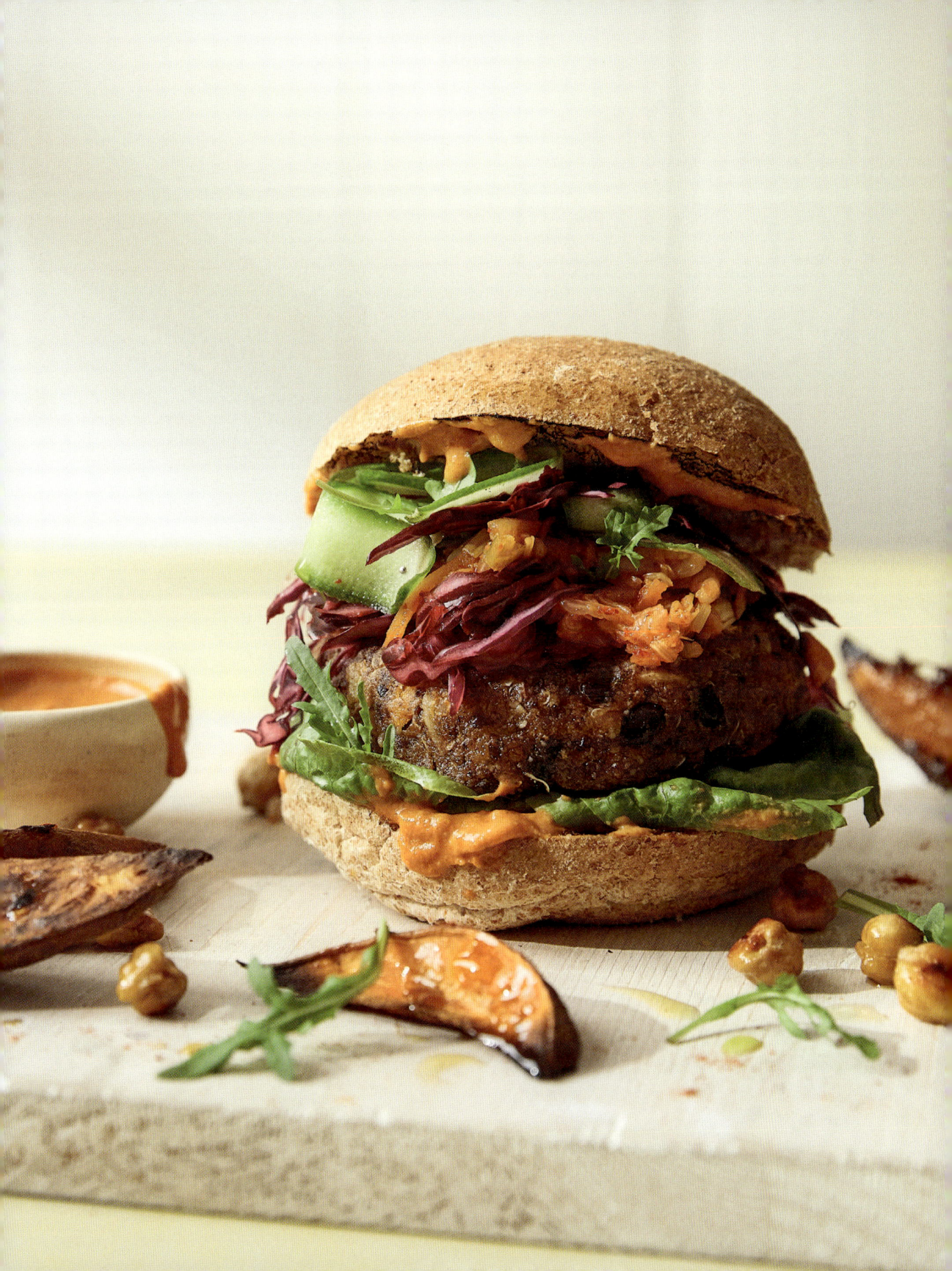

Big One-
(or Two-)
Pan Meals

Buckle up and get ready for a quick trip around the world! With influences from India, Spain, Morocco, the Middle East, and many more, this is your capsule foodie holiday served up in one large pan (plus a baking tray and a blender sauce in some cases). These can be made for meal prep, or served up family-style, so everyone can serve a portion to suit their own needs.

Winter Veg Curry

SERVES: 4
TOTAL TIME: 1 HR 15 MINS

This is my most popular recipe on social media at the time of writing. It has three main components, but once these are all made and tasting great, it comes together very easily.

The sweetness of the blended butternut squash and sweet potato with the perfectly spiced creamy sauce is definitely something to write home about. I hope you love it as much as I do!

1 tsp cumin seeds
1 tsp coriander seeds
2 tbsp olive oil
1 red onion, finely diced
4cm (1½in) piece of fresh ginger, peeled and grated
3 garlic cloves, grated
½ red chilli, deseeded and finely chopped (omit if you like less spice)
½ tbsp garam masala
1½ tsp ground coriander
1½ tsp ground cumin
½ tbsp medium or mild curry powder
½ tsp ground turmeric
2 tsp smoked paprika
½ tsp ground cinnamon
200g (7oz) fresh tomatoes, grated, or canned chopped tomatoes
240g (8½oz) chickpeas, from a can or jar, drained and rinsed
500ml (18fl oz/2 cups) vegetable stock
Salt

FOR THE ROASTED VEG
½ large or 1 small cauliflower, broken into florets, outer leaves and stem removed, smaller leaves washed
2 large or 3 medium–small sweet potatoes, skin on, cut into irregular 2cm (¾in) cubes
For the cauliflower: 1 tsp ground cumin, 1 tsp ground coriander and ⅓ tsp ground turmeric
For the sweet potatoes: 1 tsp ground cumin, 1 tsp smoked paprika, 1 tsp ground coriander, ⅓ tsp ground cinnamon
½ butternut squash, deseeded
Olive oil
Salt and black pepper

FOR THE SAUCE
30g (1oz/scant ¼ cup) cashews
280g (10oz) silken tofu
3 tbsp nutritional yeast
Juice of 1 lemon
¼ tsp salt
Black pepper
Splash of water, for blending

FOR THE TOFU
400g (14oz) extra-firm tofu
1 tbsp olive oil
2 tbsp nutritional yeast
½ tsp medium or mild curry powder
½ tsp garlic powder
⅓ tsp salt
1 tbsp lemon juice

TO SERVE
Fresh coriander leaves
Soy yoghurt
High-protein Naan (see page 206), sourdough toast, quinoa or brown rice

NOTE
Enjoy with my High-Protein Naan (page 206) or sourdough for an extra protein boost

Preheat the oven to 180°C fan/200°C/gas mark 6.

On a large baking tray, add the cauliflower florets and sweet potatoes, then drizzle with olive oil and season with spices for each vegetable and some salt and pepper.

Score the flesh of the squash in a criss-cross pattern, drizzle with olive oil, then place cut-side down on another small baking tray. Drizzle with some more oil and salt over the skin.

Roast all the vegetables for 30–35 minutes, or until taking on a nice golden colour.

In a small bowl, soak the cashews for the sauce in boiling water for 15 minutes. Drain and set aside.

In a mixing bowl, tear the tofu into irregular chunks. Whisk all the remaining tofu marinade ingredients together, then pour over the tofu and combine well. Cover and set aside.

Toast the cumin and coriander seeds in a dry frying pan, then grind in a pestle and mortar to help release their natural oils.

In a medium frying pan on a medium heat, fry the ground spices in a glug of olive oil for 30 seconds, then add the onion and a pinch of salt. Cook on a medium heat for 8–10 minutes. Add the ginger, garlic and chilli and cook for 3–4 minutes until the raw aroma of garlic and ginger has subsided. Add the spices and more olive oil, combine well, then add the grated tomatoes and another pinch of salt. Cook for about 5 minutes until the tomatoes turn a dark shade of red. Add the chickpeas and stock, bring to a slight boil, then reduce the heat and simmer for 10 minutes.

Once the cauliflower and sweet potatoes have finished roasting (they should be looking golden brown and slightly charing at the edges), remove from the oven and transfer to a bowl, BUT don't turn off the oven just yet. The butternut should be super soft and almost collapsing when you touch the skin. If it's not just yet, leave it in the oven and check regularly until it is. Then remove from the oven and leave to cool. Pop the marinated tofu on the same baking tray as the veg and bake for 10–15 minutes, or until the tofu is taking on a little char.

Once cooled, scoop out the squash flesh and add it to a blender with the remaining sauce ingredients. Blend until smooth, then add to the spicy chickpea mixture, reserving a little for garnish. Stir through half of the roasted veg, saving the rest for decoration.

Serve the curry topped with the sauce and fresh coriander, with cooling soy yoghurt and naan, sourdough toast, rice or quinoa alongside.

Protein per serving: 31g
Fibre: 16g
Plant diversity score: 15

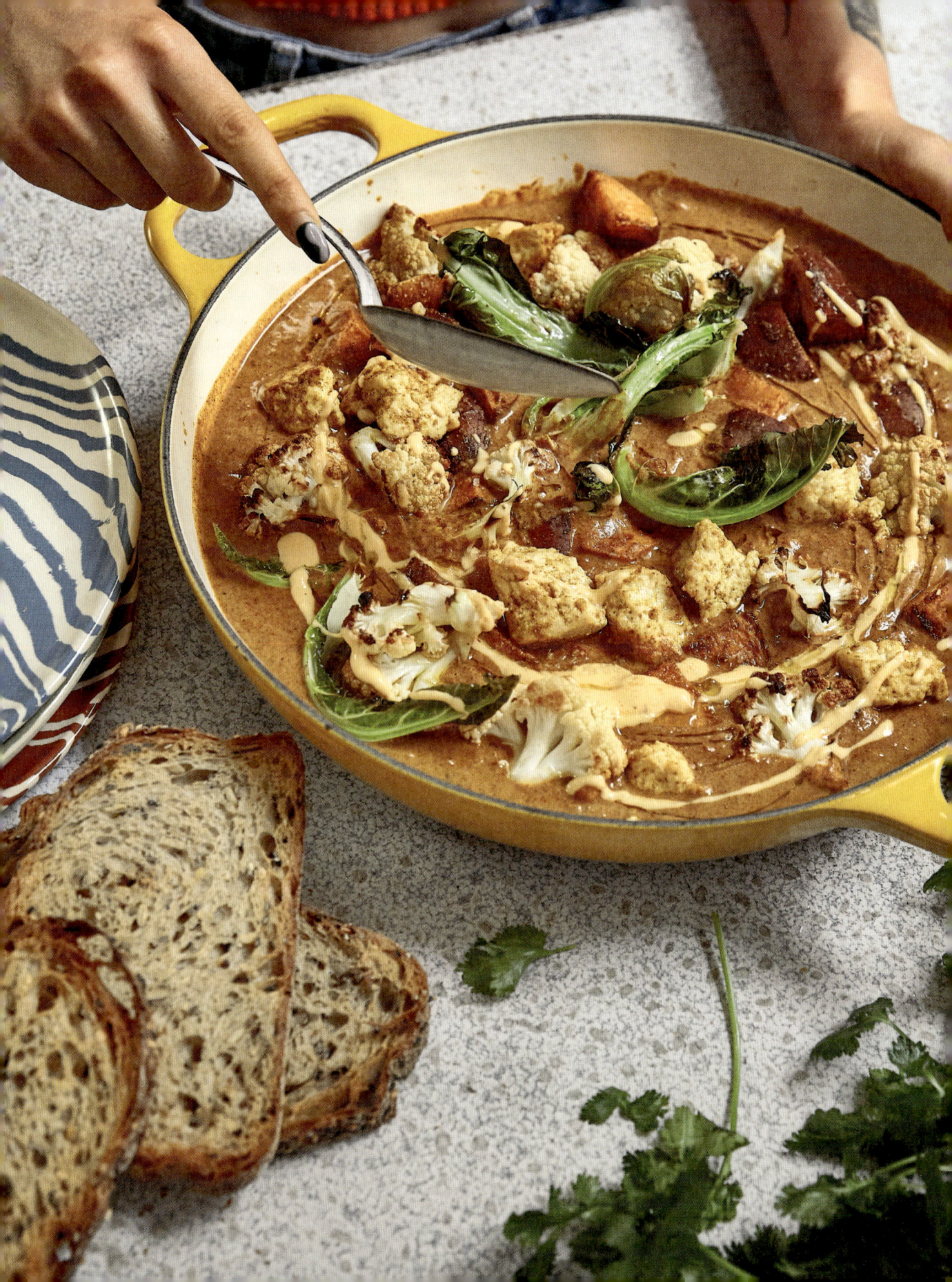

Black Bean and Sweet Potato Hotpot with Charred Sweetcorn Salsa

SERVES: 3
TOTAL TIME: 40 MINS

Earthy, spiced black beans and thinly cut crispy sweet potato rings. Perfect for a chilly night in with family or friends.

With every bean bake or bowl I develop, I think about what works flavour wise, closely followed by what new and exciting textures I can bring to a dish. Instead of mashing the sweet potato like a traditional cottage pie-style dish, thinly slicing it adds a little more bite. Served with the salty charred corn, creamy cashew sauce and sliced avo makes this the perfect party of creamy, salty and crunchy textures.

1 red onion, finely diced
Olive oil
3 garlic cloves, minced
2 tsp smoked paprika
1 tsp ground coriander
1 tsp ground cumin
½ tsp cayenne pepper
1 tbsp tomato purée
200g (7oz/¾ cup) split red lentils, drained and rinsed
1 x 400g (14oz) can plum tomatoes
600ml (20fl oz/2½ cups) vegetable stock
1 bay leaf
700g (1lb 9oz) black beans, from a jar or can
1½ tbsp natural peanut butter
200g (7oz) sweetcorn kernels, from a can (or you can cut them off fresh corn cobs)
1 very large or 2 medium sweet potatoes
Juice of 1 lime
Salt

TO SERVE
Cashew Queso (see page 219)
Sliced avocado

Protein per serving: 30g
Fibre: 24g
Plant diversity score: 8

In a medium frying pan on a low-medium heat, fry the onion in plenty of olive oil with a pinch of salt for 8 minutes until softened. Add the garlic and spices and fry for another 2–3 minutes, then add the tomato purée and mix that in. Rinse the lentils in cold water, then add them to the pan with the tomatoes, stock and the bay leaf. Bring to a bubble, then reduce the heat and simmer for 10 minutes.

Drain and rinse the black beans, then add them to the pan with the peanut butter. Mix well, then simmer on a low heat while you make the sweetcorn salsa.

Rinse, then dry the sweetcorn with kitchen paper. Add to a hot non-stick pan with olive oil and a pinch of salt and fry on a high heat for 6–8 minutes until starting to char a little. Take off the heat and carefully pour into a heatproof bowl. Taste and season more with salt if you like, tossing the kernels well.

Preheat the oven to 200°C fan/220°C/gas mark 7.

Give the sweet potato/es a good scrub and dry with kitchen paper. Carefully cut them into 3mm (⅛in) rounds.

Pour the lime juice over the beany lentil mixture and season to taste. If your pan is not ovenproof, pour the mixture into a baking dish. Place the sweet potato rounds over the top, slightly overlapping the layers. Bake for 20–25 minutes, checking halfway through cooking. The sweet potato should be nice and golden, with a very mild char if any.

Serve the bean bake family-style with the sweetcorn salsa, cashew queso and sliced avocado.

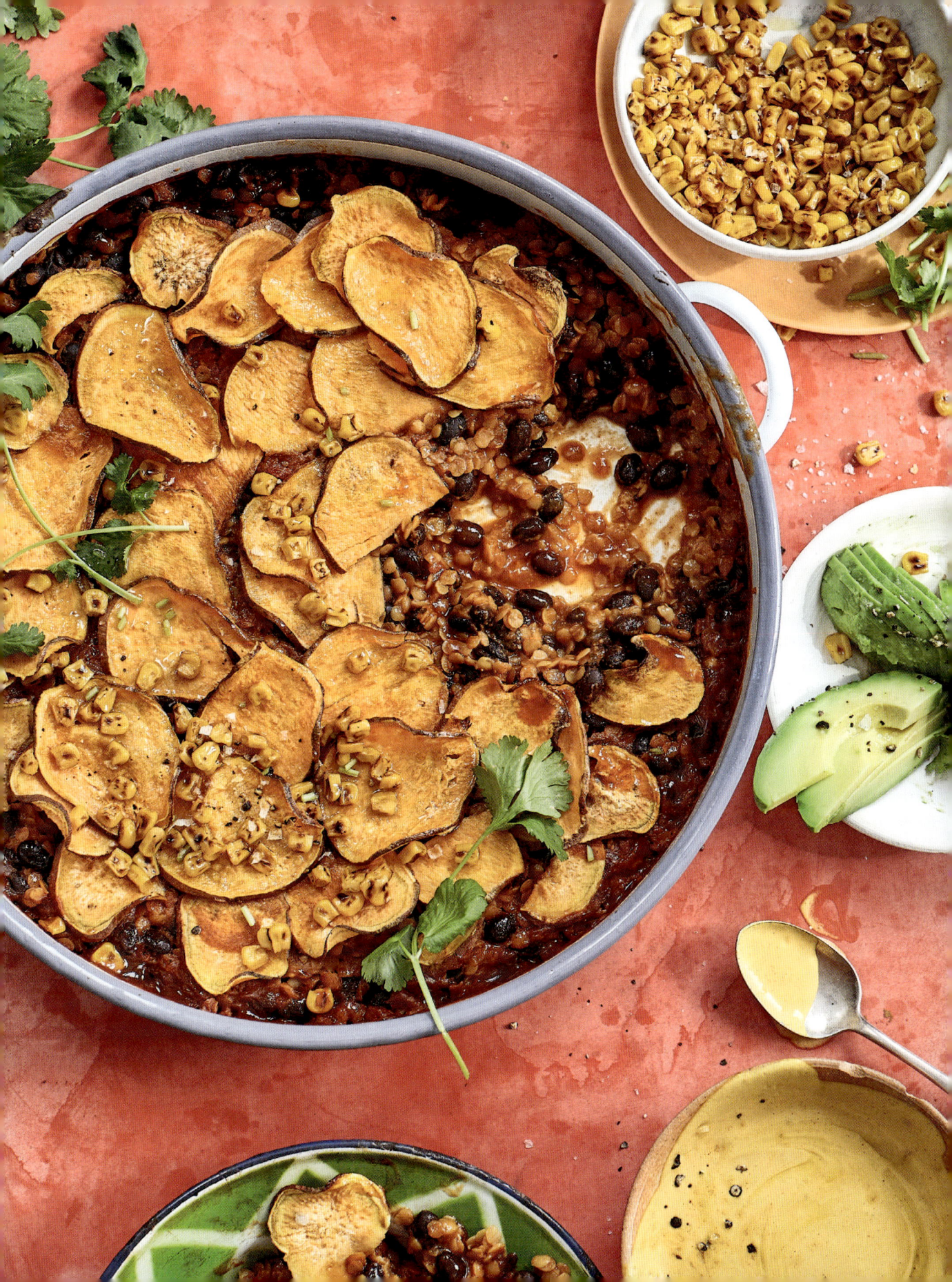

Butterbean Maghmour

SERVES 3
TOTAL TIME: 50 MINS

I was first taught to make a version of this by a Lebanese chef at a cooking class in South London called Migrateful. Migrateful is an NGO working to help refugees and asylum seekers apply for legal residency in the UK. I've changed things up to make this a high-protein dish, adding lentils and butter beans, and changing the traditional bulgur grains for quinoa, as bulgur is harder to find in supermarkets.

The method of slow cooking the whole garlic cloves so they melt into the sauce is one of my favourite things about this dish. It is simply sublime.

2 medium–large aubergines, sliced into 1cm (½in) rounds
5 tbsp extra virgin olive oil, plus more if needed
1 red onion, sliced
6 garlic cloves
1 red bell pepper, finely chopped
1 green bell pepper, finely chopped
1½ tbsp Lebanese 7-spice (if you don't have this use 1 tsp ground coriander, 1 tsp ground cumin, 1 tsp paprika, ⅓ tsp grated nutmeg, 1 clove, ½ tsp ground cinnamon, ½ tsp black pepper)
1 tsp ground coriander
1 tsp ground cumin
1 tsp smoked paprika
1 tbsp tomato purée
700g (1lb 9oz) butter beans, from a jar or 2½ x 400g (14oz) cans
200g (7oz) cooked puy lentils
1 x 400g (14oz) can plum tomatoes
Salt

Protein per serving: 32g
Fibre: 27g
Plant diversity score: 15

FOR THE QUINOA TABBOULEH
80g (3oz) cherry tomatoes, quartered
½ Persian or ⅓ English cucumber, finely chopped
100g (3½oz/½ cup) tricolour quinoa
50g (1¾oz) fresh parsley, finely chopped
20g (¾oz) fresh mint, finely chopped
4 spring onions, white and most of the green parts, finely chopped
50ml (2fl oz/3½ tbsp) extra virgin olive oil
3 tbsp lemon juice
1 garlic clove, minced
Pinch of salt

Heavily salt the aubergines, then leave in a sieve, with a bowl underneath to catch the water they will produce. Do the same with the tomatoes and cucumber for the quinoa tabbouleh, but only add a pinch of salt.

Preheat the oven to 210°C fan/230°C/gas mark 8.

Cook the quinoa according to the packet instructions. While the quinoa is cooking, arrange the aubergine rounds in a large baking dish. Give them a good dab/press with some absorbent kitchen paper on both sides. Cover with 1 tablespoon of the oil and roast for 15–20 minutes until deeply brown, flipping halfway through cooking.

In a large frying pan with a lid, fry the onion in 2 tablespoons of the olive oil on a medium heat with a pinch of salt for 6–7 minutes. Add the whole garlic cloves, the remaining 2 tablespoons of olive oil and the chopped peppers. Mix well, add a big pinch of salt, then turn the heat down to low–medium and put the lid on. Cook, undisturbed, for 10–12 minutes. Take the lid off and stir. If it's starting to stick, add some more oil, then put the lid back on and cook for another 10 minutes.

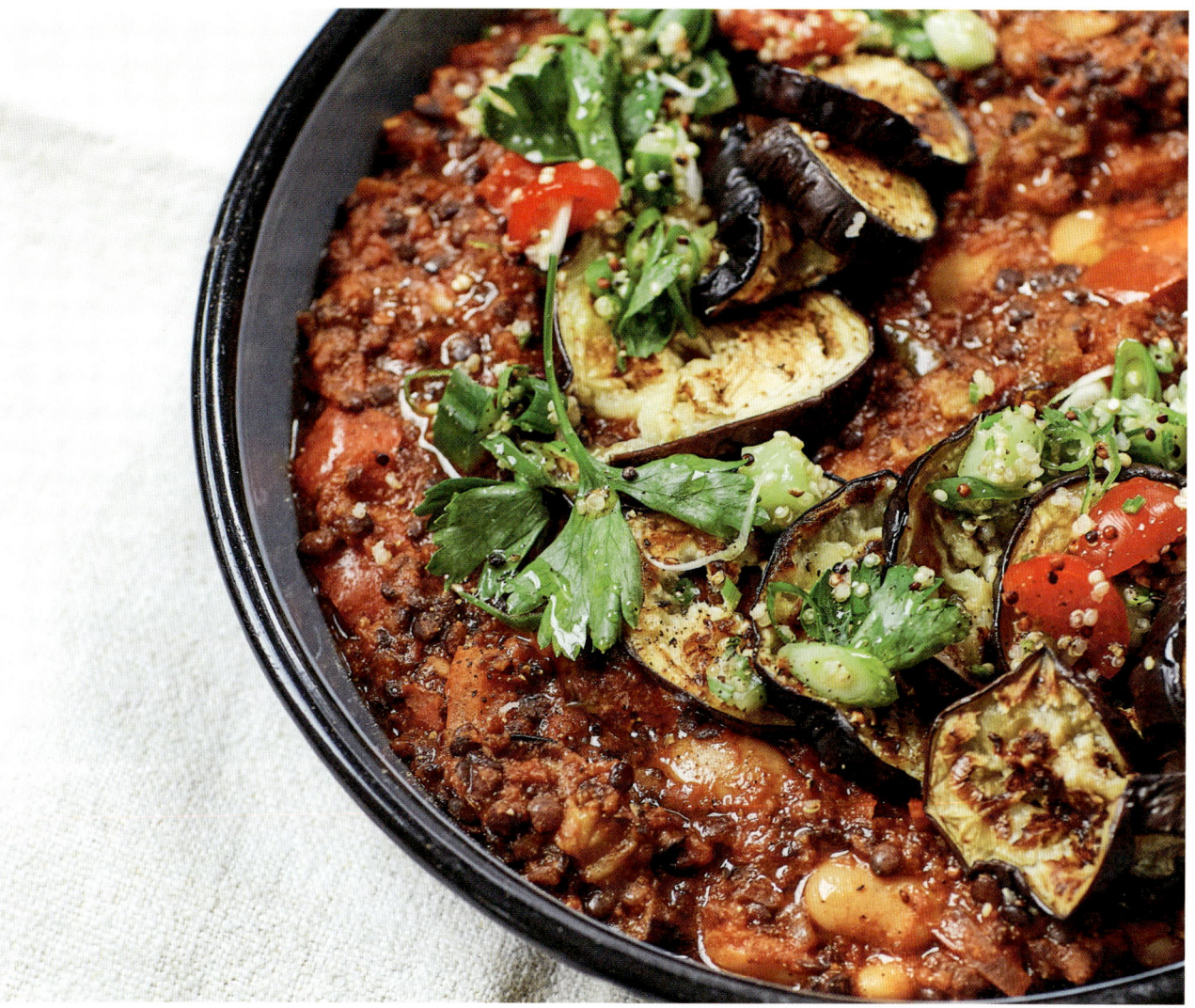

After the second 10 minutes has elapsed, the whole garlic cloves should be nice and soft. Squash them gently down into the mixture, then add all the spices and coat everything really well. Fry until fragrant, adding more oil if you need to, then add the tomato purée and cook for 2 minutes until it turns dark red.

Tip in the butter beans and lentils, then coat everything really well. Add the tomatoes, breaking them up with your hands as they come out of the can or with a wooden spoon in the pan. Fill the can up halfway with water, give it a good swill around and tip that in, too. Season to taste; I added ½ teaspoon of salt at this stage.

Bubble everything on a low–medium heat for 10 minutes so the flavours can mingle, then chop half the aubergine slices and add those to the pan.

In a medium mixing bowl, mix together all the quinoa tabbouleh ingredients.

Serve as a sharing dish, decorating the top with the remaining whole rounds of roasted aubergine.

Butter
Chickpea Curry

SERVES 4
TOTAL TIME: 45–50 MINS

This is my take on Indian Butter Chicken, a hot favourite on social media!

I highly recommend eating this with my homemade protein naan. Nothing beats a fresh, warm naan (see page 206) dipped in buttery, spiced tomato goodness.

1 large onion, diced
7 garlic cloves, minced
Thumb-sized piece of fresh ginger, peeled and grated
3 tsp ground cumin
2 tsp ground coriander
1½ tsp ground turmeric
½ tsp salt (more to taste)
4 tsp curry powder
4 tsp garam masala
3 tsp sweet smoked paprika
½ tsp ground cinnamon
2 bay leaves
1 tbsp tomato purée
2 x 400g (14oz) cans chopped tomatoes
35g (1¼oz) nutritional yeast
960g (2lb 2oz) chickpeas, from cans or jars
Olive oil
Salt and black pepper

FOR THE CASHEW CREAM
290g (10¼oz) silken tofu
Juice of 1 large lemon
½ tsp salt
80g (3oz/½ cup) cashews, soaked in boiling water for 15 minutes, then drained
50–80ml (2–2½fl oz/3½–5 tbsp) water, to loosen

TO SERVE
Fresh herbs
Chilli flakes
High-protein Naan (see page 206), rice or toasted sourdough

In a large, heavy-bottomed saucepan or shallow casserole on a medium heat, fry the onion in olive oil with a pinch of salt for about 8 minutes until caramelising. Add the garlic and ginger and sauté for another 2–4 minutes until the raw aroma has subsided. Add the spices (you may need more oil), bay leaves and cook until fragrant before adding the tomato purée and chopped tomatoes. Fill the can halfway with water and add this, too. Season to taste.

Bubble on a medium heat for 5 minutes, then turn off the heat, allow to cool and stir in the nutritional yeast. Remove the bay leaves, transfer to a bullet or food processor and blitz to a paste.

Add all the cashew cream ingredients to a bullet blender and blitz until you have a smooth consistency. Season to taste.

Return the blitzed tomato sauce to the pan, add half of the cashew cream and all of the chickpeas and stir through. Simmer for 10–15 minutes and season to taste.

Garnish with some of the remaining cashew cream, fresh herbs, chilli flakes and seeds, if you like. Enjoy with naan, rice or toasted sourdough bread.

NOTES
Add some smoked tofu (torn into small pieces) in with the chickpeas to bump up the protein content.

Protein per serving: 25g
Fibre: 20g
Plant diversity score: 10

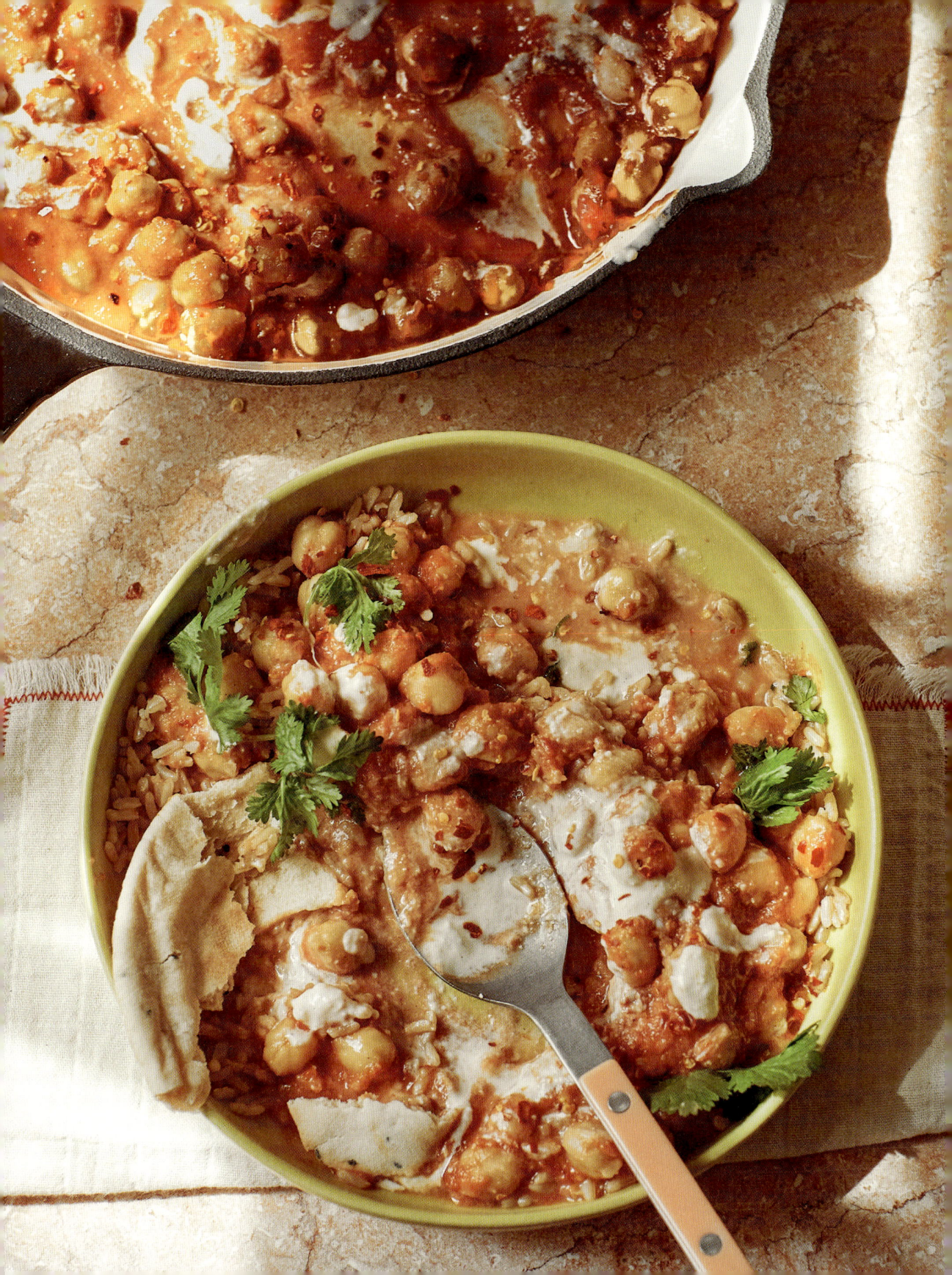

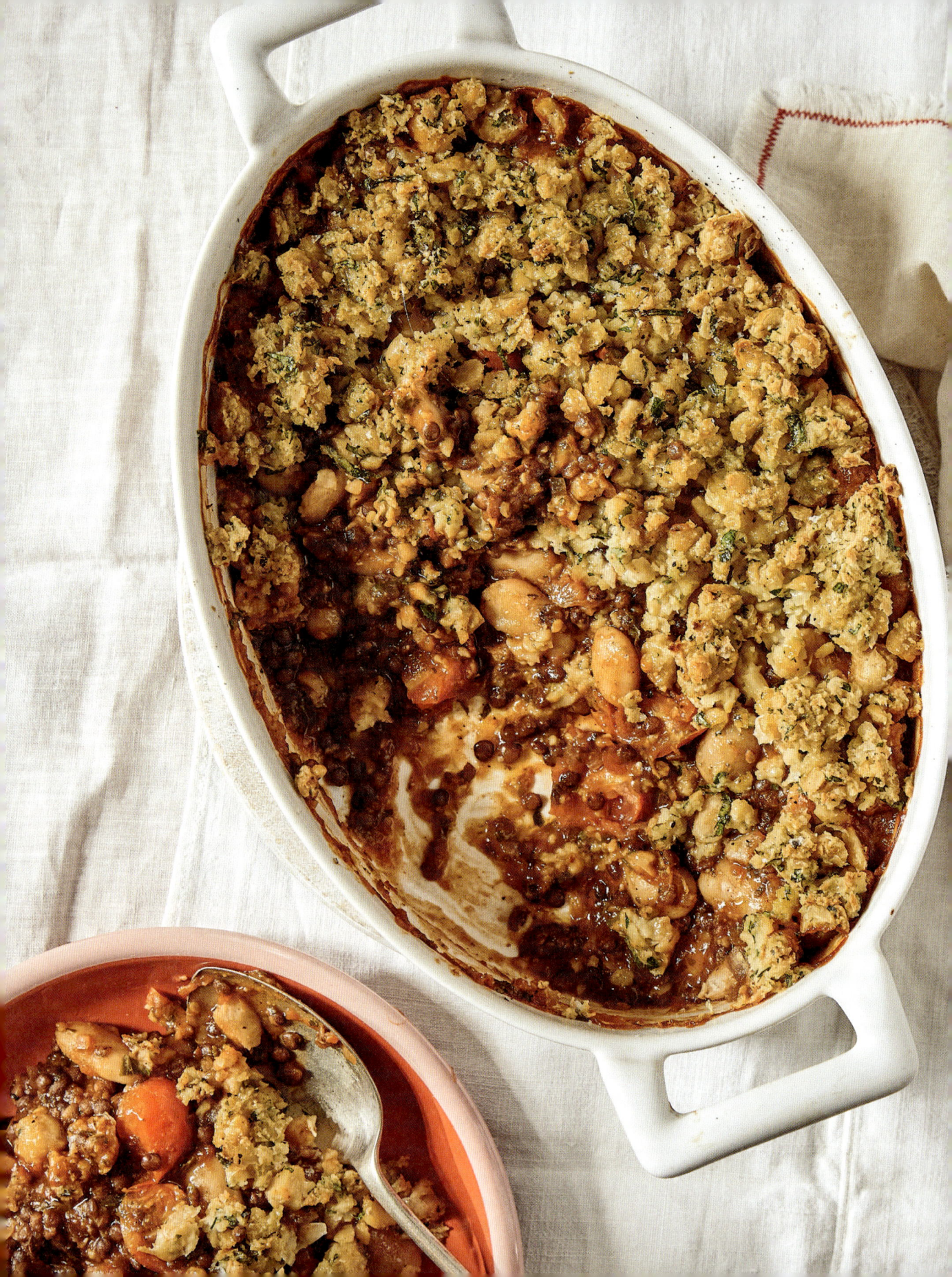

Crunchy 'Falafel' Pot Pie

SERVES: 4
TOTAL TIME: 45 MINS

If smoky, perfectly spiced beans, falafel and shepherd's pie had a baby, this would be the result. Luscious, saucy beans with a herby crunch in every bite.

½ medium brown or red onion
2 fat garlic cloves, minced
2 tsp ground cumin
1 tsp ground cardamom
1 tbsp fresh coriander stalks
1 tbsp fresh parsley stalks
200g cherry tomatoes
1 tbsp tomato purée
1 tbsp smoky harissa paste
700g (1lb 9oz) butter beans, from jars or cans, plus their juices
4 large tomatoes, grated
240g (8½oz) cooked puy lentils
½ tsp vegetable bouillon powder
Olive oil, for drizzling
Salt and black pepper

FOR THE 'FALAFEL' TOPPING
400g (14oz) chickpeas, from a can or jar, drained and rinsed
Small handful of fresh parsley, roughly chopped
Small handful of fresh coriander, roughly chopped
2 garlic cloves
½ tsp salt
Few twists of freshly cracked black pepper
2 tbsp chickpea (gram) flour
2 tbsp olive oil

TO SERVE
Sesame seeds
Fresh coriander leaves

NOTES
Serve with Quick Blender Hummus (page 214) or Tofu Feta (page 220) to bump up the protein content.

In a medium frying pan on a low–medium heat, fry the onion in olive oil with a small pinch of salt for 8 minutes.

Add the garlic and fry for another 2 minutes. Add the spices and fresh herb stalks, adding a little more olive oil if you need it. Once fragrant, add the cherry tomatoes, the tomato purée and harissa, combining everything well. Fry on a low heat for 5 minutes, then tip in the beans and their juices, tipping a little out the top of the cans first, the grated tomatoes, the lentils and vegetable bouillon powder. Add a splash of water if it's looking super thick. Bring to the boil, then reduce the heat and simmer for 10 minutes. Taste and season to your liking. Keep it on a low heat, stirring occasionally, while you prep the 'falafel' topping.

Preheat the oven to 180°C fan/200°C/gas mark 6.

In a food processor, pulse together all the falafel topping ingredients. You want a chunky crumb, so don't overmix! Season to taste. Don't worry if it tastes bitter at this point, that's the taste of the uncooked chickpea flour. It should resemble a crumble mix. If not, add a little more olive oil and pulse again.

If the pan you've been using is overproof, you can do the next step in that. If not, carefully tip the bean mixture into a baking dish. Spread the 'falafel' topping in an even layer over the beany lentil mixture, leaving some gaps for the mixture to bubble through and add texture. Drizzle some olive oil over the top. Bake for 15 minutes, then change to a grill setting and grill for 3–5 minutes to add some crunch to the topping. Do keep a close eye on it! You don't want it to burn.

Serve family-style with plenty of fresh herbs and seeds.

Protein per serving: 26g
Fibre: 22g
Plant diversity score: 9

Creamy Courgette and Butter Bean Bowl

SERVES: 3
TOTAL TIME: 1 HR

Cooking the courgettes low and slow releases the natural nutty flavour of this beautiful vegetable. As the courgettes release their water, the garlic cloves almost melt into the sauce. Coupled with the tangy cashew cream and crunchy breadcrumbs, it's a favourite on social media for a reason.

2 large courgettes, halved and cut into wonky triangles
8–10 garlic cloves, peeled
5 tbsp good-quality extra virgin olive oil
700g (25oz) butter beans from jars or cans, plus their juices
Salt and black pepper

FOR THE CASHEW CREAM
See page 219

TO SERVE
Garlicky Sourdough Breadcrumbs (see page 207)
Fresh basil leaves
Lemon zest

Preheat the oven to 160°C fan/180°C/gas mark 4.

If you're making the cashew cream, the first step is soaking cashews in boiling water, so do this now. If you have a nut allergy, you can use the same quantity of sunflower seeds instead.

Add the courgettes, garlic and olive oil to an ovenproof dish with a lid and season with salt and pepper. Toss and assemble so the fleshy side is face down. Cover and slow cook for 45 minutes, then remove the lid and cook for another 10–15 minutes until slightly browning on top. Some of the courgette chunks around the edge of the pan should have a beautiful golden layer of caramelisation, remove these and save them for garnish. If the rest of the chunks are not caramelised, it does not matter. Remove and squish these and the garlic cloves down with the back of a fork, so they release all their juices and turn into a delicious, jammy sauce.

To make the cashew cream, head to page 219.

Add the butter beans, most of their canned juices (I usually pour a little out the top beforehand), half the cashew cream and gently stir together. No need to heat.

Divide into bowls, top with the garlicky breadcrumbs (see page 207 to make), reserved caramelised courgette chunks, fresh basil and plenty of lemon zest.

Protein per serving: 30g
Fibre: 26g
Plant diversity score: 5

NOTES
Increase the protein by swapping the breadcrumbs with Crumbled Tofu or Tempeh (page 207)

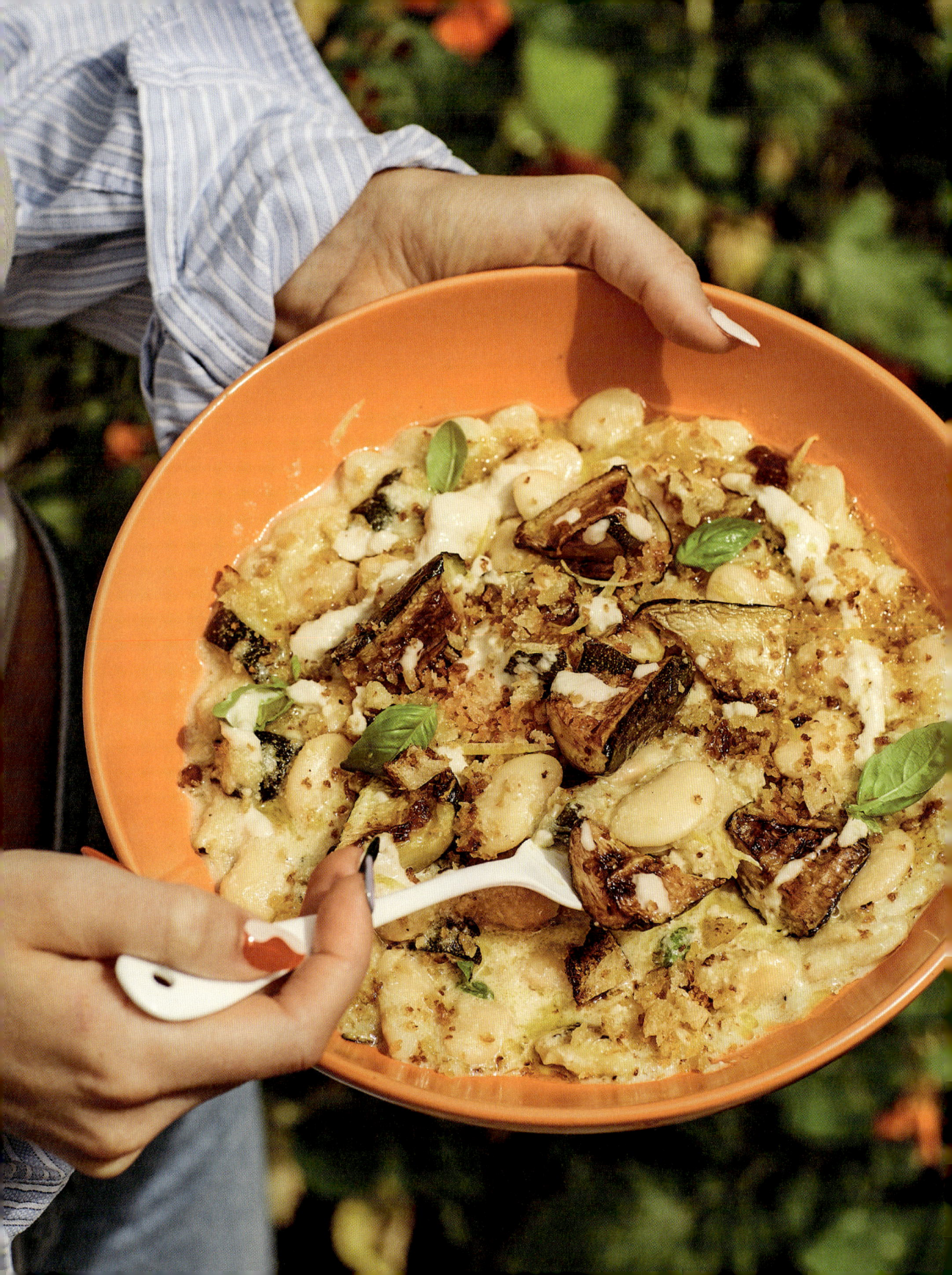

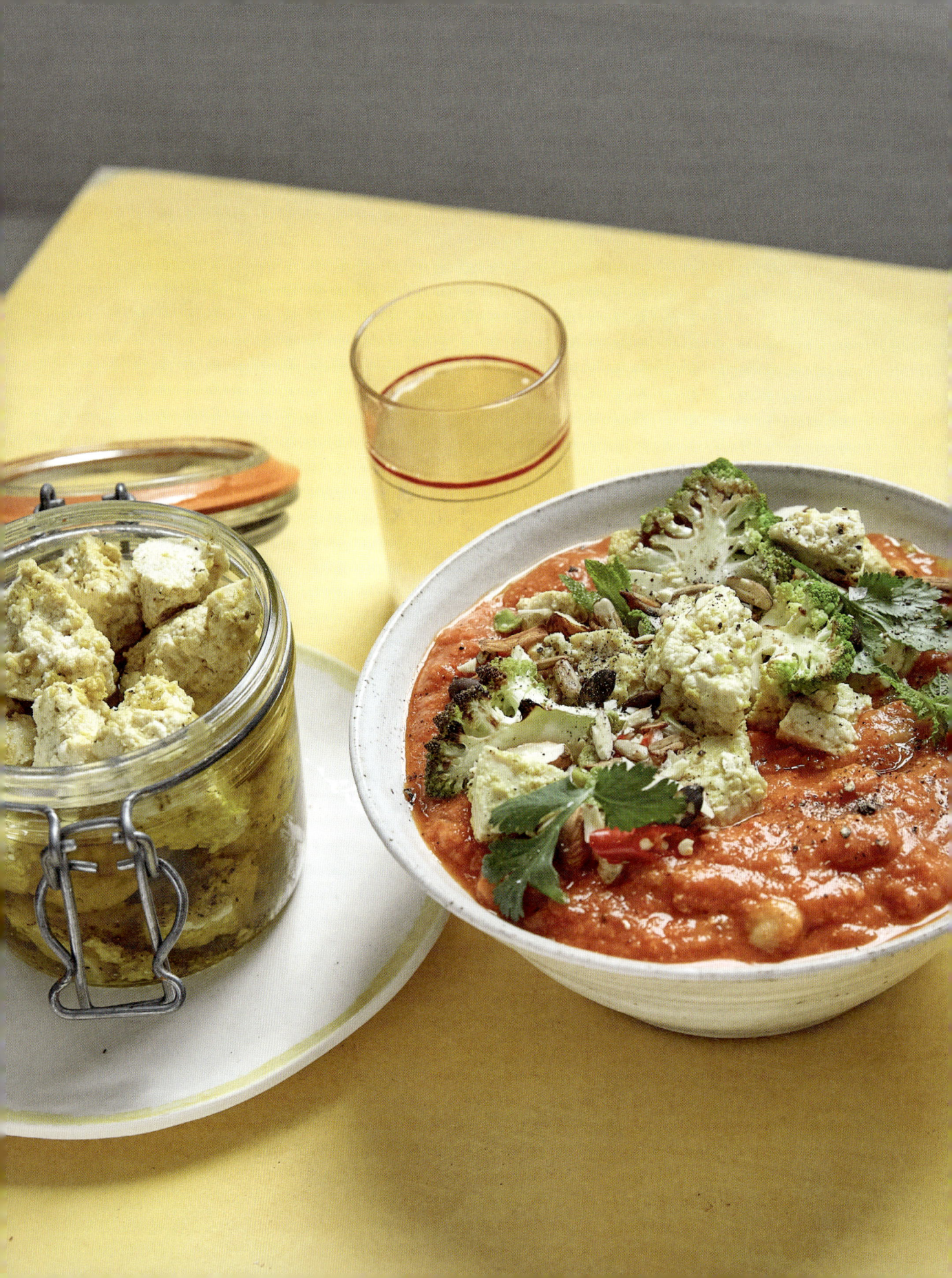

Romesco-style Chickpeas and Tamarind Glazed Veg

SERVES: 3–4
TOTAL TIME: 50 MINS

There's a fabulous vegetarian restaurant in Lisbon called Senhor Uva where they refresh their menu often to reflect the seasonal produce and have the most delicious and creative ideas I've ever come across. This is a dish inspired by their vegetable tamarind skewers. If you're ever in Lisbon, I thoroughly recommend a visit!

1 small red onion, finely chopped
Olive oil
4 garlic cloves, minced
2 tsp cumin
3 tsp smoked paprika
5 large sundried tomatoes, from a jar
2 x 400g (14oz) cans chopped tomatoes
150g (5½oz/ ⅔ cup) red split lentils
300ml (10fl oz/1¼ cups) vegetable stock
A few handfuls of chopped seasonal veg (think cauliflower, romanesco, hispi cabbage, broccoli)
2 tbsp tamarind paste
1 tbsp olive oil
½ tbsp tamari
4 roasted red bell peppers, from a jar
25g (1oz/½ cup) ground almonds
2 tbsp red wine vinegar
½ tsp chilli flakes
700g (1lb 9oz) chickpeas, from a jar or cans, drained and rinsed
Salt and black pepper

TO SERVE
A few handfuls of Tofu feta (page 220)
A small handful of almonds
Fresh herb leaves (coriander, parsley or mint)
Fresh red chilli, sliced
Cooked grain of your choice

If you haven't already made the tofu feta, do this now.

In a medium/large saucepan on a medium heat, add a good glug of olive oil and fry the onion with a pinch of salt for 8 minutes. Add the garlic, fry for another 2 minutes, then add the spices. Fry until fragrant, then add the sundried tomatoes, tinned tomatoes and ½ tsp salt, stir and simmer for 5 minutes. Add the lentils and stock, turn up the heat until it starts to boil, then cover and simmer for 10 minutes, stirring every now and then, until the lentils are cooked and soft, which should take around 15–20 mins (taste test!). Once cooked, turn off the heat and allow the mixture to cool.

Preheat the oven to 200°C fan/220°C/gas mark 7.

While it's heating, cut the seasonal veg into smaller florets, making sure to slice through the stems (so they cook quicker). Mix the tamarind paste with 1 tbsp of olive oil and the tamari, then cover the veg with the mix, using your hands to get into the crevices! Place on a baking tray and roast for 15–20 minutes until browning and soft enough to eat.

Take about half of the cooled lentil and tomato mixture and carefully add it to a blender, or just use a stick blender. Add the roasted red peppers, ground almonds, vinegar and chilli flakes. Pulse until just combined, then season to taste.

Pour it back into the pan, then add the chickpeas and mix well. Place the roasted tamarind veg artfully over the top of the dish, then scatter with tofu feta, almonds, fresh herbs and a few slices of red chilli.

Serve family-style, with your grain of choice if desired.

Protein per serving: 32g
Fibre: 24g
Plant diversity score: 8

Tempeh Paella

SERVES: 3
TOTAL TIME: 1 HR

The Spanish paella can be quite an intimidating dish to cook, so Paella police please be assured, this is not a traditional recreation, just my take!

The key to a great paella over and above the timing and delivery of spices and aromatics is the formation of the crispy rice crust, called the Socarrat. You must not stir the rice while cooking, otherwise you'll end up with fried rice. What you want is a golden, crispy layer between the rice and the bottom of the pan. This is easier to achieve with a special paella pan, however, it's not impossible to do at home. Follow the instructions carefully and you'll see.

300g (10½oz) tempeh
Olive oil, for frying
2 tbsp tamari
½ a medium onion, finely diced
1 red bell pepper, sliced
125g (4½oz) tenderstem broccoli, sliced through the stems and chopped smaller, into 2–3 cm pieces
5 garlic cloves, minced
2 bay leaves
1 tbsp smoked paprika
Pinch of ground cinnamon
Pinch of cayenne pepper
1 large pinch of saffron threads
150ml (5fl oz) tomato passata
200g arborio rice, rinsed
700ml vegetable stock
85g (5½oz) frozen garden peas
Salt

TO SERVE
Lemon wedges
Fresh parsley

Protein per serving: 27g
Fibre: 9.2g
Plant diversity score: 8

Start by prepping the tempeh. Over a medium bowl, break it apart into small chunks with your hands (or you can use a knife if you wish). Heat a glug of olive oil in a medium non-stick pan, on a medium heat. Tip in the tempeh chunks and fry with a little salt for 6–8 minutes until the tempeh starts to brown. Add the tamari and fry until the liquid has gone, making sure all pieces are evenly covered. Season to taste, set aside.

In a wide casserole dish, or a wide, sided frying pan, or a paella pan if you have one, fry the onion, red pepper and broccoli in olive oil on a medium heat with a pinch of salt for 8-10 minutes, stirring continuously, until the onion is caremelising and the veg is starting to soften. Add the garlic, bay leaves, spices, and fry for another 3 minutes. Add the passata and saffron, a big pinch of salt, and cook for 5 minutes, until the sauce starts to thicken.

Add the vegetable stock, the rice, the cooked tempeh chunks, and stir gently to combine until everything is well mixed. This is the last bit of stirring you'll do! Don't stir any more after this point, or you'll get in trouble with the Paella police. Jiggle the pan to make sure everything is nice and even, then bring the mixture to the boil, reduce to a lower heat and cook for 10 minutes, until most of the liquid is absorbed into the rice, then pop the lid on the pan and cook for a further 8–10 mins. After 8 mins, taste the rice to make sure it's cooked. If it's still a little al dente, pour a little more hot water over the top of the rice in an equal layer, place the lid back on the pan and cook for a further 5 mins.

Once the water has been absorbed and the rice is cooked, turn up the heat so you can form the layer of crispy rice on the bottom. Let it cook for 60–90 seconds, then take it off the heat and leave it to sit with a tea towel on top for 5 mins.

Squeeze lemon juice over the top and serve each bowl with a wedge of lemon and fresh parsley.

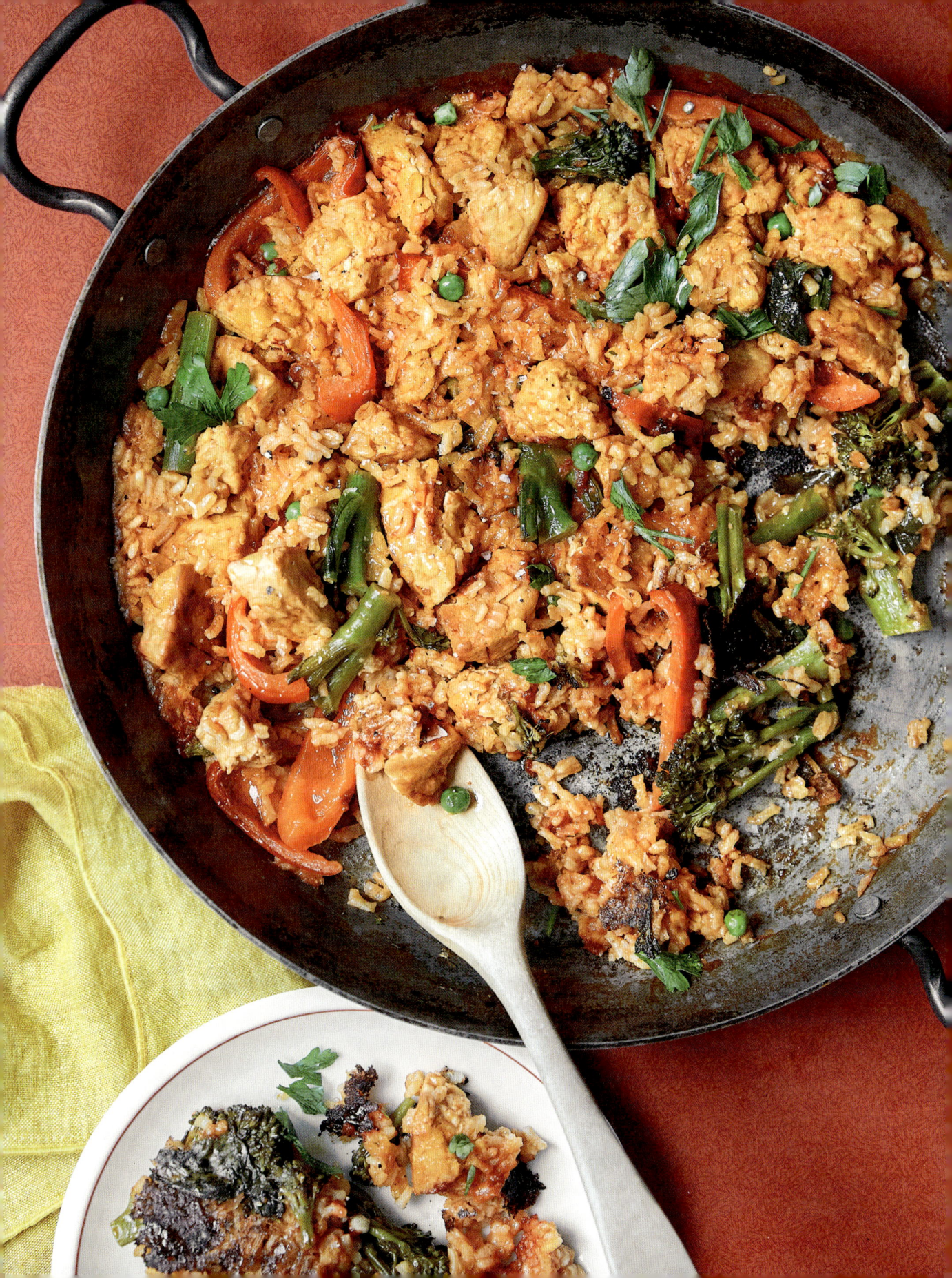

Lentil Muhammara Pasta

MAKES THREE SERVINGS

My dals are some of the most popular recipes on social media. Usually I blend squash into the sauces for some sweetness but this does tend to amp up the starchiness, so for this one I've used roasted red pepper instead. If you'd just prefer the dal on its own, omit the pasta and red wine vinegar, and adjust the water levels too if you like a soupier dal.

2 large roasted red peppers, from a jar, or roast your own 2 large fresh peppers
2 shallots, finely chopped
3 cloves garlic, minced
2 tsp smoked paprika
1 tsp ground coriander
1 tsp ground cumin
150g dried split red lentils
240g chickpeas, from a can, drained and rinsed
350ml veggie stock
40g walnut pieces, soaked in boiling water for 10 minutes
7 sundried tomatoes, from a jar
1½ tbsp red wine vinegar
Juice of half a lemon
Black pepper
300g pasta of choice

TO SERVE:
Black pepper
Some fresh leaves, parsley, coriander and/or rocket
A few toasted walnuts

—————

Protein per serving: 30g
Fibre: 14g
Plant diversity score: 9

If you're roasting fresh red peppers, preheat your oven to 180°C fan/200°C/gas mark 6. In a small roasting tray, cut the pepper in quarters around the stem, remove the pith and pips, then cover with olive oil and salt and roast cut side down for 20 mins until the skin is wrinkling and beginning to turn black. If you're using jarred, skip this step.

Start by sauteing the shallot in a large saucepan, for which you have a lid, in olive oil, on a medium heat, for 5–6 minutes, with a pinch of salt. Add the minced garlic and cook for 3 minutes more. Add the spices, fry for another minute, then add all the rinsed red lentils to the pan along with the vegetable stock. Stir well, bring the mix to the boil, then reduce to a simmer and cover, lifting and stirring occasionally, for 15–20 minutes or until the lentils are cooked. If the lentils start to dry up before they're cooked, add a splash more water. Once cooked, take off the heat and allow to cool. Whilst this is cooking/cooling, cook the pasta for 1 min less than the packet suggests. Keep a mug of pasta water.

In a medium bullet blender, add the roasted red peppers (remove the skins if you roasted your own), the sundried tomatoes, lemon juice, red wine vinegar, one tbsp extra virgin olive oil, some black pepper and half of the cooked red lentils. Pulse to a thick, paste-like consistency. Season to taste.

Drain the walnuts and roughly chop, then add to the pan with the blended mix, a splash of pasta water, the chickpeas and the cooked pasta. Mix well, then divide into bowls and serve with plenty of black pepper, and some fresh rocket, parsley or coriander and the toasted walnuts.

NOTES
Look for Durum Semolina pasta to get the protein amount listed. Find it in larger supermarkets or your local Italian deli.

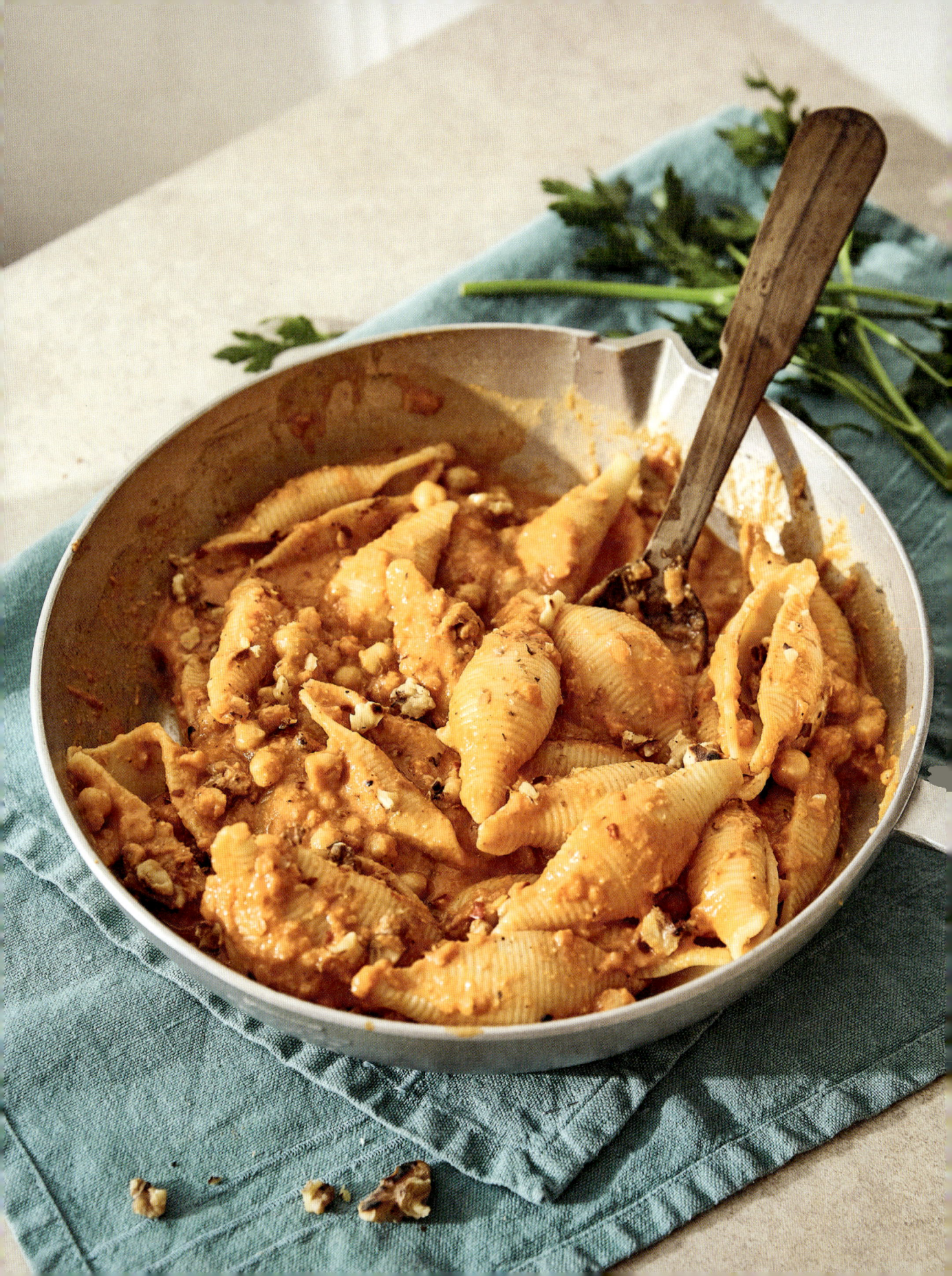

Batch Cook Preps, 3 Ways

Spend a little time on Sundays making one of these five recipes, so you can relax, knowing there's a nutritious meal to come home to from Monday - Wednesday. Option to jazz them up in three separate ways each night to keep things interesting.

Easy Black Dal

SERVES 4
TOTAL TIME: 1 HR 15 MINS
PLUS OVERNIGHT SOAKING

This Indian-inspired black dal is a lighter version of the popular Dal Makhani, a buttery, rich dal made on special occasions. We love it as the lentils are bursting with protein and fibre, making this a healthy weeknight meal. This recipe is not traditional by any means – it's a shortcut, but a good one. Feel free to sub out butter entirely and just use olive oil.

500g (1lb 2oz/2¾ cups) beluga lentils, soaked overnight, then drained and rinsed until the water runs clear
2–3 tbsp olive oil or unsalted vegan butter, plus 1 tbsp oil for the spices
1 tsp cumin seeds
1 medium brown onion, finely chopped
5 garlic cloves, minced
Thumb sized piece of ginger, peeled and grated
2 tbsp tomato purée
1 tbsp garam masala
1 tbsp ground cumin
½ cinnamon stick
2 tsp kasuri methi (dried fenugreek leaves, optional)
1 tsp mild chilli powder
Pinch of ground nutmeg
⅓ tsp ground cardamom
4 cloves
1 tbsp curry powder
2 bay leaves
500ml (18fl oz/2 cups) vegetable stock, plus more if you like a soupier dal
100ml (3½fl oz/scant ½ cup) Cashew Cream (see page 219), or soy or oat cream
Sea salt and black pepper

Protein per serving: 30g
Fibre: 24.5g
Plant diversity score: 9

FOR THE TEMPER (optional)
1 tbsp olive oil
1 garlic clove, finely sliced
½ tsp cumin seeds

TO SERVE
Fresh sliced red chilli
Fresh coriander leaves
Nigella seeds (optional)

Cook the soaked lentils for about 45 minutes, or until soft but still holding their shape well.

In a wide casserole dish or dutch oven, heat the olive oil over a medium–low heat, then fry the cumin seeds for about 1 minute until fragrant. Add the onion and a pinch of salt and fry for 8 minutes until nice and soft.

Add the garlic and ginger and cook for 3–4 minutes until the raw aroma has subsided. Now for the spices and the flavour! Add 1 tablespoon of olive oil in the centre of the pan, then all the spices, bay leaves and 1 teaspoon of salt. Fry for 1 minute, then add tomato purée and coat everything really well.

Add the lentils and the stock. Mix well, then season to taste. Bring to the boil, then reduce and simmer for at least 30 minutes. I recommend using a full hour if possible, so the flavours really get to know each other.

When you're happy with the overall taste, remove the bay leaves and cinnamon stick, crumble in the kasuri methi leaves if using and mix well. Allow the dal to cool, then blitz around one-third to half the mixture with a stick blender, or if you don't have a stick blender scoop out some of the dal with a cup measure or mug and transfer into a small blender. Pulse until chunky, then pour back in. Mix well, then pour in the cream. I like to gently mix so there are streaks of creamy white and darker lentils, and I reserve a little to decorate the dal but this is personal preference!

Now is the time for the temper, which is optional but recommended. In a small frying pan or saucepan, heat the olive oil and add the garlic and cumin seeds and fry for 30 secs or until the garlic starts to brown off. Remove from the heat and pour the contents straight from the frying pan over the dal, so the hot oil sizzles on contact.

Gently fold in, then top with the chilli, fresh coriander and nigella seeds (if using).

NIGHT 1
Eat with wholemeal rice, roti or High-protein Naan (see page 206) and Easy Zingy Slaw

FOR THE EASY ZINGY SLAW
Small handful of rocket leaves
Small handful of shredded green cabbage leaves
½ tbsp olive oil
½ tbsp apple cider vinegar
Pinch of salt

Add all the zingy slaw ingredients to a small bowl and gently combine. Set aside until ready to serve.

NIGHT 2
Layer over crispy smashed new potatoes with plenty of fresh herbs and Omega-3 Boost (see page 209).

FOR THE CRISPY NEW POTATOES
200g (7oz) new potatoes
Olive oil, for drizzling
Sea salt and black pepper

Put the new potatoes in a large saucepan and cover with at least 5cm (2in) of cold water. Boil until the bubbles start to roll, then set a timer for 5 minutes. When the time's up, test with a fork if the potatoes are soft in the middle, then drain and set aside. If not, wait another minute or so.

Preheat the oven to 180°C fan/200°C/gas mark 6 and line a large baking tray with baking parchment or a silicone mat. Place the boiled potatoes on the tray and use a heavy-bottomed glass to squish them down into a smashed shape. Don't over squish, you want them to hold together, but don't underdo it either! Liberally drizzle olive oil over them, sprinkle with sea salt and black pepper. Bake for about 20-25 minutes, or until they're nice and crispy.

NIGHT 3
Pop the dal in a wholemeal tortilla wrap or roti and fold to make a burrito with some cooked brown rice and pink pickled onion (see page 206).

NOTES
If you want to speed up the cooking time, you can use already cooked beluga lentils. These come in pouches (I like the Merchant Gourmet ones) and you will need about 5 x 250g pouches for this recipe.

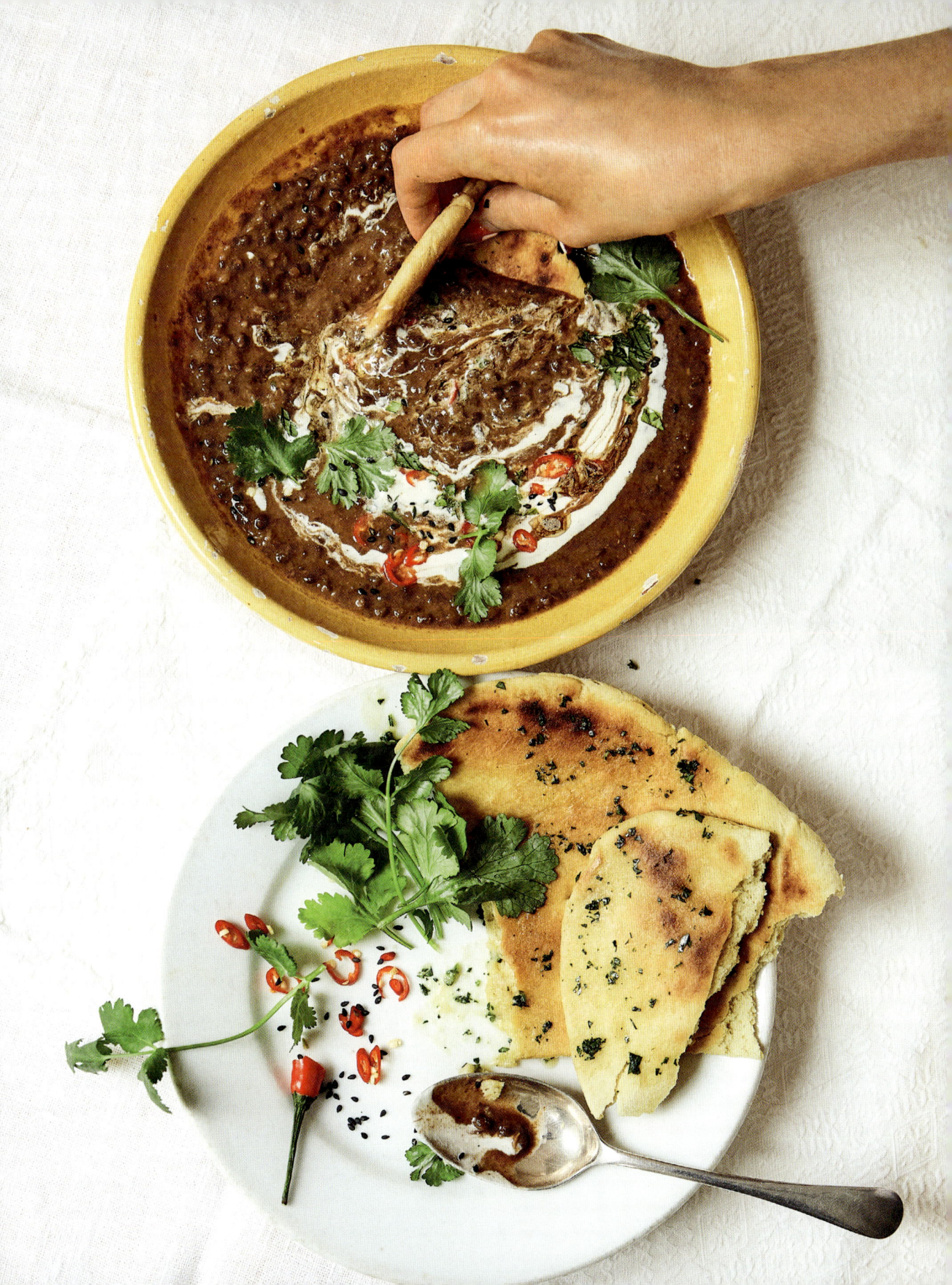

Cuban-style Stewed Black Beans

SERVES 4
TOTAL TIME: 45 MINS

A nice warming bowl of spiced black beans are always my go-to on colder nights. Perfect nourishing comfort food!

Olive oil, for frying
2 large red onions, finely chopped
2 red bell peppers, finely chopped
2 green bell peppers, finely chopped
2 celery stalks, finely chopped
1 tbsp finely chopped coriander stalks
6–8 garlic cloves, minced
½ red chilli, finely chopped (adjust depending on your spice tolerance, or leave out)
1 tbsp ground coriander
1 tbsp ground cumin
1 tbsp dried oregano
4 bay leaves
4 x 400g (14oz) cans black beans, plus their juices
250ml (9fl oz/1 cup) vegetable stock
1½ tbsp red wine vinegar
4 tbsp nutritional yeast
Salt and black pepper

Cover the bottom of a large casserole or heavy-bottomed saucepan with olive oil, then cook the onions, peppers and celery with a pinch of salt on a medium heat for 8–10 minutes until most of the steam subsides and the veg start to caramelise. Add the chopped coriander stalks, garlic and chilli and cook for another 3–4 minutes.

Add the spices, ½ teaspoon of black pepper, dried oregano and bay leaves. Fry, using a little more olive oil if you need it, for 1-2 minutes until nice and fragrant, and the vegetables are suitably covered in spices.

Go in with all the beans and their juices, the nutritional yeast, and the stock. Bring to the boil, then simmer, uncovered, for 20–30 minutes.

Season to taste, then take off the heat and add the red wine vinegar.

NIGHT 1

Enjoy the beans with crispy kale and a slice of sourdough bread for dipping.

FOR THE CRISPY KALE
3 large handfuls of kale, washed and destemmed
Olive oil, for drizzling
1 tbsp nutritional yeast
½ tsp maple or agave syrup
Salt

Preheat the oven to 160°C fan/180°C/gas mark 4.

Add the kale to a baking tray, drizzle with oil and season with salt. Bake for 6–8 minutes. Remove the tray from the oven, scatter over the nutritional yeast and drizzle with the agave or maple and mix again. Return to the oven for a further 4–6 minutes until the leaves are crispy.

Protein per serving: 24g
Fibre: 24.5g
Plant diversity score: 9

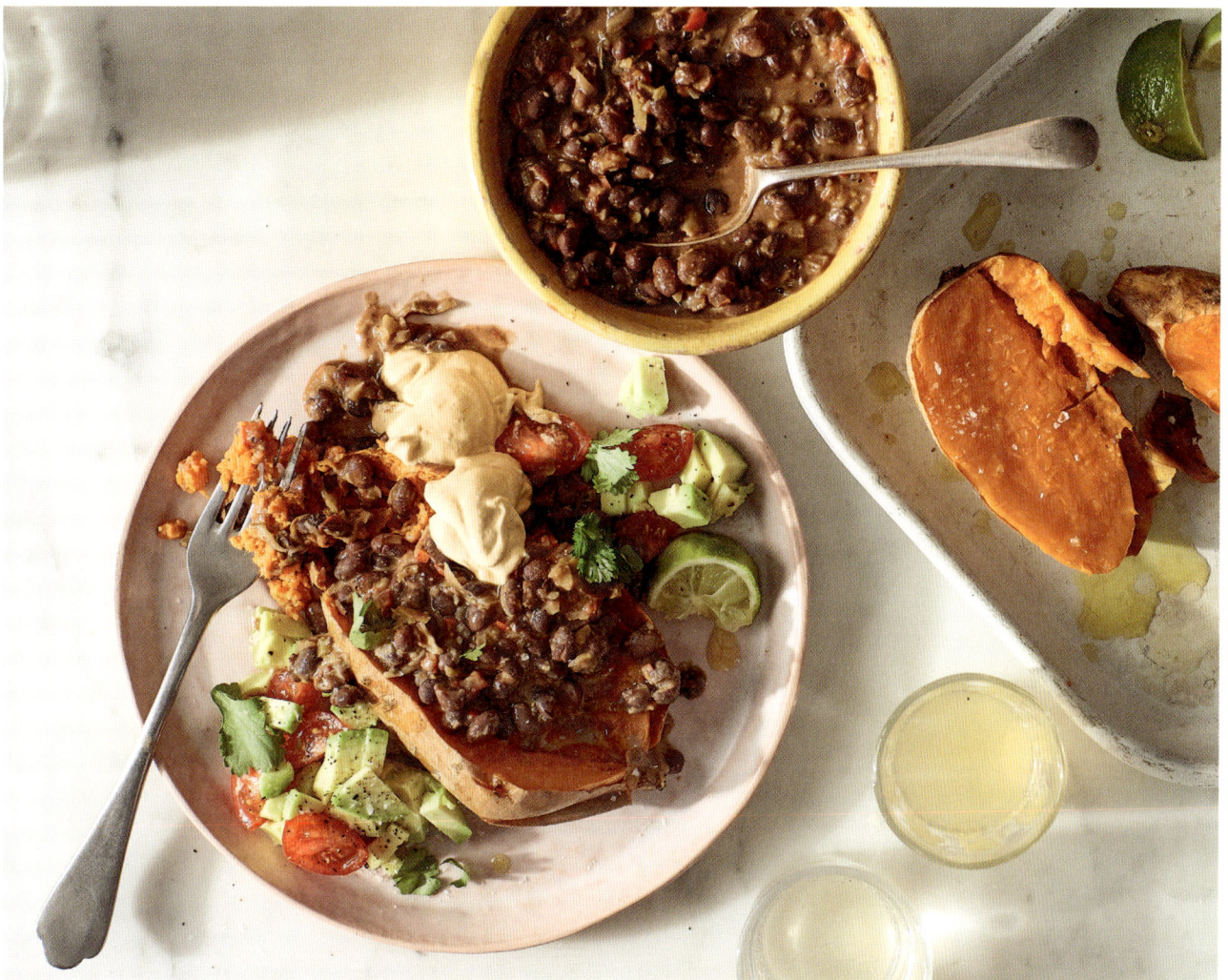

Roast sweet potato, use the beans as a filling and top with cashew cream (see page 219), tamari seed sprinkle (see page 208) and fresh coriander.

FOR THE ROAST SWEET POTATO
2 medium sweet potatoes
Olive oil, for drizzling
Salt

Preheat the oven to 180°C fan/200°C/gas mark 6.

Wash and prick the sweet potatoes a few times with a fork. Microwave on high for 4–5 minutes to soften, then transfer to a baking tray. Drizzle with olive oil, sprinkle with salt and bake for 30–35 minutes until soft.

Cook quinoa in vegetable stock according to the packet instructions, dress with lemon juice, olive oil and fresh herbs, then serve with the remaining beans and some crispy, garlicky breadcrumbs for crunch (see page 207).

NOTES
Bump up the protein content with 100g Tofu Feta per person (page 220), a cooked grain, or large slice of wholemeal sourdough.

The Ultimate Lasagne

SERVES 4–6
TOTAL TIME: 1 HR 20 MINS

Lasagne needs no introduction, so here's my tried and tested high-protein version for you to bookmark. (According to many recipe testers on social media, you'll want to come back again and again!)

1 x 250g (9oz) pack spelt lasagne sheets
400g (14oz) fresh spinach
Vegan mozzarella (optional, or use Cashew Parm, see page 221)

FOR THE TOMATO, CHICKPEA, AND AUBERGINE SAUCE
4 medium aubergines
4 tbsp olive oil
1 garlic bulb, plus 5 cloves, grated
1 large white onion, diced
1 tbsp fresh thyme leaves
1 tbsp dried oregano
3 tbsp tomato purée
6 sun-dried tomatoes, finely chopped
2 x 400g (14oz) cans plum tomatoes
500ml (18fl oz) passata
1 tbsp balsamic vinegar
2 x 400g (14oz) tins cooked puy or green lentils
Salt and black pepper

FOR THE 'BÉCHAMEL'
560g (1lb 4oz) silken tofu
2 tbsp sweet white miso paste
½ tsp ground cumin
½ tsp grated nutmeg
Juice of 1 lemon
80g (3oz/½ cup) cashew nuts, soaked in boiling water for 15 minutes
6 tbsp nutritional yeast

TO SERVE
Fresh basil leaves
Olive oil
Sprinkle of Cashew Parmesan (see page 221)

Preheat the oven to 180°C fan/200°C/gas mark 6.

In a medium baking dish, prick the aubergine skins with a fork a few times, then drizzle and rub a little olive oil over their skins and salt. Roast until the aubergines skins have expanded and a knife slides in very easily. If it doesn't slide in easily, leave them in for another few minutes. Once done and the aubergine flesh is very soft, take them out and leave them to cool whilst you start the sauce.

In a large frying pan on a medium heat, cook the onion with a pinch of salt for 6–8 minutes until translucent, then add the garlic, thyme and oregano. Cook for a further 2–3 minutes, then add the tomato purée and sun-dried tomatoes. By this point, the aubergines should be done. Cut them in half and scoop out the flesh, mash it well with a fork and add to the pan with 1 teaspoon of salt. Combine everything together, making sure there are no big lumpy bits. Add the tomatoes, passata, more salt to taste, then simmer for 15 minutes while you blend all the ingredients for the 'béchamel' sauce. When the sauce is ready and seasoned to your liking, remove from the heat and stir in the balsamic vinegar and lentils.

In a 30cm wide casserole ovenproof dish or similar sized baking dish, layer the lasagne, starting with the lentil, aubergine and tomato sauce, then lasagne sheets, 'béchamel' sauce and spinach. Repeat until all ingredients are used up, finishing with a layer of 'béchamel' sauce, a few large blobs of tomato sauce and vegan mozzarella (if using).

Bake for 35–40 minutes, or until the top layer starts to go crispy and char in places.

Top with fresh basil, olive oil and cashew parm.

Serve the lasagne with a kale, cucumber, onion and tomato side salad with a punchy vinaigrette.

FOR THE KALE SIDE SALAD
2–3 large handfuls of kale, chopped
2 large salad tomatoes, cut into wedges
½ cucumber, chopped into half-moons
1 small finger-sized wedge of red onion, thinly sliced
1 tbsp sprouted seeds (optional)
3–5 Kalamata olives, pitted and chopped

FOR THE PUNCHY VINAIGRETTE
2 tbsp olive oil
1 tbsp red wine vinegar
1 tsp Dijon mustard
½ garlic clove, grated
½ tsp maple or agave syrup
Pinch of salt and pepper

In a small bowl, whisk the ingredients for the vinaigrette together. Season to taste.

In a mixing bowl, combine all the veg with the vinaigrette and toss gently to combine. Serve straight away!

Protein per serving: 27g
Fibre: 17g
Plant diversity score: 10

Serve with miso butter garlic bread and fresh lettuce leaves.

FOR THE MISO BUTTER GARLIC BREAD
1 large garlic bulb
Olive oil, for drizzling
1½ tbsp vegan butter, softened
1½ tsp white miso paste
1½ tbsp nutritional yeast
Small handful of chopped fresh chives or chopped parsley
1 fresh baguette
Salt and black pepper

Preheat the oven to 180°C fan/200°C/gas mark 6.

Cut the garlic bulb in half and drizzle both halves with olive oil and season with a little salt. Wrap them in foil and roast for 15–20 minutes.

In a small bowl, mix the softened butter, miso, nutritional yeast, some salt and pepper, the fresh herbs and the garlic (squeeze out the cloves from the roasted bulb once it's cooled).

Cut the baguette in half and spread a thick layer of the miso garlic butter on top, then bake for 6–8 minutes or until slightly golden.

Serve with seasonal greens, lightly sautéed with shallot, chilli and garlic, dressed with a lemon and caper vinaigrette.

FOR THE SAUTÉED SEASONAL GREENS
1 tbsp olive oil
1 small shallot, finely sliced widthways
1 large handful of asparagus, woody ends snapped off, green beans, topped and tailed, or broccoli, florets broken and sliced through the stem
1 small garlic clove, finely chopped
Juice of ½ lemon
Pinch of chilli flakes
1 tbsp capers, plus 1 tbsp of their brine
Salt and black pepper

In a frying pan on a medium heat, heat the oil, then add the shallot and cook for 5 minutes. Add the veg, garlic and some salt and pepper, then cook for another 5 minutes or until the veg is fork tender. Remove, serve and dress with the lemon juice, chilli flakes, capers and caper brine.

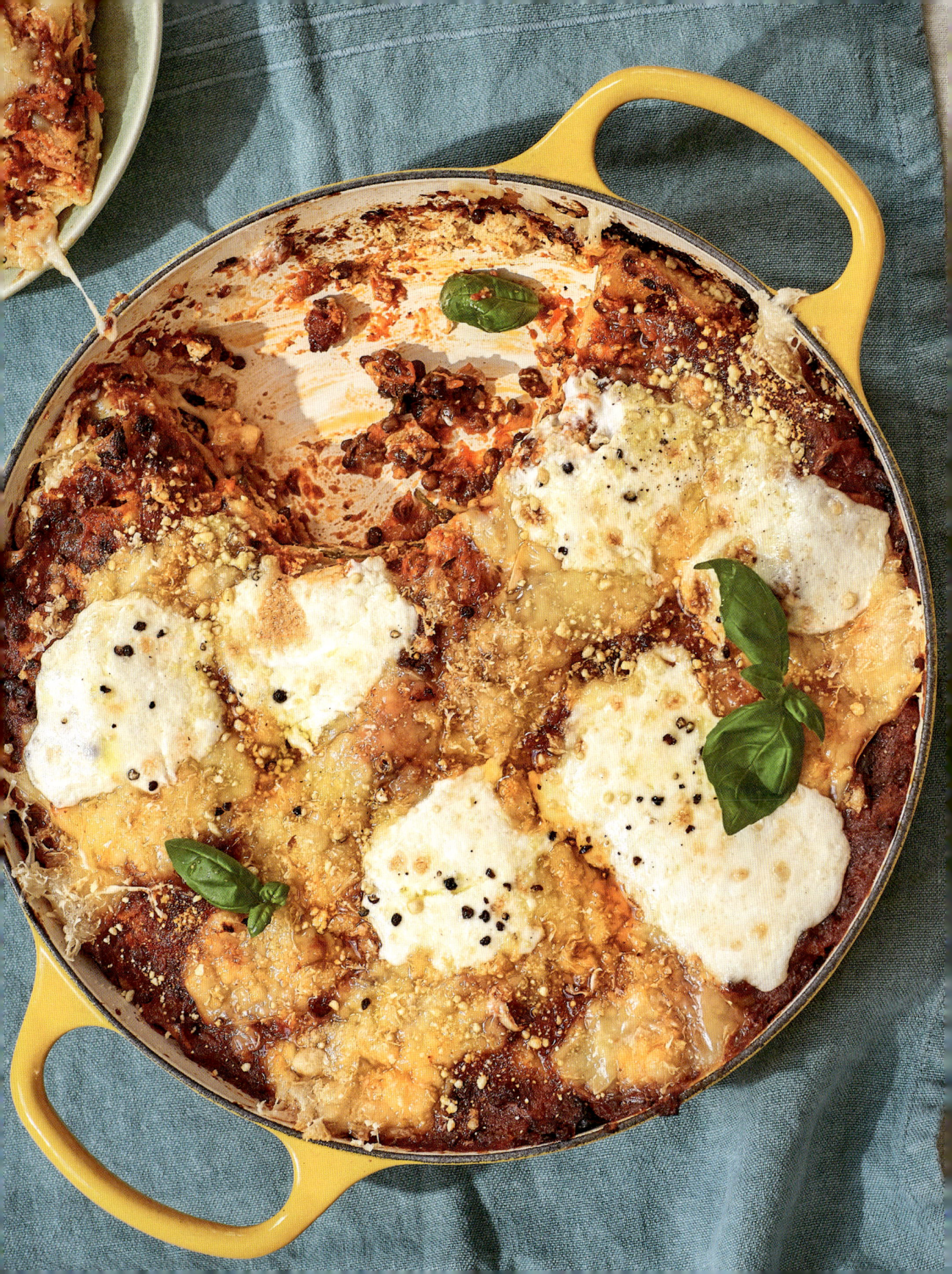

Mega Squash Chilli

SERVES 6
TOTAL TIME: 1 HR

It wouldn't be a meal prep chapter without a winning chilli. If you've never tried adding coffee and dark chocolate to yours, you're in for a treat.

1 medium butternut squash, unpeeled if organic, deseeded and cut into rough 1–2cm (½–¾in) cubes
1 medium red onion, diced
3 celery stalks, finely chopped
1 red bell pepper, roughly chopped
1 yellow bell pepper, roughly chopped
2 tbsp finely chopped coriander stalks
5 garlic cloves, minced
1 red chilli, finely chopped
2½ tsp ground cumin
2 tsp ground coriander
1½ tbsp smoked paprika
¼ tsp cayenne pepper (optional)
1 x 400g (14oz) can black beans, plus their juices
1 x 400g (14oz) can kidney beans, plus their juices
2 x 400g (14oz) cans plum tomatoes
2 x 400g (14oz) cans brown lentils
40ml (1½fl oz/scant 3 tbsp) coffee
15g (½oz) dark chocolate (about 1–2 squares)
Squeeze of lime juice
Salt and black pepper

TO SERVE
100g Tofu Feta (see page 220)
Quick-pickled Onion (see page 206)
Guacamole (or sliced avocado
Cashew Queso (see page 219)
Chilli flakes
Fresh coriander leaves
Omega-3 Boost (see page 209)
Toasted sourdough or cooked quinoa

Protein per serving: 32g
Fibre: 20g
Plant diversity score: 14

Preheat the oven to 180°C fan/200°C/gas mark 6.

Add the squash to a baking tray and drizzle with olive oil and season with salt and pepper. Roast for 35–40 minutes until soft.

Cover the bottom of a hot casserole or large saucepan with 4 tbsp olive oil and heat it until a little bit of onion sizzles on contact. When ready, fry the onion, celery and peppers with a pinch of salt for 10 minutes until greatly reduced in volume. Add the coriander stalks, garlic and chilli and fry for another 2–3 minutes. Add the spices and ½ teaspoon of salt and continue to fry for 2 minutes.

Add the beans and their juices and stir to combine. Add the tomatoes, breaking them up with a spatula, then fill their cans up halfway, swill around and add that tomatoey water in, too. Season to taste.

Bring to the boil, then reduce the heat and simmer for 20 minutes to let the flavours mingle together and the chilli thicken up.

Add the coffee, dark chocolate and two-thirds of the roasted squash, saving some of the crispier bits for garnish.

Top with the tofu feta, pink pickled onions, more squash, guac or sliced avo, cashew queso, chilli flakes and fresh coriander.

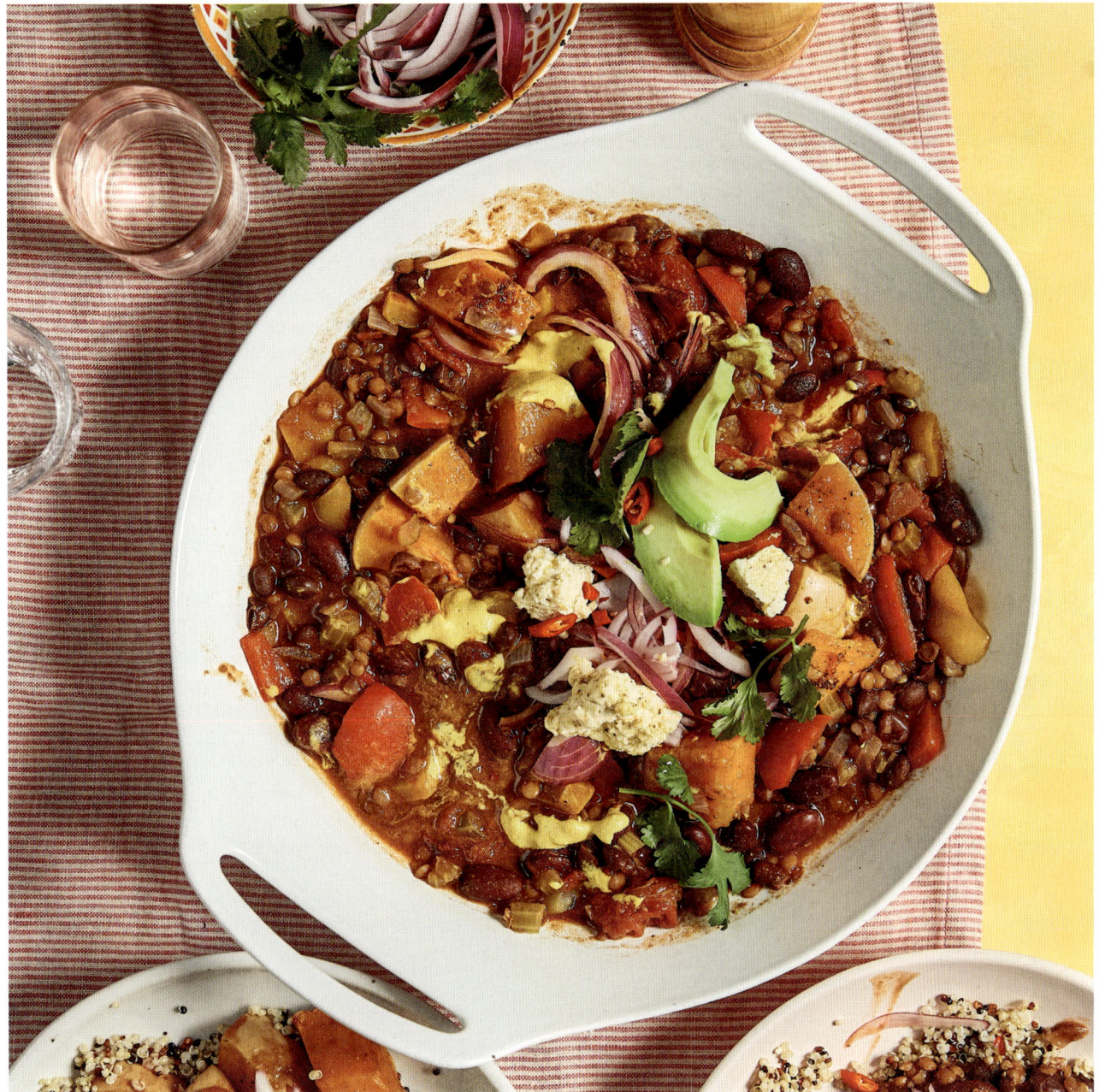

<table>
<tr><td>

NIGHT 1

Enjoy with the tofu feta, other various toppings, and some sourdough toast.

</td><td>

NIGHT 2

Make it into a minestrone! Cook up a small pasta shape of choice and add this to your chilli bowls along with fresh herbs and more tofu feta.

</td><td>

NIGHT 3

Cook a batch of seasoned quinoa or other grain of choice mixed with chopped coriander and parsley leaves, mixed in with a glug of olive oil, 1 tbsp lemon juice and salt to taste.

</td></tr>
</table>

Very Healthy Triple Legume Stew

SERVES 4
TOTAL TIME: 1 HR

Inspired by Harira, a Moroccan, tomato-based soup with chickpeas and sometimes pasta, this dish is a nutritional powerhouse, perfect for freezing and easily repurposed in many ways. I've included three here, but feel free to get creative – add roasted veg, tofu, seeds and plenty of fresh herbs to jazz it up throughout the week.

It's a great recipe to double up and freeze leftovers too. Your future self will thank you!

Olive oil, for frying
1 medium white onion, finely chopped
1 carrot, peeled and finely chopped
2 celery stalks, finely chopped
4 garlic cloves, minced
1 tbsp grated fresh ginger
1 tsp ground coriander
1 tsp ground cumin
½ tsp ground turmeric
½ tsp ground cinnamon
½ heaped tbsp ras el hanout
Pinch of cayenne pepper
1 tsp smoked paprika
2 tbsp tomato purée
2 x 400g (14oz) cans chopped tomatoes
800ml (1⅓ pints/3¼ cups) vegetable stock
150g (5½oz/⅔ cup) red split lentils, rinsed
150g (5½oz/¾ cup) green lentils, rinsed
100g (3½oz/½ cup) quinoa
600g (1lb 5oz) chickpeas, from jars or cans, drained and rinsed
Juice of ½ lemon
Salt and black pepper

In a casserole or large saucepan, warm a layer of olive oil and when a piece of onion sizzles on contact, add all the onion, celery, carrot and a small pinch of salt. Cook on a medium heat for 8–10 minutes until the onion is translucent and the veg reduced in volume. Add the garlic and ginger and cook for another 2 minutes, then add ⅓ tsp black pepper and ½ teaspoon of salt along with some more oil if it's looking dry.

Now add the spices, fry until fragrant, then add the tomato purée and mix again. Tip in the cans of tomatoes, then fill their cans halfway with water, swill the juice around and tip that in, too. At this point, you can scoop out some of the soup and blend it for a smooth texture or use a stick blender to pulse a few times. When this is done, add the stock and stir through.

Bring to the boil, stirring continuously, then turn down to a simmer and add the lentils. Cook for about 30 minutes, stirring regularly, until the lentils are softer.

Add the quinoa and chickpeas and continue to cook for 15 minutes, or until the little spiral separates itself from the quinoa grain. Then you know it's done.

Season to taste with the lemon juice, salt, and pepper.

Protein per serving: 22g
Fibre: 22g
Plant diversity score: 11

NOTES
Serve with Crumbled Fried Tofu or Tempeh (page 207) or Soy Free Tofu (page 210) to increase the protein.

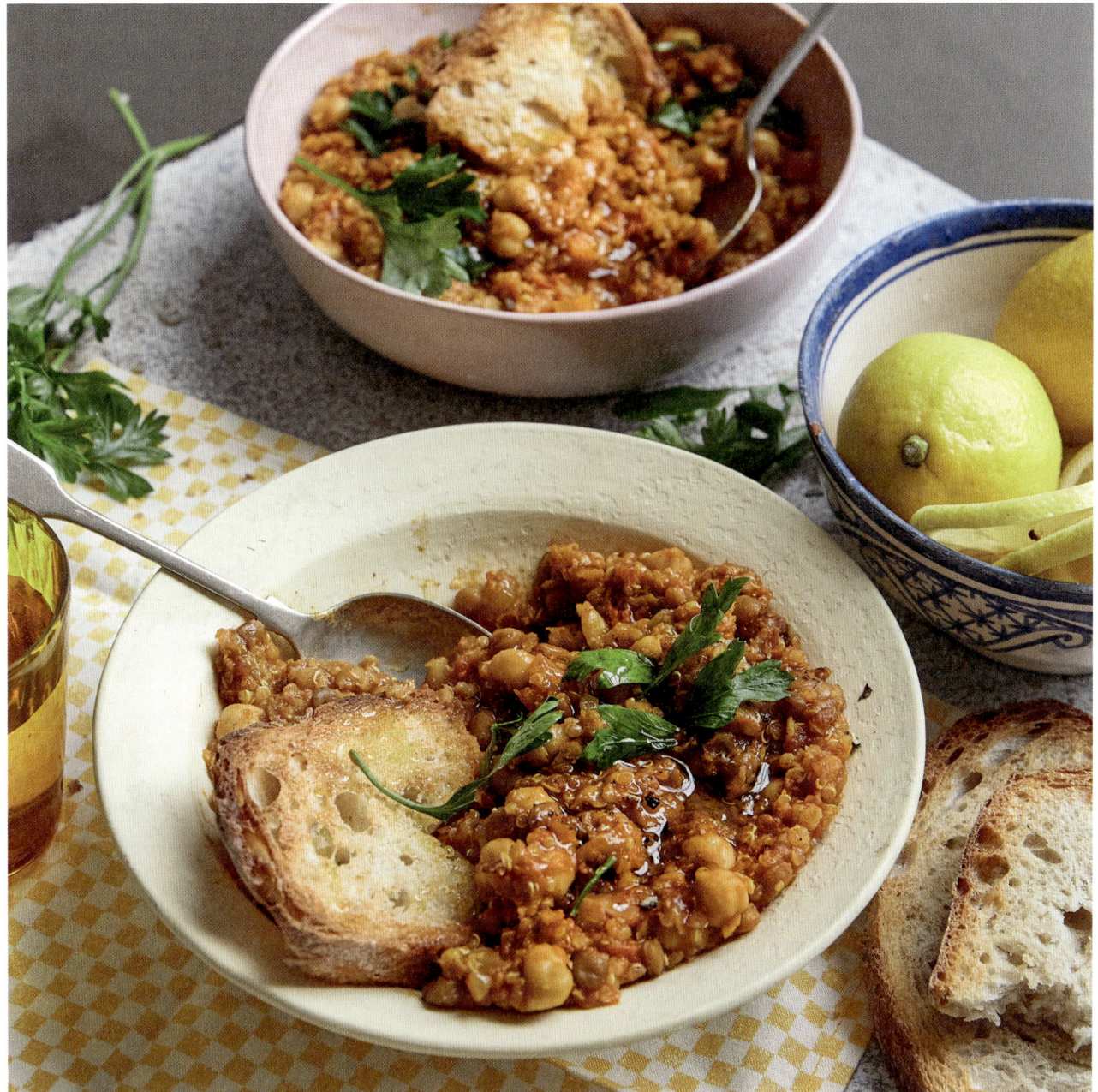

NIGHT 1

Serve with cashew cream (see page 219), fresh coriander, a drizzle of olive oil, freshly cracked black pepper and a slice of sourdough toast.

NIGHT 2

Roast a sweet potato and generously ladle the stew over the cooked flesh, serve with fresh herbs and salad.

NIGHT 3

Eat with couscous mixed with chopped dried apricots, chopped mint leaves, along with a glug of olive oil, 1 tbsp lemon juice and salt to taste.

Protein Layering

Let me introduce you to protein layering, where you can pick and choose the mini recipes in this chapter to bulk out your meals with nutrient-dense protein rich ingredients like Tofu Stracciatella-style Balls (see page 222) (put on pastas, bean bowls and loaded toasts), crunchy seed and nut toppers (pages 208–209), homemade wholefood 'sausages' and 'meatballs' (pittas, wraps, on beany mash, pastas and more), and my homemade plant-based cheeses to add creaminess to any dish.

I also have two recipes for soy-free tofu alternatives: Red Lentil Tofu and Chickpea Tofu (see pages 210–211). These are great if you're allergic to soy, as you can replace most of the tofu elements throughout the book with them.

And, finally, if you look at a recipe and think 'Hmmm, I need more protein in this', these recipes are your solution. Check out the table on page 22 to see how nutrient dense each of these ingredients are and choose the most appropriate option to hit your goals.

High-protein Naan

MAKES 4 NAAN
TOTAL TIME: 40 MINS

Perfect for curries, dips, salads, bean bowls, or even just a tasty snack.

135g (4¾oz/scant 1 cup) spelt flour
135g (4¾oz/1 cup) plain flour
1 tsp bicarbonate of soda
½ tsp sea salt
100g (3½oz) silken tofu
3 tbsp soy yoghurt
2 tbsp olive oil
1 tbsp water

FOR THE GARLIC BUTTER
3 tbsp melted vegan butter or olive oil
2 garlic cloves, grated
½ tsp sea salt
Small bunch of fresh parsley leaves, very finely
  chopped

In a mixing bowl, sift the flours, bicarbonate of soda and add the salt. Gently mix.

In a small blender, blend the silken tofu and yoghurt together. Make a well in the dry ingredients, then pour in the tofu mixture, along with the olive oil and water. Knead with your hand until a ball forms. If it's too dry, add a splash more water. If it's too wet, add a touch more flour. You want it to be dry and spring back a little when you touch it. Cover with a damp tea towel and set aside to rest for 20 minutes.

Once rested, dust the work surface with a little flour, then divide the dough into 4 equal pieces and roll each one into a ball. Roll out each ball with a rolling pin, or if you don't have one, a clean bottle of wine or vinegar will do.

To make the garlic butter, in a small bowl, mix the vegan butter with the garlic cloves, salt and fresh parsley. Set aside.

Heat a dry non-stick frying pan on a medium-high heat. Place a piece of the rolled dough on the frying pan and cook for about 2 minutes until you see it start to smoke a little. Wiggle the pan and move the naan as it's cooking to avoid burning it. Flip and cook the other side for a few minutes, until browning in places (the amount of browning/charring is a personal preference, I like mine charred in some places!).

Remove from the pan, brush with garlic butter and leave to rest in a lined bowl or basket, covered with a clean tea towel (so the steam from the hot pan puffs up the naan and makes it fluffy). Repeat with the remaining rolled dough.

Quick-pickled Red Onion

TOTAL TIME: 5 MINS

Great for jazzing up salads, stews, bean bowls and more – particularly leftovers!

½ red onion, finely sliced widthways
Juice of 1 lime
½ tsp salt
½ tsp sumac (optional)

In a small bowl, add all the ingredients and pinch together for 2 minutes with your hands until you hear the onion slices start to 'pop', which is the sound of the enzymes breaking down. This will produce the pinky colour of the onion. Leave in the fridge to pickle for 30 minutes, but you can also eat them straight away and they will still have a nice bite to them.

Store in an airtight container for up to 1 week.

Protein per serving: 5g
Fibre: 3.2g
Plant diversity score: 9

Protein per serving: 0.5g
Fibre: 0.5g
Plant diversity score: 1.5

Crumbled Tofu or Tempeh

TOTAL TIME: 15 MINS

100g extra firm tofu or tempeh per person
1 tbsp olive oil or sesame oil
1 tbsp tamari or soy sauce
1 garlic clove

If using extra firm tofu, give it a good squeeze with your hands, wrapped in kitchen roll or a clean tea towel, to draw out any excess moisture. Crumble the tofu or tempeh into a non-stick frying pan with your hands, you want small-ish pieces, about ½–1cm in length. Heat and add 1 tbsp olive oil or sesame oil, add a pinch of salt, then fry until golden (about 7–8 mins). Add the tbsp tamari or soy sauce and the minced garlic clove and fry for 4–5 minutes more, until the liquid has been soaked up by the crumbs. Season to taste and enjoy on top of bean bowls, pastas, stews and more to bump up the protein and add extra umami flavour.

Garlicky Sourdough Breadcrumbs

MAKES 5 SERVINGS
TOTAL TIME: 15 MINS

The perfect crispy topping to pastas, bean bowls and salads.

1 large slice of sourdough or wholemeal bread, stale or fresh
2 tbsp olive oil
1 tsp garlic powder
Pinch of salt, plus more to taste

In a blender or food processor, blend the slice of bread into very fine breadcrumbs. If you're using sourdough, it might not be possible to get super fine breadcrumbs, depending on the hydration of the dough, so pulse until you start to see it clump a little, then stop.

In a non-stick frying pan on a medium heat, heat the olive oil and fry the breadcrumbs with the garlic and salt for up to 8–9 minutes until very crispy and golden. You'll need to move the crumbs regularly with a spatula or wooden spoon, add more oil if you need to, and season to taste. Once crisped up (they should make a crunchy sound when you eat them), transfer to a plate, lined with kitchen paper.

Store in an airtight container, lined with fresh kitchen paper and use within 2–3 days.

Protein per serving, tofu: 16g
Fibre: 2g
Protein per serving, tempeh: 20g
Fibre: 8.3g

Protein per serving: 1.9g
Fibre: 1g
Plant diversity score: 1

Nut and Seed Toppings, 3 Ways

The key to a great meal is varying the texture. These crispy meal toppers add a satisfying crunch to pastas, soups, salads, beany dishes and more. Keep a large jar on the counter so it reminds you to dip in and give your meal a little crunchy protein boost.

Nutty, Noochy Crumb

MAKES 12 SERVINGS
TOTAL TIME: 12 MINS

60g (2¼oz/⅓ cup) almonds
60g (2¼oz/⅓ cup) cashews
50g (1¾oz/½ cup) walnuts
20g (¾oz/1½ tbsp) pine nuts
3 tbsp nutritional yeast
1½ tsp tamari

Add all the nuts to a small blender and pulse 2–3 times to break down. Alternatively, roughly chop by hand.

To a dry frying pan, add all the nutty mix and toast on a medium–high heat for 5–6 minutes, moving constantly so they don't burn. You're looking for a slight browning off in colour. Once you start to see this, take them off the heat and add the nutritional yeast and tamari. Toss in the residual heat until the liquid is absorbed, and no visible nutritional yeast flakes remain. Pour the nuts onto a plate to cool off, then, once cool, store in a dry, airtight jar or container for up to 3 weeks.

Store these sprinkles in plain sight on your kitchen counter, then you'll be more likely to use them! A serving of 6–8g (¼oz) is recommended, meaning you'll be adding around 3–4g (⅛oz) protein to your meals, plus lots of nutrients and taste.

Protein per serving: 3.5g
Fibre: 1.6g
Plant diversity score: 5

PROTEIN LAYERING

Quick Dukkah

MAKES 12 SERVINGS
TOTAL TIME: 15 MINS

1 tsp cumin seeds
1 tsp coriander seeds
½ tsp fennel seeds
60g (2¼oz/scant ½ cup) hazelnuts
50g (1¾oz/½ cup) pecans
50g (1¾oz/½ cup) almonds
60g (2¼oz) Crispy Roasted Legumes (see page 78, optional)
Small pinch of cayenne pepper
½ tsp salt
5 tbsp sesame seeds

Toast the cumin, coriander and fennel seeds in a dry frying pan for 30–60 seconds until fragrant. Add to a pestle and mortar and roughly bash. Pour into a small mixing bowl.

In the same frying pan, toast the hazelnuts, pecans and almonds for 3–4 minutes until slightly browning, adding the sesame seeds halfway. Remove, set aside to cool, then, when cooled, pulse them a few times with the crispy chickpeas (if using) in a small blender. You want a fine crumb, so about 6–8 pulses should do it. Add the nuts and seeds to the same bowl as the spices.

Add the cayenne, and salt, mix well, then season to taste with salt and pepper. Store in an airtight container for up to 2 weeks.

Protein per serving: 2.3g
Fibre: 1.6g
Plant diversity score: 5

Omega-3 Boost

MAKES 12 SERVINGS
TOTAL TIME: 15 MINS

200g (7oz) mixture of pumpkin seeds, sunflower seeds, flaxseeds
½ tsp tamari
Small pinch of cayenne pepper (optional)

Preheat the oven to 140°C fan/160°C/gas mark 3 and line a large baking tray with baking parchment.

Tip the seeds onto the lined tray, then add the tamari and cayenne (if using). Mix well, then bake in the centre of the oven for 16–18 minutes, stirring halfway through cooking.

Store in an airtight container or jar for up to 3 weeks.

Protein per serving: 2.4g
Fibre: 1.6g
Plant diversity score: 5

Soy-free Tofu, 2 Ways

Soy-free crew, I gotchu. These are two very low-effort ways (no overnight soaking!) of making a tofu alternative, which you can use as a sub for most of the tofu recipes in this book, (bar the cheeses!). Use in curries, stir-fries, bean or pasta dishes, or simply enjoy them on their own with some yum dipping sauce.

NOTE:
These tofus will not tear apart in quite the same way or hold their shape like extra-firm, or firm tofu would. Always cut the shapes with a sharp knife and fry first in the cornflour and seasoning before you use them.

Neither of these are a suitable replacement for silken tofu, instead of this, you can use plant-based yoghurt, coconut milk or diluted cashew cream.

Red Lentil Tofu

MAKES 2 SERVINGS
TOTAL TIME: 1 HR

100g (3½oz scant ½ cup) red split lentils
1 tbsp nutritional yeast
½ tsp salt
300ml (10fl oz/1¼ cups) water

Pour the red lentils into a medium, heatproof bowl and cover with plenty of boiling water (the lentils will start to expand, so pour a good 10cm/4in over them!) Soak for 45 minutes.

Once soaked, drain the lentils, rinse them, and add to a blender with the nutritional yeast, salt and water. Blend until no lumps remain and you have a smooth, salmon-coloured liquid.

Heat a medium heavy-bottomed saucepan or casserole on a medium heat, then pour in the lentil mixture and whisk for 5–7 minutes until it's thickened to a smooth paste. The mixture should be thick enough to stick to the whisk in globs. If it isn't thick enough, keep heating and whisking.

Grab a glass food storage container or silicone mould (5 x 5 in is a perfect size, however it doesn't have to be square, a rectangle is fine) and pour the mixture in. Smooth it out on top so it's even, then leave to cool for 1 hour in the fridge.

Once cooled, pop the lid on and store in the fridge for up to 5 days. When you're ready to eat it, upturn the container onto a chopping board and slice into rough 2cm (¾in) cubes (or any other shape of choice). Make sure to coat the red lentil tofu in cornflour, spices of choice and seasonings before either baking, air-frying or pan-frying. I like to fry mine in plain cornflour, then add a splash of tamari towards the end as the edges start to crisp up nicely.

Protein per serving: 7.3g
Fibre: 8.4g
Plant diversity score: 1.25

PROTEIN LAYERING

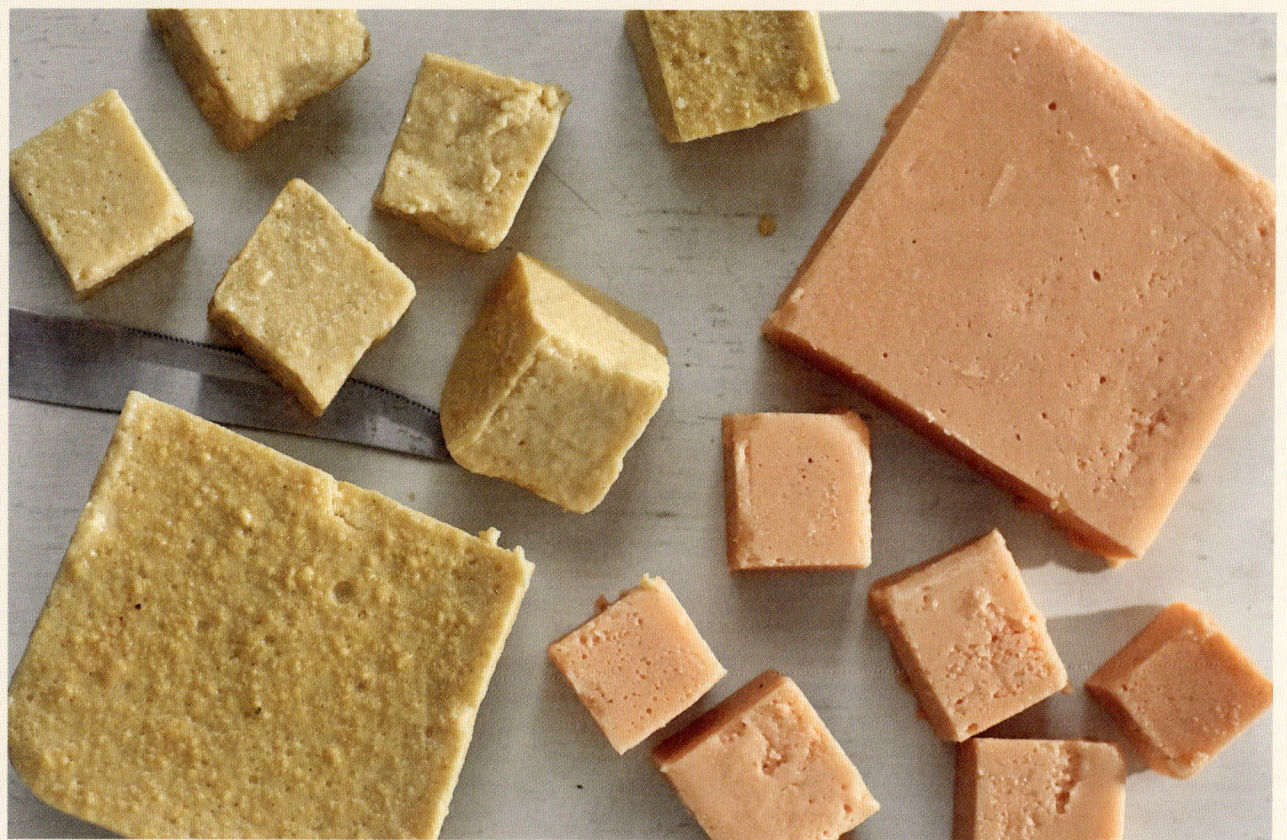

Chickpea Tofu

MAKES 2 SERVINGS
TOTAL TIME: 20 MINS

100g (3½oz/generous 1 cup) chickpea (gram) flour
½ tsp salt
1 tbsp nutritional yeast
200ml (7fl oz/¾ cup) water

To a mixing bowl, add the chickpea flour, salt, nutritional yeast and water. Whisk to combine.

In a heavy-bottomed saucepan, bring 200ml (7fl oz) water to the boil. Turn down the heat and pour in the chickpea flour mixture. Now, this is the part where you whisk very quickly for 5 minutes, otherwise the chickpea mix will start to stick to the bottom of the pan and be a bit of a pain to clean off. You're looking for a thick, glossy texture which is still pourable, but only just pourable! Once this has been achieved, take it off the heat.

Immediately pour the mixture into a glass food container and smooth out the top with the back of a spoon, so it's nice and even.

Leave to set in the fridge for at least 1 hour, then you should be able to use it right away. After one hour, test to see if it lifts cleanly away from the side of the container with a knife, if not, leave to set for longer. Carefully upturn it onto a chopping board and give it a little wiggle to release. Cut it into 2cm (¾in) cubes, or your shape of choice, then either use right away or store in the fridge for up to 4 days.

When you're ready to cook it, experiment with baking, pan-frying or air-frying! Just make sure to give it a coating of cornflour, so the edges get nice and crispy. I like to pan-fry in olive oil, then add a little tamari towards the end of cooking for some salty, umami goodness.

Protein per serving: 14g
Fibre: 6.7g
Plant diversity score: 1.25

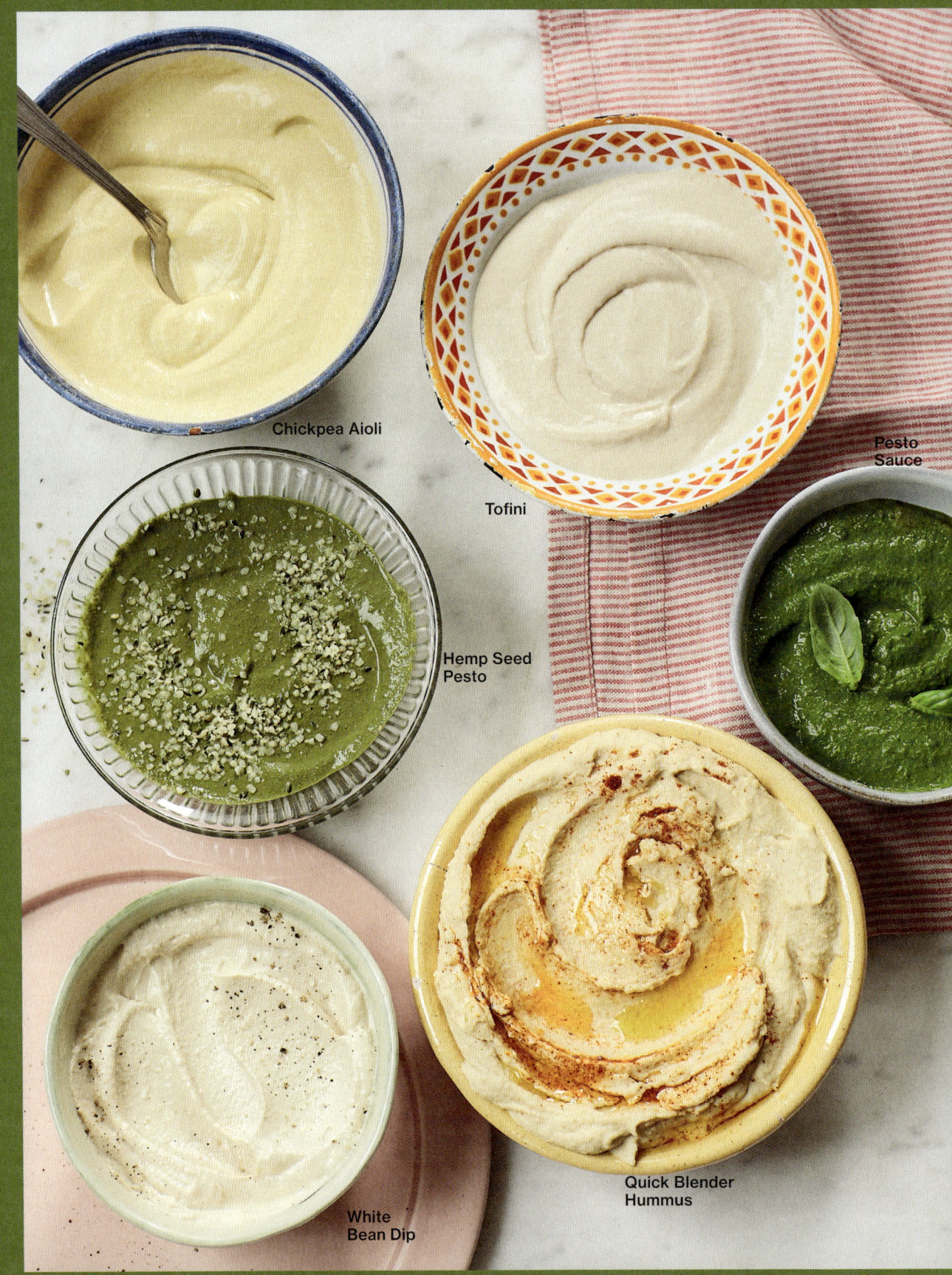

Chickpea Aioli

Tofini

Pesto Sauce

Hemp Seed Pesto

White Bean Dip

Quick Blender Hummus

Simple Sandwich Sauces

Chickpea Aioli

MAKES 6 SERVINGS
TOTAL TIME: 15 MINS

All of these sauces are extremely versatile, full of good, high-protein and high-fibre ingredients, can be made quickly and used to jazz up sandwiches, roasted veg and more.

200g (7oz) chickpeas, from a jar or can
3 garlic cloves
1 tsp Dijon mustard
2–3 tbsp lemon juice
50ml (2fl oz/3½ tbsp) olive oil
Pinch of salt
A little water, if needed to loosen

Add all the ingredients to a small blender cup and blend until silky smooth. Season to taste with salt. Keeps in an airtight container or jar in the fridge for up to 5 days.

Tofini

MAKES 6 SERVINGS
TOTAL TIME: 15 MINS

250g (9oz) firm smoked tofu
3½ tbsp good-quality runny tahini
2 garlic cloves
Pinch of salt and black pepper
Juice of 1 medium lemon
50ml (2fl oz/3½ tbsp) water

In a small blender cup, blend all the ingredients together until a smooth consistency is reached. Season to taste.
   Use as a spread for underneath roasted seasonal veg, or in sandwiches as a spread. Keeps in an airtight container in the fridge for up to 4 days.

Protein per serving: 6g
Fibre: 1.1g
Plant diversity score: 3

Protein per serving: 2.4g
Fibre: 1.8g
Plant diversity score: 3

Quick Blender Hummus

MAKES 4 SERVINGS
TOTAL TIME: 15 MINS

1 x 400g (14oz) can chickpeas, plus 1 tbsp aquafaba
(their canning liquid), leave a small handful for
garnish
3 tbsp good-quality runny tahini
1 tbsp lemon juice
2 garlic cloves
½ tsp sea salt, plus more to taste
Pinch of ground cumin
1 small ice cube

TO SERVE (optional)
Olive oil
Fresh parsley or coriander leaves
Smoked paprika

Add all the ingredients, except the ice cube, to a
blender cup, blend until very smooth. As the mixture
is very thick, you'll need to do this in 2–3 second
bursts, taking the blender cup off and shaking it in
between each blend, or taking off the lid and pushing
everything off the sides with a silicone spatula
or spoon. If it's really not blending, add another
tablespoon of aquafaba or water. I actually take the
whole blender and give it a little rock back and forth
as it's blending, which can help, but be mindful of
your appliance!

Once it's looking silky smooth, taste, season, adding
more lemon for brightness, more tahini for depth,
adjusting salt levels to your personal preference, and
blend again. Once happy with the taste and texture,
add the ice cube and blend again to make it soft
and airy.

Transfer to a shallow bowl or plate, grab a large,
clean spoon, confidently place it in the centre of the
hummus and move it up and down a few times, like it's
bouncing on a trampoline. At the bottom of the third
bounce, smoosh it a little up and out to the side, then
turn the plate or bowl with your other hand in a few
circles, until you get an artistic whipped 'well' shape
on the plate, with steep-ish sides. Gently remove the
spoon, resist touching it any more, then decorate with
olive oil in the centre, some of the leftover chickpeas
from the can, some fresh parsley or coriander, and a
little sprinkle of smoked paprika, if you desire.

Dig in with crackers, warm pitta, veg sticks, slather
it on sandwiches, eat with roasted veg, in pasta
sauces ... endless possibilities!

It'll keep for 3–4 days in the fridge, if stored in an
airtight container with a little olive oil on top to seal it.

Protein per serving: 5g
Fibre: 4g
Plant diversity score: 4

PROTEIN LAYERING

White Bean Dip

MAKES 4 SERVINGS
TOTAL TIME: 15 MINS

240g (8½oz) butter beans or cannellini beans, from a
  jar or can, drained and rinsed, plus 2 tbsp of
  their juices
3 tbsp good-quality runny tahini
3 garlic cloves
1 tbsp lemon juice
1½ tsp white miso paste or ½ tsp sea salt
1 ice cube

In a food processor, blend all the ingredients, except
the bean juice and ice cube, until smooth. The texture
will depend on the quality of your beans, some will be
harder, some mushier, some starchier, which is why
we reserve the 2 tablespoons of canning liquid. If
the mixture is looking dry, add some of that liquid, ½
tablespoon at a time as bean dips tend to get drippy
and liquid-y quite quickly. You don't want it
too viscous!

  Season to taste, remembering that adding more
lemon juice will make it runnier too, so if it's looking
too thick and needs more lemon anyway, forgo the
canning liquid for more lemon juice instead.

  Finish with the ice cube to whip things up nicely.
Plate up as you would hummus (see page 214) and
dig in with warm pitta, crisps, crackers, veg batons, or
use it as a plating sauce for roasted seasonal veg, or
in sandwiches as a sauce.

  Keeps in an airtight container in the fridge for up to
4 days.

Protein per serving: 5g
Fibre: 4g
Plant diversity score: 4

Pesto Sauce

MAKES 4 SERVINGS
TOTAL TIME: 10 MINS

2 large handfuls (about 50g/1¾oz) of fresh basil
1½ tbsp pine nuts, toasted (optional)
2 tbsp olive oil
½ tsp sea salt
Juice of 1 lemon
1 tbsp nutritional yeast
2 tsp water

Blend all the ingredients together in a small blender or
food processor, season to taste, adding more lemon
or salt if needed.

  Keeps in an airtight container or jar in the fridge for
up to 5 days, if sealed with olive oil.

NOTE
Bulk out the sauce with fresh spinach or
kale to make it into a super green sauce!
If you want to retain the bright green
colour, blanch the greens first (immerse
them in boiling water for 1 minute, then
in ice water for 2 minutes and squeeze
dry). Adjust the seasoning if you plan on
upping the greens, and you may need to
add more water, too.

Protein per serving: 3g
Fibre: 1.5g
Plant diversity score: 4

Hemp Seed Pesto

MAKES 4 SERVINGS
TOTAL TIME: 10 MINS

2 large handfuls (about 50g/1¾oz) of fresh basil
1½ tbsp pine nuts, toasted (optional)
2 tbsp shelled hemp seeds
2 tbsp olive oil
½ tsp sea salt
Juice of 1 lemon
1 tbsp nutritional yeast
2 tsp water

Pulse together until just combined, in a small blender.
Try not to overblend. Season to taste, adding more
lemon for acidity if needed.
   Keeps in the fridge in an airtight container or jar,
sealed with olive oil, for up to 5 days.

Protein per serving: 4g
Fibre: 1.5g
Plant diversity score: 4

90s Baby Beanburger

MAKES 7–8 BURGERS
TOTAL TIME: 35 MINS

If I had to make a mood board of my childhood, bean burgs and those sweetcorn nuggs would definitely take up a lot of space. Bean burgers I can still get behind, nuggs, questionable.

Here's my take on the ultimate sweet potato, black beans and quinoa burger, reimagined for today!

PS. When making the burgers, definitely double up! It's a great idea to have some of these on hand in the freezer when you need a quick healthy meal.

100g (3½oz/½ cup) quinoa
Vegetable stock, for the quinoa
1 large sweet potato
Olive oil, for drizzling
1 x 400g (14oz) can black beans, drained and rinsed
3 spring onions, finely chopped
3 garlic cloves, minced
50g (1¾oz/scant ½ cup) walnuts
40g (1½oz/¼ cup) almonds
40g (1½oz/¼ cup) cashews
20g (¾oz) hemp seeds
1 tbsp tamari
½ tsp sea salt, plus more to taste
1 tbsp tomato purée
1 tsp ground cumin
1 tsp ground paprika
1 tsp ground coriander
1–2 tbsp oat flour

Protein per burger: 10g
Fibre per burger: 7g
Plant diversity: 9

Preheat the oven to 160°C fan/180°C/gas mark 4.

Cook the quinoa in a little (I use 1 tsp of vegetable bullion powder) vegetable stock, according to the packet instructions.

Meanwhile, wash the sweet potato and prick the skin with a fork a few times. Put on a small baking tray, drizzle with oil and salt, then bake for 35 minutes, or until soft inside (test with a sharp knife, it should go in easily and without much resistance!)

While the sweet potato is roasting, in a food processor, add all the remaining ingredients, except the quinoa. When the quinoa is ready, add half. Once the sweet potato has softened and cooled, peel back the skin, scoop the flesh out and add it to the food processor.

Process until you have a chunky, well mixed wet dough, then scoop it out into a bowl and add the rest of the quinoa. If it's too wet to shape with your hands, add another tablespoon of oat flour. It may stick to your hands a little but still be easy to work with. Touch it lightly, don't press too hard!

Shape into 7–8 medium, 2cm (1in) deep discs and bake for about 20 minutes until browning at the edges.

When you take them out, they will still be a little soft, which is normal. They will firm up as they cool. Leave for about 20 mins until you plan to use!

These will keep for up to 1 week in the fridge in an airtight container, and will freeze for up to three months (pre-cooking). If you freeze once cooked they may go crumbly on thawing.

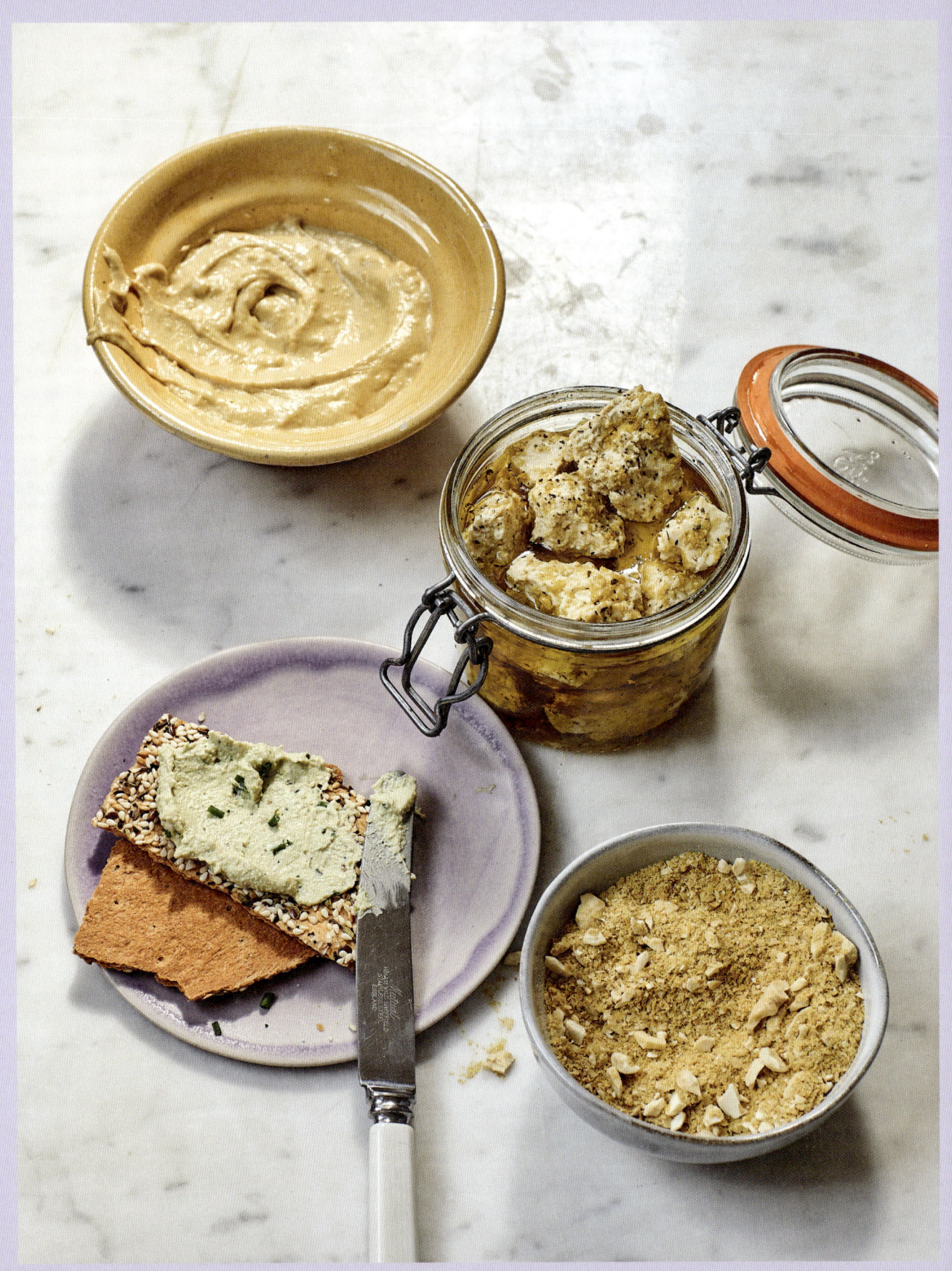

DIY 'Cheeses'

These are my go-to DIY cheese replacements I use weekly. I don't often buy vegan cheese, not any of the supermarket varieties anyway, as I find they rely on coconut or starch bases which don't agree with me!

When I do buy vegan cheese, I go for the independent brands such as La Fauxmagerie, Kinda Co. and Julienne Bruno® (just to name a few!).

Make no mistake, these recipes are super tasty, but they're not meant to imitate dairy cheese to a tee. To be honest, I don't want that either, but when a traditional recipe calls for cheese, these DIY methods step up to the plate and will do more than scratch any cheesy itch you may be feeling. I'd say they're in a league of their own – easy to make, healthy and tasty.

Don't worry, none of these methods require straining, overnight soaking, any funny moulds or obscure ingredients. Truth be told, I lack skill and patience for all this, so if you're anything like me, these recipes will be useful!

Cashew Cream

MAKES 6 SERVINGS
TOTAL TIME: 15 MINS

100g (3½oz/⅔ cup) cashews, quick-soaked in boiling water for at least 15 minutes
3 tbsp nutritional yeast
Juice of 1 large lemon
½ tsp sea salt
Pinch of ground black pepper
2 garlic cloves
60–80ml (2–3fl oz) water, for blending to desired consistency

ADD-INS FOR CASHEW QUESO
1 tsp smoked paprika
Pinch of ground turmeric
Optional pinch of chilli powder

In a small, high-speed blender, add all the ingredients and blend together until a silky smooth consistency is achieved. Taste and adjust the salt and acidity as needed. Store in an airtight jar or container in the fridge for up to 4 days.

Protein per serving: 5g
Fibre: 1.5g
Plant diversity score: 4

Tofu Feta

MAKES 2 SERVINGS
TOTAL TIME: 10 MINS

200g (7oz) extra-firm tofu
2 tbsp nutritional yeast
2 garlic cloves, minced, or 2 tsp garlic granules
2 tbsp olive oil
½ tbsp dried oregano
Juice of 1 lemon
½–1 tsp salt

Squeeze the tofu in kitchen paper to draw out any excess water. In a mixing bowl, break the tofu apart into small, irregular chunks with your hands. Add the remaining ingredients and gently toss to combine. Season to taste. Pour into an airtight container and store in the fridge for up to 4 days.

Tofu Cream Cheese

MAKES 6 SERVINGS
TOTAL TIME: 10 MINS

200g (7oz) firm tofu
2 tbsp lemon juice
1 tbsp apple cider vinegar
2 garlic cloves
1 tsp onion powder
1½ tbsp white miso paste
3–4 tbsp soy milk, depending on the consistency and the power of your blender
1 tbsp nutritional yeast
20g (¾oz/1½ tbsp) cashews, soaked in boiling water for 15 minutes
2–3 tbsp fresh finely chopped chives for stirring in after it's blended
1 tsp sea salt
Black pepper

Squeeze the tofu in kitchen paper to draw out any excess water. Add all the ingredients to a blender and blend until a thick, paste-like consistency is achieved. You may need to pause the blending and use a spatula to scrape the mixture down the sides every now and then and/or add more milk if the mixture is struggling to blend. Season to taste, spoon into an airtight container or sterilised jar and store in the fridge for up to 5 days.

Add the chopped chives on top when serving, or stir these into the blended mix.

Protein per serving: 19.8g
Fibre: 2.75g
Plant diversity score: 4

Protein per serving: 7g
Fibre: 1g
Plant diversity score: 6

Cashew Parmesan

MAKES 8 SERVINGS
TOTAL TIME: 2 MINS

50g (1¾oz) nutritional yeast
40g (1½oz/¼ cup) cashews
1 tsp garlic powder
½ tsp sea salt

In a small bullet blender, add all the ingredients and pulse 2–5 times until a fine, Parmesan-like crumb texture is achieved. Season to taste.

Store in a jar at room temperature for up to 2 weeks.

Protein per serving: 4g
Fibre: 1g
Plant diversity score: 2

Tofu Stracciatella-style balls

MAKES 4 SMALL–MEDIUM BALLS
TOTAL TIME: 1HR 15 MINS

Soft Italian cheese is something I really missed after going fully plant-based. It adds a lot to a dish, the creamy texture melts beautifully into pasta sauces, salads and beany bowls. I am also obsessed with the beautiful pattern olive oil makes when it's carefully drizzled over the cheese. Sublime.

Here's my plant-based, high-protein take on the delicate cheesy balls. I've tried to make it as faff-free as possible, meaning you're more likely to make them! There's a little skill involved in tying up the balls in clingfilm without breaking them (long nail girlies, I'm looking at you) but it's definitely worth it.

You'll need 4 small bowls, large squares of cling film or some pliable wraps, and some elastic bands or string to tie them up, so check you have all this before you start.

150g (5½oz/1 cup) cashews
300g (10½oz) silken tofu
2 tbsp lemon juice or apple cider vinegar
500ml (18fl oz/2 cups) soy milk
1 tsp salt
2½ tbsp cornflour
3 tbsp nutritional yeast
Olive oil, to serve
Black pepper, to serve

Soak the cashews in boiling water for 20 minutes, then drain.

To a blender cup, add the drained cashews and all the remaining ingredients. Blend until very smooth.

Pour into a large saucepan. Whisk on a medium heat for 5–6 minutes until the mixture thickens enough to make trails with the whisk. Turn off the heat and leave to cool.

While it's cooling, prep 3 small bowls ready for the mixture, placing a large square of clingfilm on top of each one and an elastic band by the side. Divide the cooled mixture equally between the 3 bowls. Carefully gather the edges of the clingfilm and tie the bundles up with the elastic bands.

Grab a bowl, add some ice and cold water. Plop the balls in and leave for 5 minutes. Remove from the water, return to the bowls and then transfer to the freezer. Be careful to drain the water off the balls before they go in the freezer, otherwise you'll end up with pools of frozen water in the bottom of the bowls.

Remove from the freezer after about 40 minutes. They should be firm enough to hold their shape but soft enough to give when you poke them. Untie the clingfilm and carefully place the ball on your plate of food (you might have to upturn them straight from the wrap). Serve with olive oil and black pepper.

NOTE

If you leave the balls in the freezer for longer than 40 minutes, or you're not planning on serving them all that day, the balls will discolour and look a little yellow-ish. That's quite normal, when you begin to thaw them, this will disappear.

I suggest thawing them in the fridge for 30 minutes before eating. Check every 5 minutes or so to see if they are ready – you want the texture to give when it is touched but not completely collapse.

They will keep for up to 1 week in the freezer.

Protein per serving: 17g
Fibre: 3.5g
Plant diversity score: 3

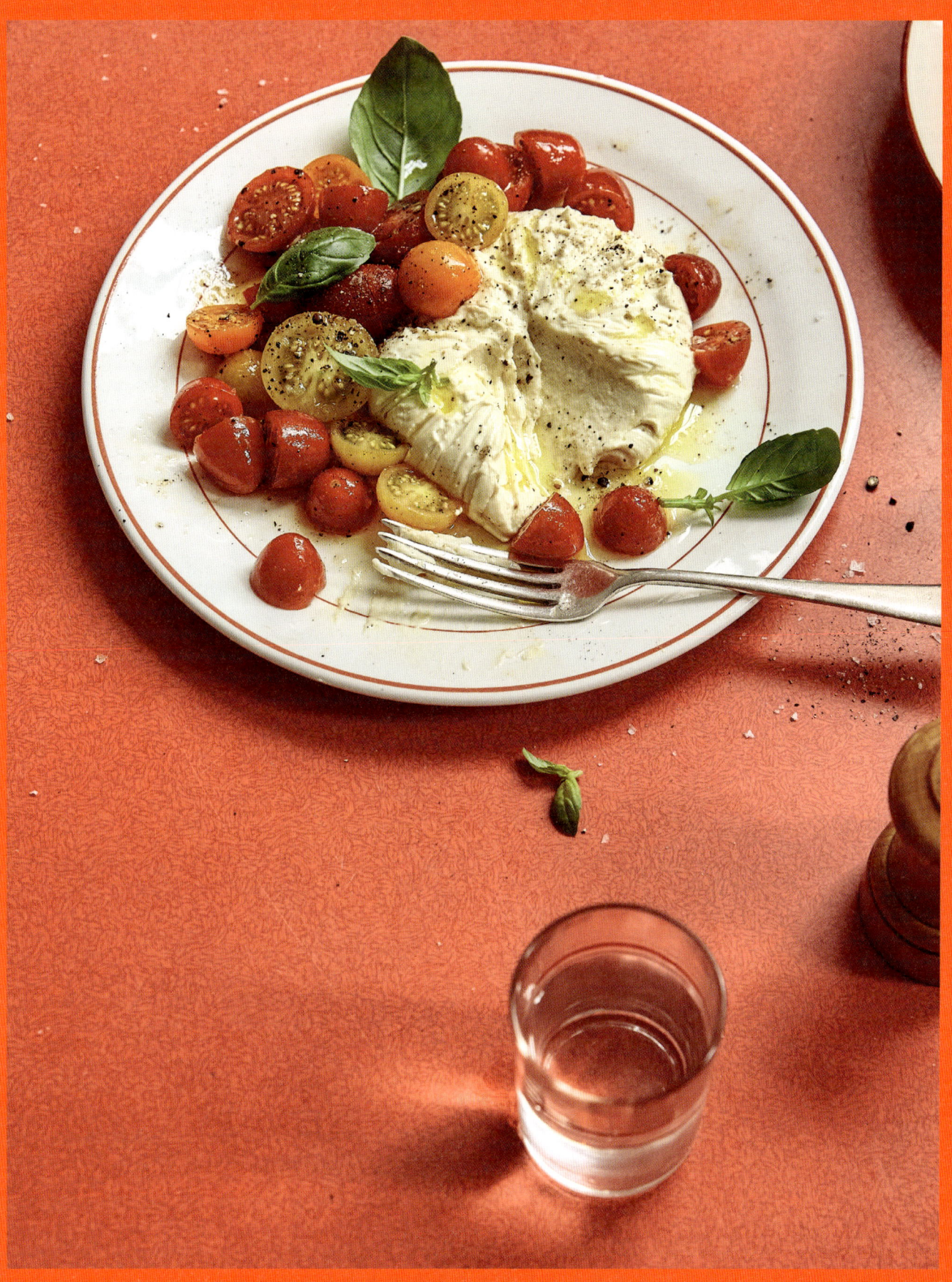

Homemade 'Sausages'

MAKES 8 SAUSAGES
TOTAL TIME: 40 MINS

These make it into my top five recipes in the book. Now, don't expect them to taste anything like a meat replacement, but do expect some wholesome, protein-rich goodness that will add another flavour/texture profile to your dish. I tried many combinations of legumes and grains for these, but to be honest nothing beats using a slice of stale sourdough bread. It acts as a spongy binder, adds depth and is great for avoiding food waste.

I honestly suggest you double up and freeze half for a rainy day, so you only have to whip up some mash or grill some veg and enjoy with a wholemeal grain for a tasty, healthy meal.

2 tbsp ground flaxseed
6 tbsp warm water
1 small white onion, finely chopped
Olive oil, for frying
3 large garlic cloves, minced
½ tsp fennel seeds
1 tsp smoked paprika
1 tsp ground cumin
1 tbsp tomato purée
100g (3½oz) sourdough or wholewheat bread
1 x 400g (14oz) can brown lentils, drained and rinsed
1 tsp wholegrain mustard
½ tsp salt

In a small bowl, cover the ground flaxseed with the warm water and set aside for it to thicken.

In a medium frying pan on a medium heat, sauté the onion in olive oil with a small pinch of salt for 8 minutes. Add the garlic and fry for another 2–3 minutes. Add the spices and a little more oil if you need it, then toast them for 1–2 minutes. Add the tomato purée and combine everything together, cook for a further 2 minutes, take off the heat and allow to cool.

In a food processor, pulse the bread a few times until the crusts break down. Add the flax mixture, the cooled onion mix, lentils, mustard and another pinch of salt. Blend everything up until well combined, but don't obliterate the mix, keep it a little 'grainy'. Season to taste, adding a little more mustard or salt and pepper if you think it needs it.

Once happy, shape the mixture into 8 sausage shapes with your hands (you can wet them a little so the mix does not stick), then pop them into the fridge for 30 minutes to firm up.

If you're eating them straight away, pan-fry in olive oil for a few minutes each side until they start to brown, or brush with olive oil and bake for 8–10 minutes at 180°C fan/200°C/gas mark 6.

If not eating straight away, store them in an airtight container in the fridge for up to 4 days, or freeze for up to 1 month.

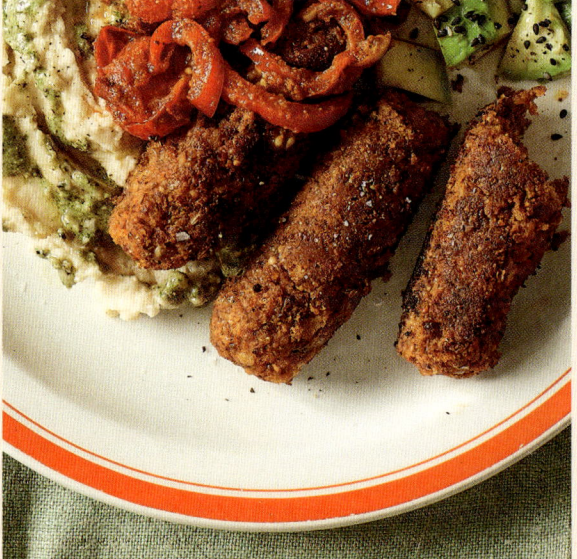

Protein per 2 sausages: 6.5g
Fibre: 6.7g
Plant diversity score: 6.5

Homemade 'Meatballs'

MAKES 12 BALLS
TOTAL TIME: 35 MINS

I like to call these 'Savoury energy balls', perfectly spiced, packed with flavour and all the good stuff. You'll see I've combined chickpea flour, black beans and cooked quinoa – meaning you get a good amino acid spread.

I chose to include these over falafel because they bind together better, meaning you can bake them and not have to worry about them falling apart. I find with falafel I have to deep-fry, which is a lot of faff in a home kitchen.

The possibilities for use are literally endless. Put them in pitta with salad, on spaghetti, in a power bowl, pack them in a lunchbox as an on-the-go snack with some hummus or red lentil sauce, you can even deconstruct them (break them down into crumbs) and put them on bean bowls or bakes.

The mix will freeze for up to 6 weeks; just make sure to portion it out into balls and separate with greaseproof paper.

2 tbsp ground flaxseeds
6 tbsp warm water
60g (2oz/½ cup) chickpea (gram) flour
150g (5½oz/¾ cup) cooked quinoa
1 x 400g (14oz) can black beans, drained and rinsed
50g (1¾oz/½ cup) walnuts
3 garlic cloves, minced
1 tsp smoked paprika
2 tbsp nutritional yeast
1 tsp ground coriander
½ tsp salt
Black pepper

In a small bowl, cover the ground flaxseeds with the warm water and set aside for it to thicken.

In a food processor, add all the ingredients and pulse to combine, but don't blend it to a paste. The mixture should stick together when you firmly press it between your fingers. Season to taste.

Preheat the oven to 180°C fan/200°C/gas mark 6.

Shape into 12 balls, about golf ball-sized and place on a lined baking tray. Drizzle with olive oil and bake for 12 minutes, or until slightly browning. Store in the fridge for up to 4 days.

Protein per 4 meatballs: 12g
Fibre: 9g
Plant diversity score: 6

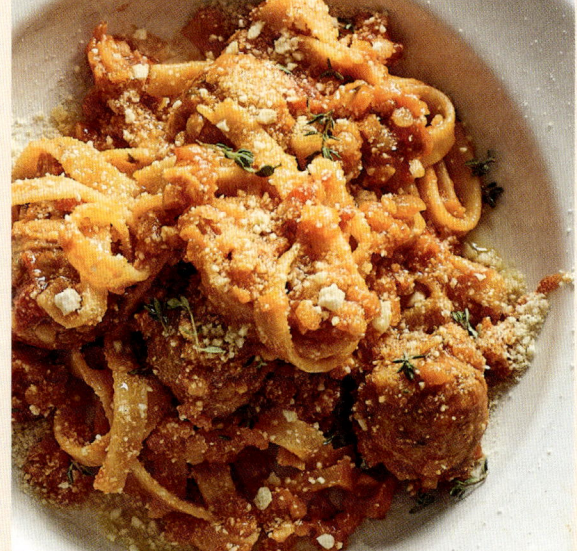

It's All About Balance

Have a sweet tooth? Following a healthy lifestyle doesn't mean you have to give up what you love, far from it. I tend to follow the 80:20 rule, which helps me to keep a balanced mindset about eating. Indulging in the occasional sweet treat is a healthy way to live, and if you restrict yourself from enjoying the things you love, aside from being unhappy, you'll be more likely to 'fall-off-the-wagon' and ditch the lifestyle altogether.

Nutty, Fudgy Protein Brownies

MAKES 12 BROWNIES
TOTAL TIME: 40 MINS,
PLUS COOLING TIME

Decadent and indulgent with a healthy touch, this is a brownie recipe you'll keep coming back to. I like my brownies less sweet, so if you have more of a sweet tooth, add a touch more maple syrup or an extra Medjool date.

3 tbsp ground flaxseeds
7 tbsp warm water
6 Medjool dates, pitted
500ml (18fl oz/2 cups) soy milk
100ml (3½fl oz/scant ½ cup) maple syrup
70g (2½oz/½ cup) cacao powder
85g (3oz/⅔ cup) oat flour
1 tsp bicarbonate of soda
Pinch of sea salt
2 heaped tbsp chocolate vegan protein powder
100g (3½oz) mixed nuts, pulsed once or twice in a blender or roughly chopped (I used hazelnuts, walnuts and pecans)
100g (3½oz) dairy free chocolate chips

Preheat the oven to 160°C fan/180°C/gas mark 4 and line a 23cm (9in) square baking tray with baking parchment or lightly grease a silicone tray.

In a small bowl, cover the ground flaxseeds in the warm water and set aside.

In a small blender, add the dates, milk and maple syrup. Whizz until super smooth.

In a medium mixing bowl, add the cacao, oat flour, bicarb, salt and protein powder. Mix to combine. Pour in the date mixture along with the flaxseed gel, mix until well combined, but don't overmix. Fold in the nuts and three-quarters of the chocolate chips, then pour into the baking tray and top with the remaining chocolate chips.

Bake in the centre of the oven for 25–26 minutes. When you take them out, the brownie will be wobbly in the middle. Leave to cool for 30 minutes, before putting in the fridge for at least 1 hour to cool, firm up and get that lovely crinkle topping.

Cut into squares and enjoy! These keep for up to 4 days in the fridge.

Protein per serving: 6g
Fibre: 5g
Plant diversity score: 7

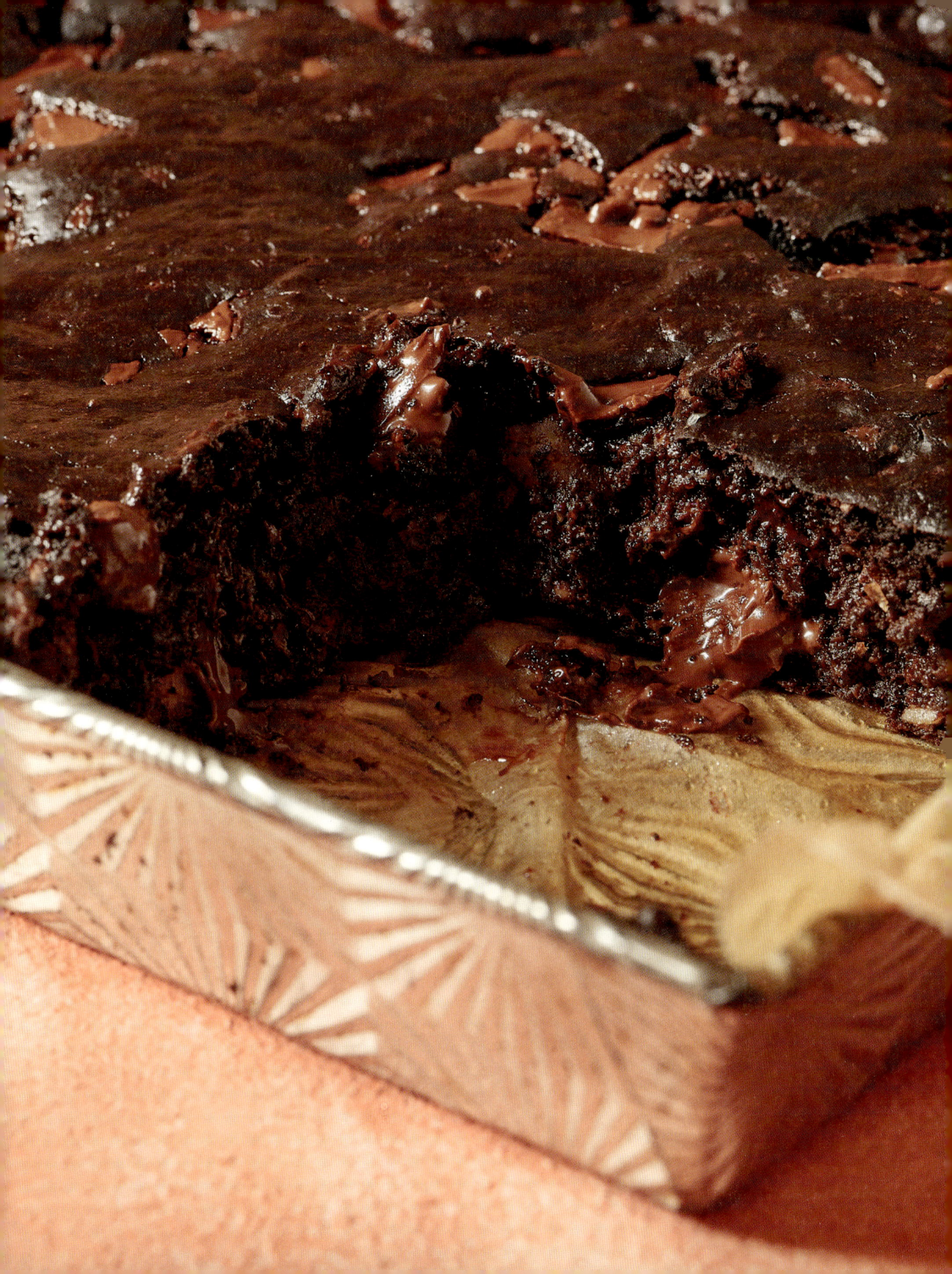

Plant Diversity Flapjacks

MAKES 8 FLAPJACKS
TOTAL TIME: 40 MINS, PLUS COOLING

Every good cook has to have a killer flapjack recipe up their sleeve, and this is mine. I love how much plant diversity you can fit in these. Feel free to swap things out and add additional seeds, just make sure to use the slightly smaller rolled oats as opposed to jumbo, as this will ensure the flapjacks stick together, and please, let them cool down properly before you cut them up! Cutting when warm makes them crumbly.

175g (6oz/1¾ cups) rolled oats
2 tbsp oat flour
25g (1oz/2 tbsp) pistachios
25g (1oz/2 tbsp) cashews
25g (1oz/2 tbsp) almonds
25g (1oz/¼ cup) pecans
2 tbsp hemp seeds
2 tbsp chia seeds
60g (2oz) sultanas
2 tbsp goji berries
½ tsp baking powder
150ml (5fl oz) maple syrup, plus extra to glaze
1 ripe banana – about 100g (3½oz)
140g (4½oz) peanut butter
Pinch of sea salt
80g (3oz) dark chocolate, melted

Preheat the oven to 140°C fan/160°C/gas mark 3 and line a medium, high-sided baking tray or a square tin with baking parchment.

In a large mixing bowl, mix the oats, oat flour, all the nuts, seeds and dried fruit, the salt, and baking powder.

In a blender cup, add the maple syrup, peanut butter and banana. Blend until smooth, then pour into the dry ingredients and stir well to combine, making sure everything is covered and sticky.

Pour the mixture into the lined tray and press down with a rubber spatula to ensure everything is even. Bake for 20–22 minutes – when the edges start to turn a light brown, you know it's ready.

Remove from the oven and leave to cool completely, then brush over a little maple syrup with a pastry brush if you like – this will give the flapjacks a nice sheen.

Slice into bars, then melt the chocolate over a bain marie or in the microwave in bursts, drizzling it over the flapjacks and leaving it to cool before tucking in.

They will keep for up to a week in an airtight container. I prefer to keep them at room temperature or bring them to room temperature before I eat.

Protein per serving: 13g
Fibre: 5.3g
Plant diversity score: 12

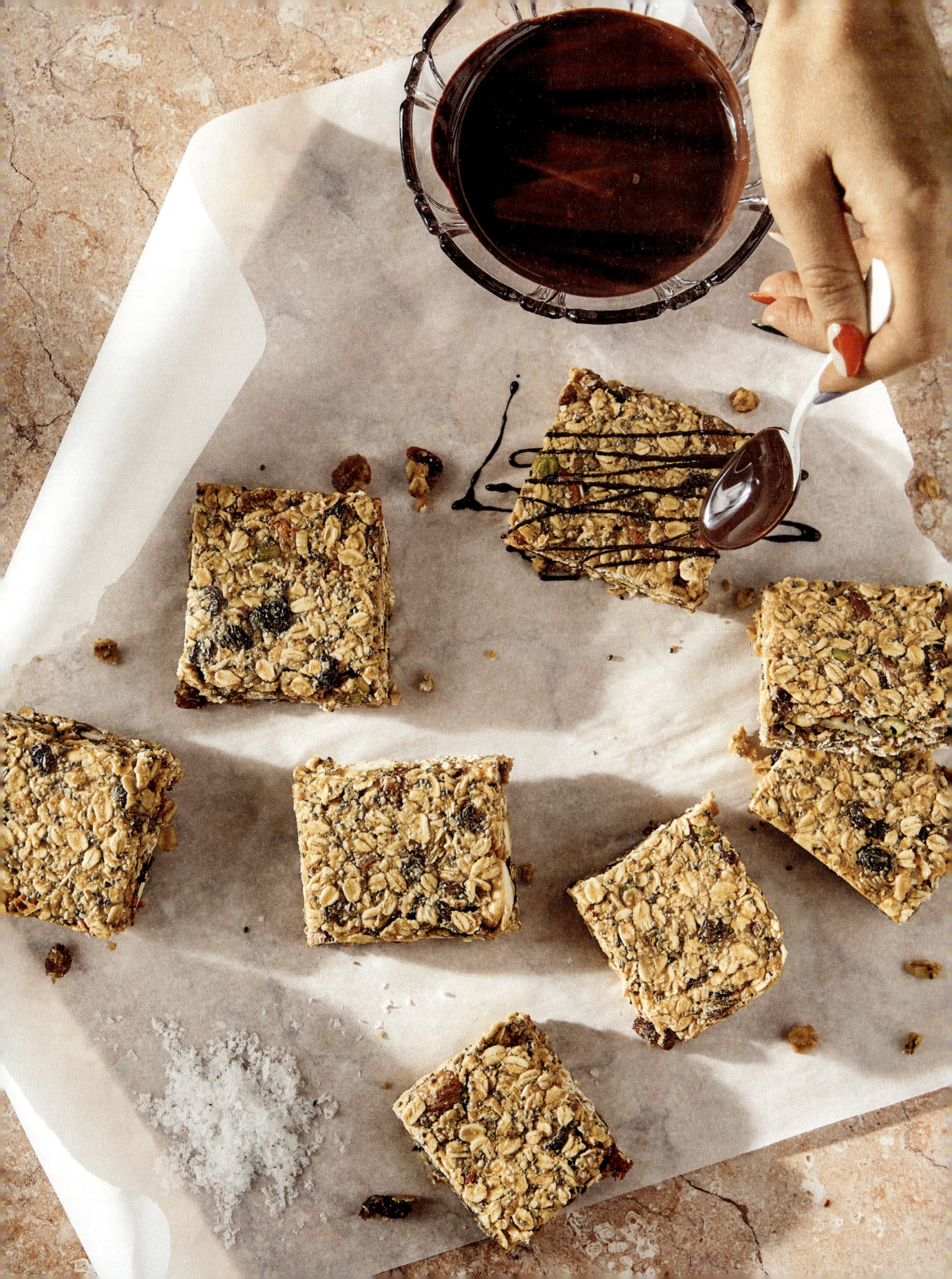

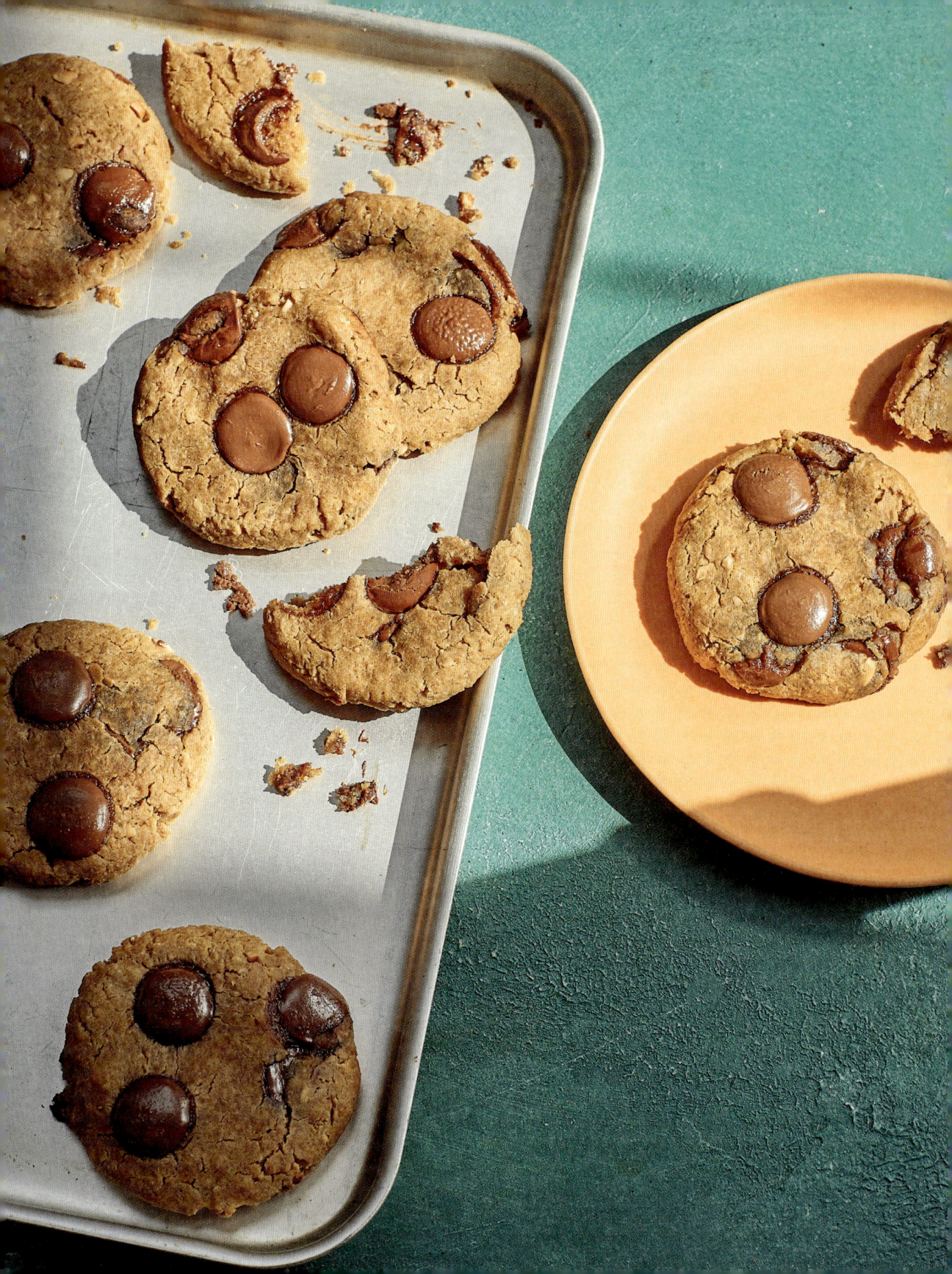

Chunky Chickpea Cookies

MAKES 8 COOKIES
TOTAL TIME: 25 MINS

Chickpeas are wonderfully versatile and delicious balls of goodness! Honestly, I think they might be the most versatile legume. In this book, I've made them into tofu, crispy salad toppers, hummus, sauces, aioli, soups, stews, sandwich fillings and now cookies!

You can eat this cookie dough raw too, if that's your vibe. Just be mindful that it's quite sticky, so a cookie scoop is recommended for the portioning part so you can get them nice and even.

100ml (6 tbsp) maple syrup
1 x 400g (14oz) can chickpeas, drained and rinsed
140g (5oz) natural crunchy peanut butter
35g (1¼oz/¼ cup) spelt flour
½ tsp bicarbonate of soda
1 tsp vanilla extract
½ tsp baking powder
80g (3oz) dairy-free chocolate chips

Preheat the oven to 160°C fan/180°C/gas mark 4.

In a small blender, whizz the maple syrup and chickpeas until no chickpea lumps remain. Add the peanut butter, flour, bicarb, vanilla and baking powder, and mix again.

If this is too tough for the blender, decant to a mixing bowl and mix everything together, then fold in most of the chocolate chips (do this in the bowl even if everything has already been blended together), reserving a large handful for the top of the cookies.

Use a tablespoon or cookie scoop to make 8 balls and gently press them down into flat discs. Top with the reserved choc chips and bake for 12–13 minutes in the middle of the oven.

When they come out, you can gently shape them with a circle cookie cutter so they look even. Just place it over the cookie and move it in a quick, smooth circular motion a few times.

Leave them to cool completely before eating, so they can firm up.

Protein per serving: 7.3g
Fibre: 3.3g
Plant diversity score: 3.5

Pastel de Nata

MAKES 8–10 TARTS
TOTAL TIME: 40 MINS

I lived in Lisbon for two years, so it seemed rude not to include a recipe for the famous Portuguese custard tarts. The origin of Pastéis de Nata dates back to the 18th century, where they were created by monks at the Jerónimos Monastery in the parish of Santa Maria de Belém in Lisbon. As the monks were previously based in France, they picked up a liking for pastries – and they also needed to use up the egg yolks they were separating from the whites used to starch clothing in those days. And so, the Pastel de Nata was born!

This is my plant-based adaptation, using a few shortcuts.

125ml (4½fl oz) soy milk
60g (2oz) caster sugar
Lemon peel
Cinnamon stick
30g (1oz) cornflour
1 sheet ready to roll puff pastry
100ml (3½oz) double soy cream
100g (3½oz) silken tofu
70g (2¼oz) cashews, soaked in boiling water for
   15 minutes
2 tsp vanilla essence
Icing sugar, to dust
Cinnamon, to dust

Protein per serving: 2.8g
Fibre: 0.5g
Plant diversity score: 3.5

Start by soaking the cashews in boiling water.

Now infuse the milk. In a small saucepan on a low heat, heat the milk, lemon peel, cinnamon stick, and sugar. Don't boil it, just gently heat, stirring regularly for 6–7 mins, until the sugar has been dissolved. Take off the heat and allow the mix to cool. Take the pastry out of the fridge, allowing it to come to room temp (wait 3–4 mins)

On a lightly floured surface, carefully roll out the pastry with your hands. Roll it up again, lengthways this time (rolling from the longer side) nice and tightly (so there are no air gaps between layers, there will of course be one on the first turn) so you have a longer sausage shape. Chop the rolled up sheet into 1-ish inch pieces, like you would when making gnocchi. Pop them into a lightly greased cupcake tray, so the spiral on each is touching the bottom of the tray, then, with the back of your fingers (or you can use the back of a spoon) carefully push down and shape the mix to fill each hole, so the pastry becomes the cupcake case. They don't have to be perfect, just make sure they don't stick up above the sides. If they do, carefully cut the excess off with a pair of kitchen scissors. Pop these in the fridge whilst you finish off the filling.

Back to the infused milk, which should be cool by now. Remove the peel and cinnamon stick. Take 2 tbsp of the infused milk, and add this to the cornflour. Whisk until a thick paste-like consistency is reached, adding a little more milk if you need to.

In a blender cup, or high speed blender, blend the tofu, cream, soaked cashews, vanilla, turmeric. Add to the pan with the cornflour slurry. Heat gently, whisking continuously, until thickened and your whisk starts to makes thick trails in the mixture, it should have the same consistency as thick custard.

IT'S ALL ABOUT BALANCE

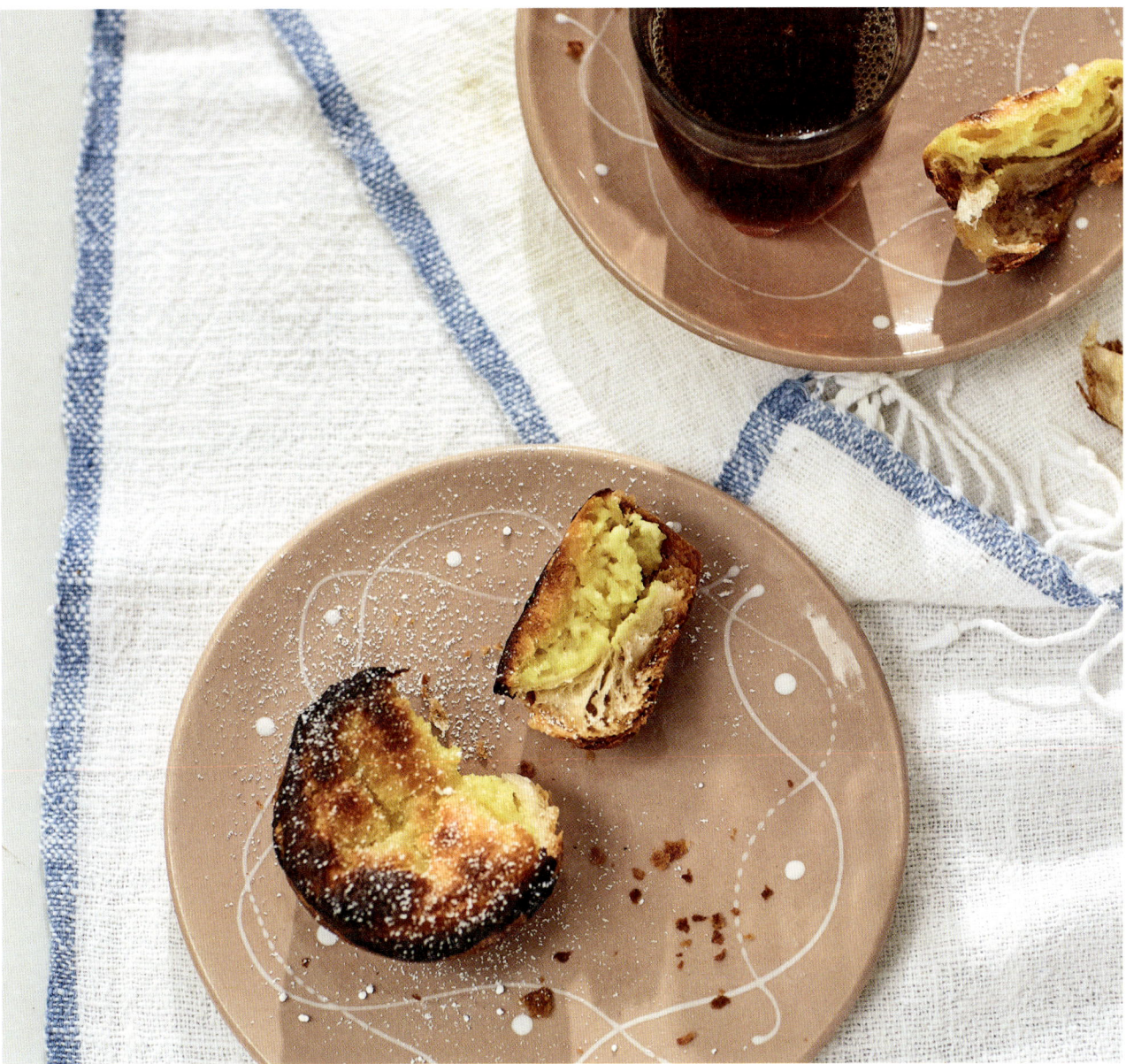

At this point, preheat your oven to 200°C fan/220°C/ gas mark 7. Give the mixture a stir before you fill each pastry case ¾ of the way, leaving a little well in the centre if you like and carefully, with the back of a teaspoon, gliding the mix up to the edges of the pastry so it resembles a more traditional pastel de nata.

Bake for 16 minutes, checking every now and then to make sure they're all cooking evenly, rotating the tray if not. The custard will expand slightly in the oven, but will drop once cooled. If you have no blackened or darker spots at the 16 minute mark, leave for another minute or so, or until you start to see them turn brown in places. Keep a close eye, they may burn quickly. Once out of the oven, you can flick them with little speckles of water so they get a glossy texture when drying. Serve with icing sugar and extra cinnamon, if you like.

Decadent Dark Choc and Orange Pudding

For 15 minutes work (minus the setting time), these taste absolutely incredible. Perfect for dinner parties, quick desserts, or even mixed into overnight oats.

280g (10oz) silken tofu
70ml (2½fl oz/¼ cup) soy milk
4 tbsp cacao powder
60ml (4 tbsp) maple syrup
1 tsp vanilla extract
Pinch of sea salt
Juice of ½ large orange, plus 1 tbsp orange zest
180g (6oz) dark chocolate

TO SERVE
Orange slices
Dark chocolate shavings
Orange zest

In a food processor, blend the silken tofu, soy milk, cacao, maple syrup, vanilla, sea salt and orange juice and zest.

Melt the chocolate in a bain-marie (a heatproof bowl over a saucepan of warm water – make sure the bowl doesn't touch the water!) or in a microwave in 15-second bursts. If melting in a microwave, stir the chocolate well every 15 seconds and don't microwave it until it's all liquid. Stop short of there being a few solid lumps of chocolate, which will melt as you stir a little. This will ensure you don't burn the chocolate.

Pour the chocolate into the blender as it runs on a low setting. Taste and adjust the sweetness to your liking, adding more maple if you desire. Pour into 4 decorative glasses and leave in the fridge to set for at least 4 hours.

Before serving, decorate with the orange slices, dark chocolate shavings and orange zest.

Protein per serving: 7.6g
Fibre: 5.3g
Plant diversity score: 5

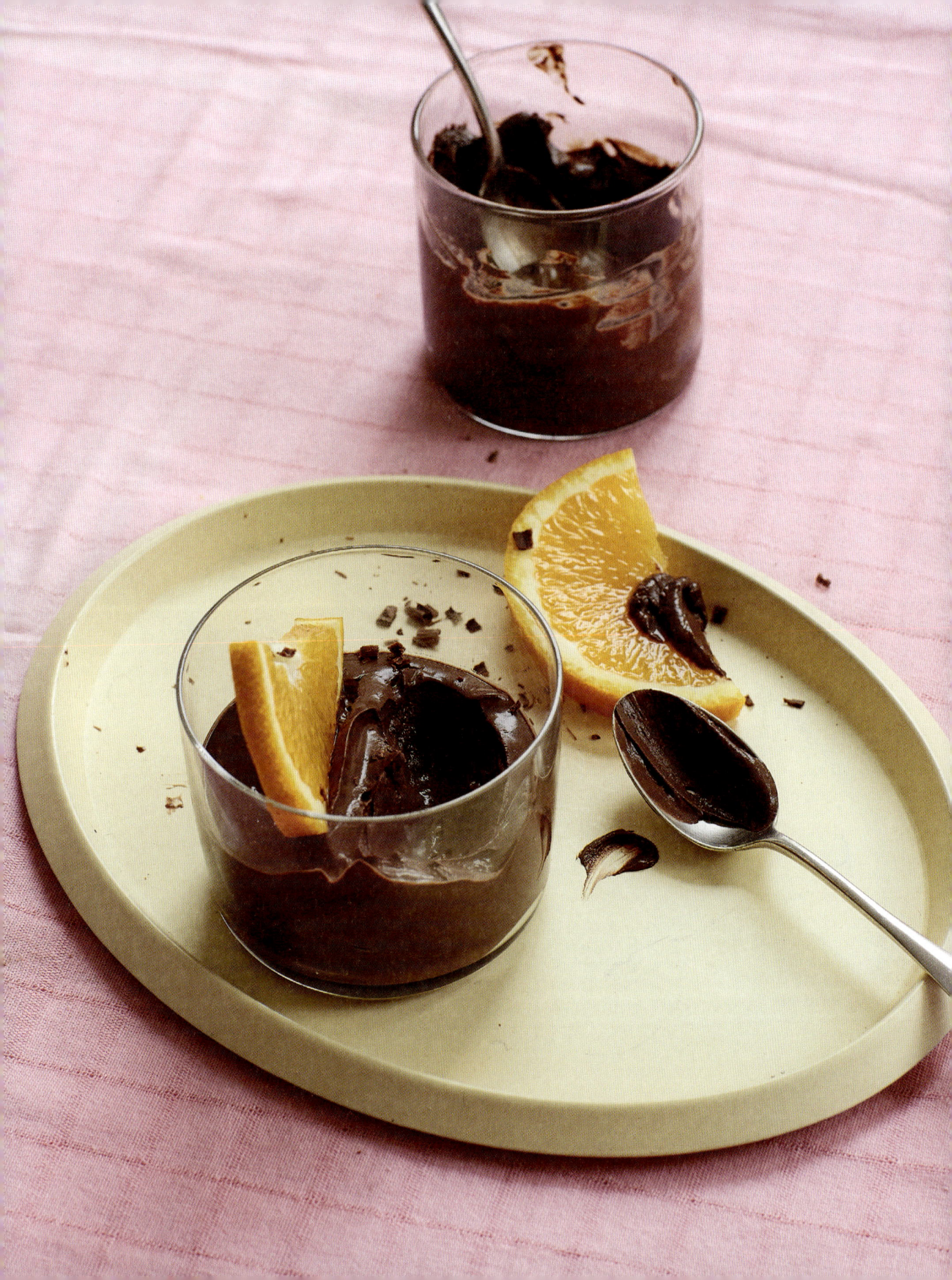

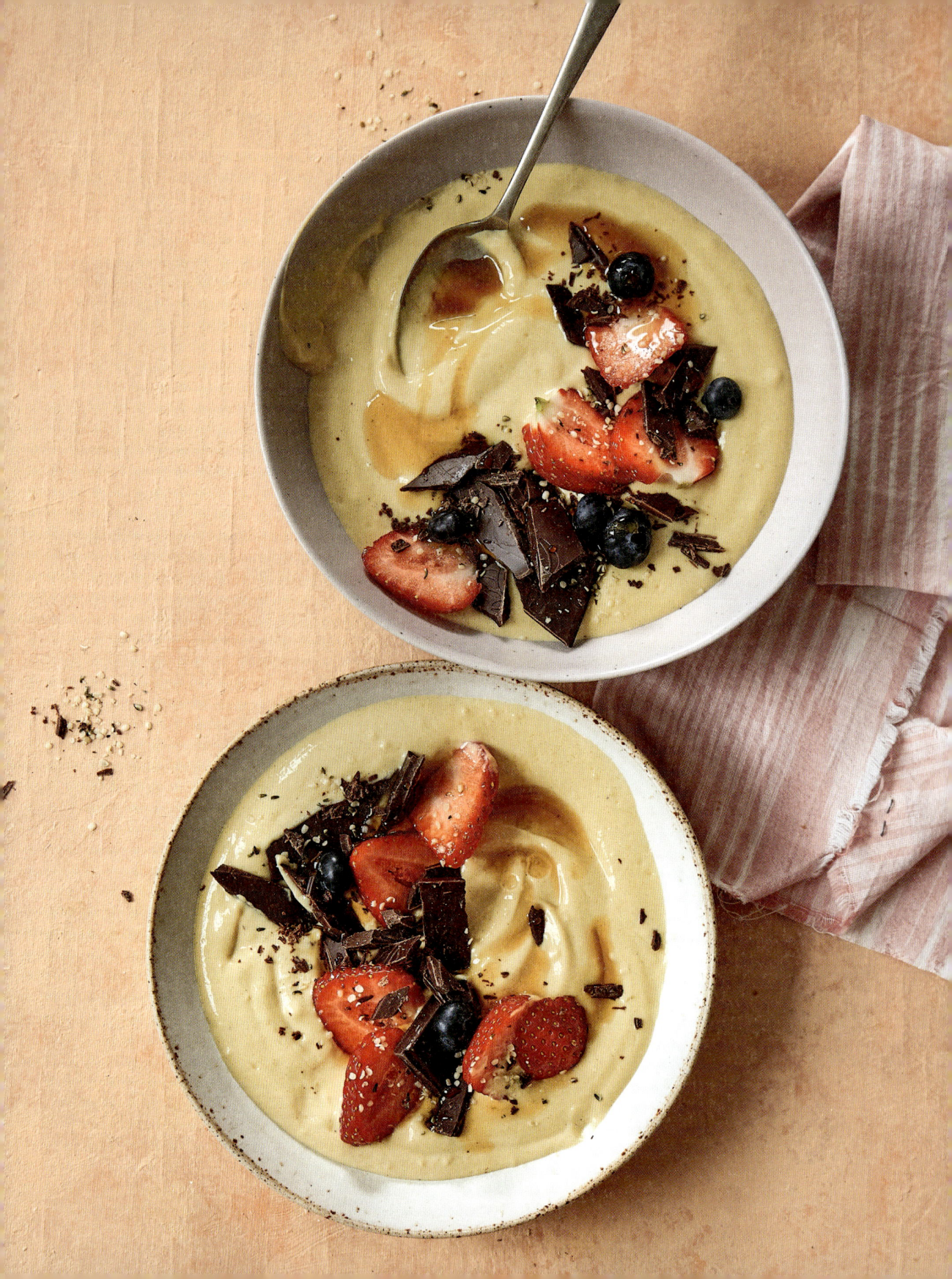

High-protein Yoghurt Bowl Top-up

SERVES 1
TOTAL TIME: 5 MINS

A perfect way to top up your protein intake for the day. Jazz it up with berries, seeds or even a slice of banana bread to make it more appropriate for your goals.

100g (3½oz/scant ½ cup) soy yoghurt
1 scoop (30g/1oz) vegan protein powder of your choice
1–2 tbsp plant milk

FOR THE OPTIONAL TOPPINGS
Fresh berries
Granola
Dark chocolate
Hemp seeds
Maple syrup

In a small mixing bowl, add the yoghurt and protein powder and mix together well with a spoon. Add the plant milk to make it runnier if you desire; this will depend on the thickness of yoghurt you're using.

Swirl into a bowl and add your toppings.

Protein per serving: 26.9g
Fibre: 8.5g
Plant diversity score: 6

Marzipan Truffles

MAKES 12 TRUFFLES
TOTAL TIME: 50 MINS
PLUS SETTING

I have a thing for marzipan, and these balls of goodness satisfy that craving perfectly.
  They're super easy to make and will impress guests!

100g (3½oz/1 cup) ground almonds
100g (3½oz/¾ cup) icing sugar
3 tbsp agave syrup
1 tbsp water
12 hazelnuts (optional)
100g (3½oz) dark chocolate

FOR THE COATING (OPTIONAL)
Freeze-dried raspberry pieces
Hemp seeds
Cacao nibs
Sesame seeds

In a food processor, add the ground almonds and icing sugar. Pulse for about 8–10 pulses until well combined.

In a large mixing bowl, combine the almond and sugar mixture, the agave and water. Bring the mix together with both hands and shape into a ball. Continue mixing/kneading until you have a smooth, pliable ball. Wrap it and pop in the fridge for 30 minutes.

Once cooled, take it out, unwrap and begin to shape the individual truffles. You want them a little bigger than a marble. At this point, if you want to fill them with the hazelnuts, flatten the mixture with your thumb while shaping, place the nut in the centre and close the marzipan mix around it. Lightly roll into a smooth ball using your palms. Place on a baking tray or completely flat plate lined with baking parchment. Repeat until all the mixture has gone, you should have 12 balls!

When you're ready, melt the dark chocolate in a bain-marie (a heatproof bowl over a saucepan of warm water – make sure the bowl doesn't touch the water!) or in a microwave in 15-second bursts. If melting in a microwave, stir the chocolate well every 15 seconds, and don't microwave it until it's all liquid, stop short of there being a few solid lumps of chocolate, which will melt as you stir a little. This will ensure you don't burn the chocolate.

With a fork and teaspoon, lower the truffles into the melted chocolate and cover all exposed areas. Try to drain off most of the excess chocolate after the ball is covered; this will ensure you don't have big puddles around your truffles, which can impact their final appearance.

Once all truffles are covered you can decorate them with a few freeze-dried raspberry pieces, hemp seeds, cacao nibs or even sesame seeds. Vary the toppings a little so you've got a nice array of colours.

Leave to set in the fridge for at least 1 hour. Once ready, these will last in an airtight container in the fridge for up to 7 days.

Protein per serving: 3g
Fibre: 2.2g
Plant diversity score: 4

IDEA
These would be great to prepare with children.

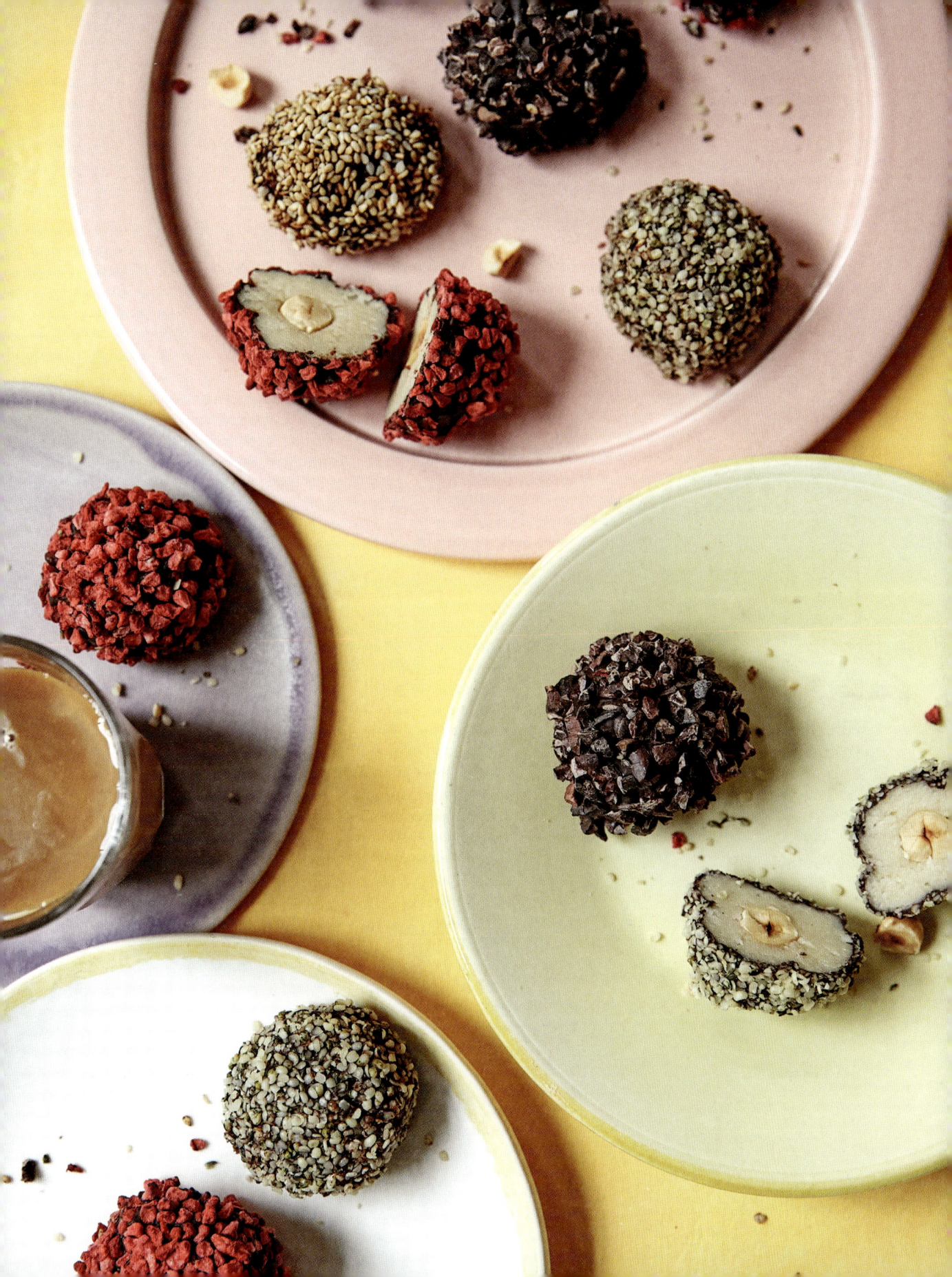

Will's Millionaire Protein Slice

MAKES 9 BARS
TOTAL TIME: 40 MINS

Probably my favourite dessert in this book and it needs no introduction, really! The shortbread base is mostly oats, soy milk and unflavoured protein powder, which you can't taste at all in the overall bite. High-protein dessert heaven!

FOR THE BASE
120g (4oz/1 cup) oat flour
Pinch of salt
4 level tbsp unflavoured vegan protein powder
60g (2oz/¾ cup) desiccated coconut
120ml (4fl oz/½ cup) soy milk
1 tsp vanilla extract
1–2 tbsp water

FOR THE 'CARAMEL'
15 Medjool dates, pitted
3 heaped tbsp peanut butter
3½–4 tbsp water

FOR THE CHOCOLATE TOPPING
120g (4oz) dark chocolate
1 tsp coconut oil

Put the dates in a small bowl, then cover them with boiling water and set aside for 10 minutes.

Preheat the oven to 140°C fan/160°C/gas mark 3 and line a 25 x 15 x 7cm (9in) tin with baking parchment.

Start with the base. In a medium mixing bowl, add all the dry ingredients, mix well, then add the soy milk and vanilla. Give it a good stir to bring it all together, it will look very scraggy at this point and won't be holding together, but that's OK. Add the water, a tablespoon at a time, kneading with your hands until you get a ball.

In the lined loaf tin, push the mixture down in an even layer with your hands and the back of a spoon. Make sure it's super even and packed down. The more even it is at the sides, the cleaner the layers will look. Prod the layer with a fork a few times, then bake for 10 minutes.

Drain the soaked dates and add them to a blender with the peanut butter. Blend until smooth and there are no large pieces of dates, smaller ones are fine though. Add a tablespoon of water at a time to the blender if necessary to help it blend.

Layer the date peanut caramel evenly over the base, using the back of a spoon to help it spread evenly. Pop this in the fridge while you melt the chocolate for the next layer.

Melt the dark chocolate and coconut oil in a bain-marie (a heatproof bowl over a saucepan of warm water – make sure the bowl doesn't touch the water!)

Protein per serving: 8g
Fibre: 8g
Plant diversity score: 6

IT'S ALL ABOUT BALANCE

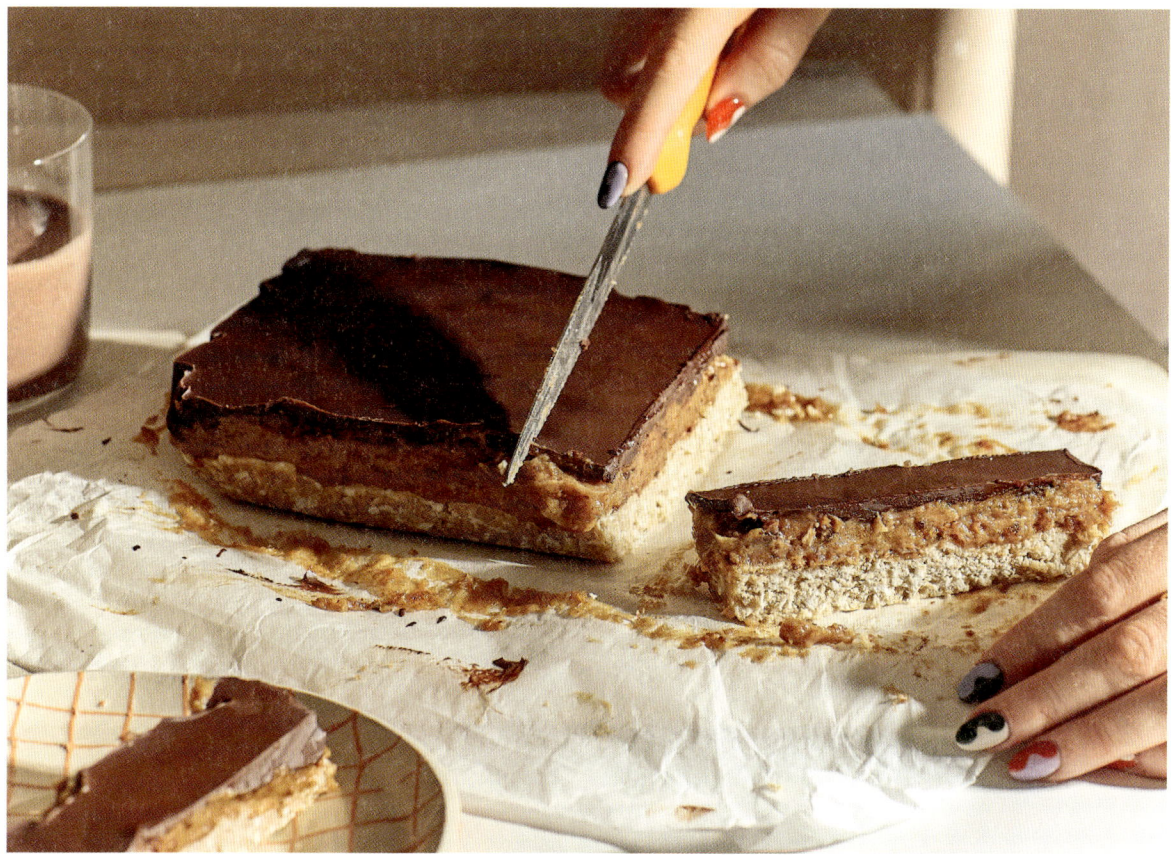

or in a microwave in 15-second bursts. If melting in a microwave, stir the chocolate well every 15 seconds and don't microwave it until it's all liquid. Stop short of there being a few solid lumps of chocolate, which will melt as you stir a little. This will ensure you don't burn the chocolate.

Pour the chocolate over the date caramel layer and tip it to ensure the chocolate covers the entire layer. Gently smack the tin down on the work surface to remove any bubbles. Pop in the fridge for 25 minutes.

When the chocolate is almost set (make sure you can see no visible wet patches and it's not too runny), cut widthways into bars with a clean, sharp kitchen knife to get those even layers. Wash the knife in between each cut to get perfect-looking bars!

NOTES

If the chocolate has set already, no worries. You can still get clean cut edges without cracking the layer by submerging the knife in a mug of boiling water for 3–4 seconds, shaking to remove the drips, then letting it sit without pressure on the cut line for about 15–20 seconds. The residual heat will melt the chocolate without pressure and potential cracking.

Melt-in-the-middle PBJ Choc Lava Mug Cake

The perfect, high-protein dessert for one.

2 tbsp spelt flour (or buckwheat or plain flour)
1 tbsp cacao powder
½ tsp baking powder
1 tbsp coconut sugar
Pinch of sea salt
1 tbsp coconut oil, melted
75ml (2½fl oz/⅓ cup) soy milk
1 tbsp natural peanut butter
1 tbsp raspberry or strawberry jam
1 square of dark chocolate
1 tbsp chocolate protein powder

FOR THE TOPPING (optional)
Hemp seeds
Fresh berries
Peanut butter

In a mug, mix the flour, cacao, baking powder, sugar, protein powder and sea salt. Pour in the melted coconut oil and soy milk, and stir well. Put the peanut butter on top of the dark chocolate square, add the jam on top and nestle it in the middle of the mix, so you can't see any poking above.

Microwave on medium for 45–60 seconds. It should be a little wet when it comes out, that's fine. You don't want it too dry. Serve with toppings of your choice.

Protein per serving: 26g
Fibre: 11g
Plant diversity score: 11

IT'S ALL ABOUT BALANCE

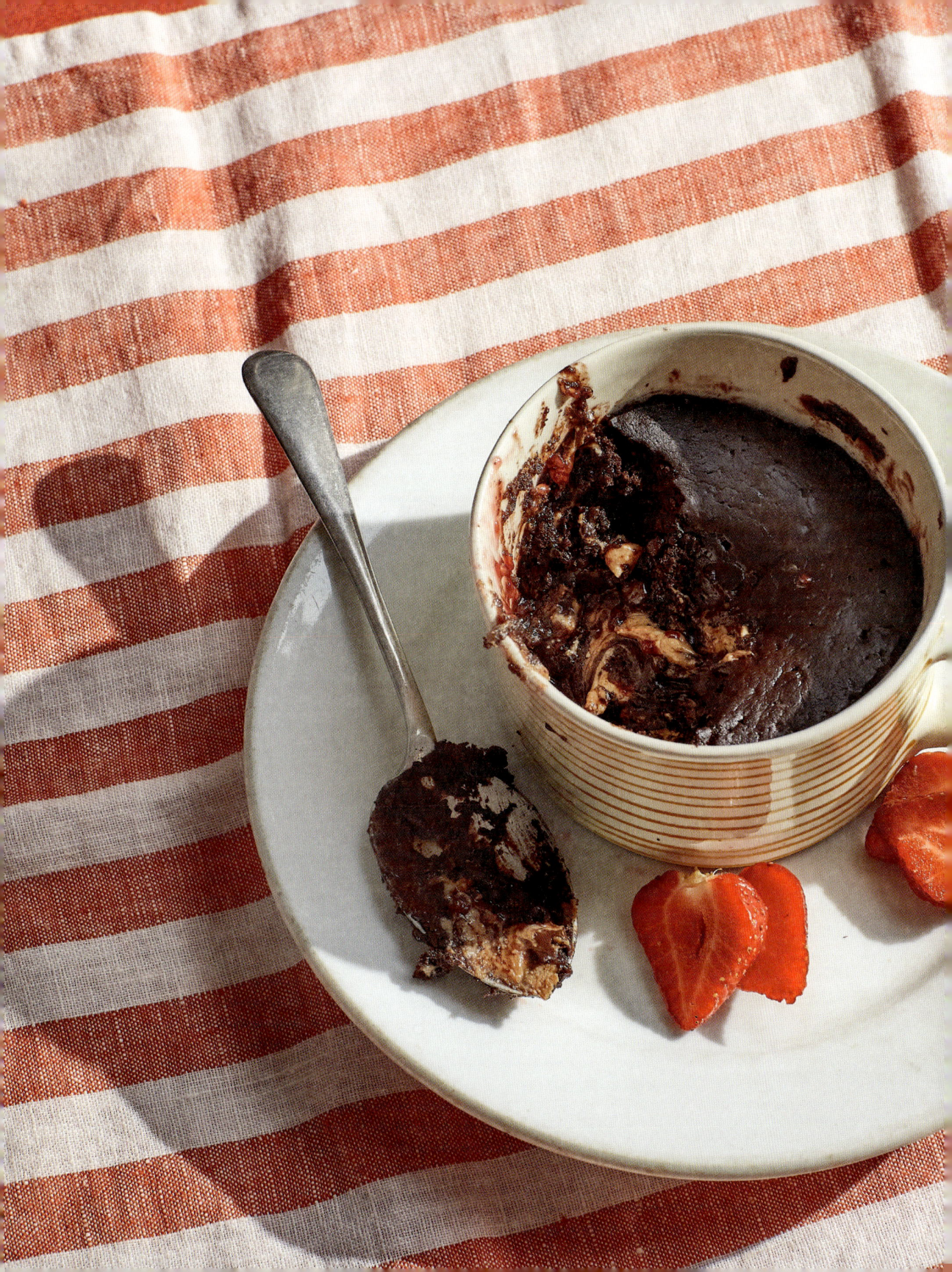

Tofoffee Tart

MAKES 8 SLICES
TOTAL TIME: 25 MINUTES

Tofu, like you've never seen it before! I made this to celebrate my 30th Birthday, as I'm not a huge sponge cake fan. It was perfect.

FOR THE 'SHORTBREAD' BASE
120g (4oz/1 cup) oat flour
4 level tbsp unflavoured vegan protein powder
60g (2oz/ ¾ cup) desiccated coconut
Small pinch of sea salt
½ tsp ground cinnamon
120ml (4fl oz/ ½ cup) soy milk
1 tsp vanilla extract
1–2 tbsp water

FOR THE 'CARAMEL' MIDDLE
15 Medjool dates, pitted
3 heaped tbsp peanut butter
3½–4 tbsp water (add a tbsp at a time)

FOR THE WHIPPED TOFU 'CREAM'
400g (14oz) firm tofu
2 tbsp lemon juice
Zest of 1 lemon
2 tbsp maple syrup or agave
1 tbsp olive oil
Pinch sea salt
2–4 tbsp water (add a tbsp at a time)

3 bananas, sliced fairly thinly at an angle
50g (1¾oz) dark chocolate, grated or shaved

If your dates are not squishy, soak them in boiling water for at least 10 mins.

Preheat your oven to 160°C fan/180°C/gas mark 4.

In a medium mixing bowl, add all the dry ingredients for the base, mix well, then add the soy milk and vanilla. Give it a good stir to bring it all together. Add the water a tablespoon at a time, kneading with your hands until you get a ball.

In a circular tart tin with a detachable bottom, push the mixture down in an even layer with your hands and the back of a spoon. Make sure it's super even and packed down. The more even it is at the sides, the cleaner the layers will look. Prod the layer with a fork a few times, then bake for 10 minutes.

Drain the soaked dates and add them to a blender with the 3 tbsp peanut butter. Blend until smooth and there are no large pieces of dates, smaller ones are ok! Add a little splash of water to the blender if necessary to help it blend.

Layer the date peanut caramel evenly over the shortbread base, using the back of a spoon to help it spread evenly. Pop this in the fridge whilst you whizz up all the ingredients for the whipped tofu cream. Season to taste, add a little more lemon or liquid sweetener if you want to. It should be super creamy, so blend it for a while.

Slice the banana and layer this over the top of the date caramel. Dollop the tofu cream over the top and lightly style it with the back of a spoon. Grate the chocolate over the top, slice like a pizza and dig in.

Protein per slice: 12g
Fibre: 10.5g
Plant diversity score: 8

IT'S ALL ABOUT BALANCE

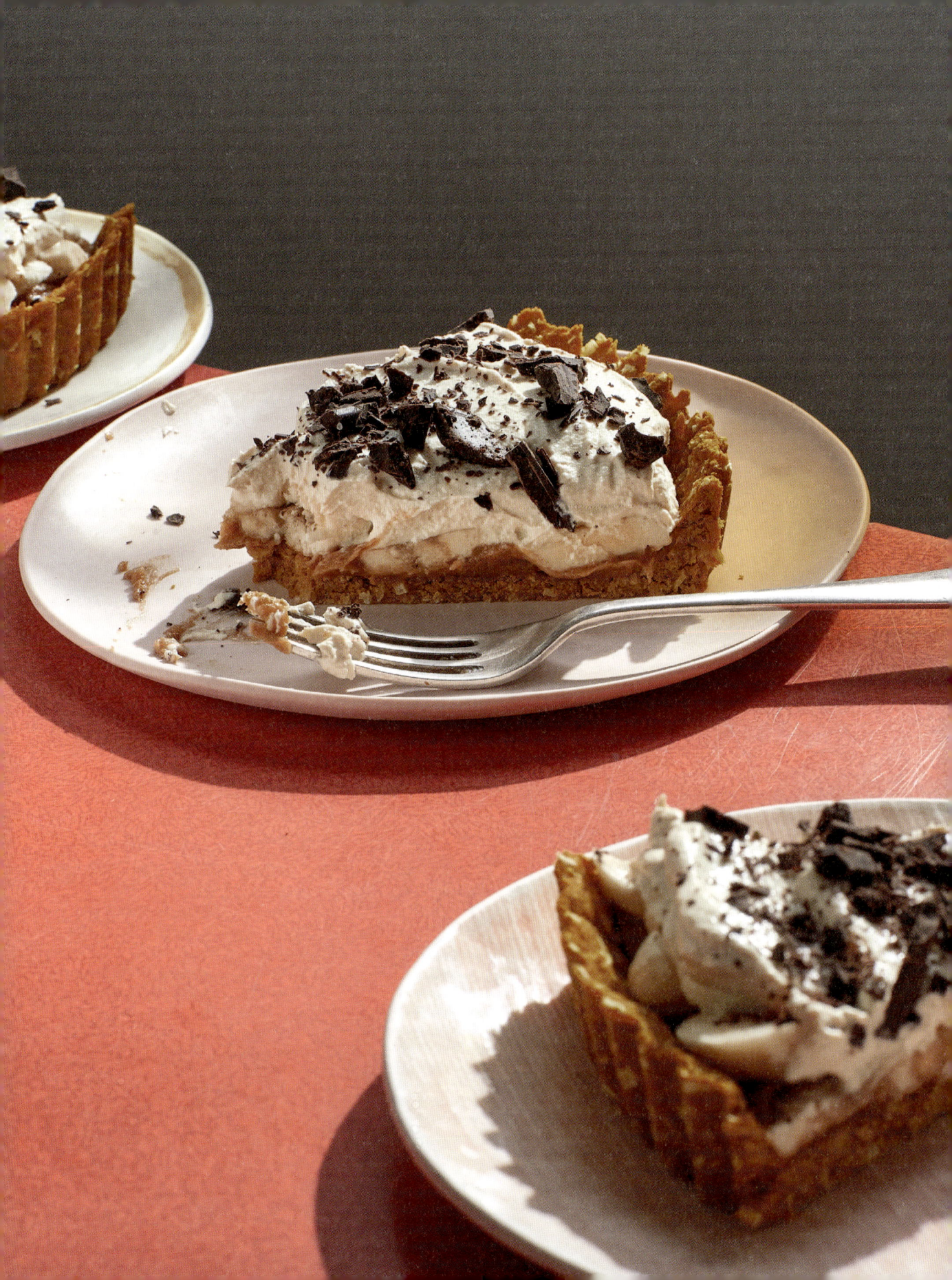

Index

Note: page numbers in bold refer to illustrations.

INDEX

Acknowledgements

I'll start by saying I never thought I would see the day where this would be ME writing an acknowledgments page, and the only reason I am is because of YOU, and this community, so, thank you, from the bottom of my heart, for following me, for loving these recipes and my philosophy on eating well. I have only ever wanted to do some good in the world, and make a positive impact. I believe this book can do just that, so please share it with friends, family, colleagues. I would love for it to be a firm fixture in your kitchens for years to come.

For all those who made this book possible, from the first meeting right up until now, I am so, so grateful for you. Firstly, to Bev of the wonderful Bev James Management, you are an icon and a legend; thank you for believing in me and taking this on. To Tom and Aoife, I appreciate EVERY FIBRE of your beings, you are simply the best. Your belief in me, your enthusiasm for this book, for my mission, for being there every step of the way, and for being my rocks throughout the process. I know it hasn't always been plain sailing, I have a tendency to only see the bits I can improve, and not what has been achieved, so I can't thank you enough for your patient, professional, warm candour over the past year. This book wouldn't be here without you.

To Issy, my day-to-day agent, and my friend, thank you for being an ear to my woes, for believing in me, and for putting up with my stream-of-consciousness WhatsApps – I appreciate you more than you know.

For the fabulous team at Yellow Kite; Nicky Ross my brilliant commissioning editor, thanks for pushing me in the right direction and believing in this book right from the start. Charlotte Macdonald, my project editor, for putting up with my wobbles, steering the ship throughout with your wisdom, feedback and patience – all with smiles and warmth – you truly are a gem. Claire Rochford, for your brilliant eye for design, thanks for distilling what was probably quite a hectic and very unusual brief (Hackney Deli, followed by an afternoon at the Tate, followed by a 90s rave, anyone?). For the sales and marketing team, and to every person who touched this project in some way at Hodder and Stoughton, I am truly thankful for all your incredible hard work.

To the real artists of this book, my photographer Lizzie Mayson, and assistant Ollie Grove, what a joy it was to watch you work. The final result is better than I ever could have imagined. Thank you for your talent, attention to detail, and great company.

To Flossy McAslan and Rosie Reynolds, and Louie Waller on props, thank you for making my recipes look better than I ever could have imagined, and letting me peer into the world of food styling – what fun! Thank you for being flexible, adapting to changes, attentive and wonderful to be around.

To Maisie, Omar and Sophie, thank you for cooking my recipes beautifully, and for your gorgeous company. Those shoot weeks were some of the best times for me, I hope you loved them too.

Now, the more personal thank-you's. To my friends, for your unwavering support, to Katie, for opening your home to me and putting up with many a tearful evening, recipe testing, and for all your hugs and kind words.

To everyone who said I couldn't do something great with my life, thank you for giving me the fuel I needed to light the fire.

And finally, to Will, my partner. Four years ago, before I met you, I barely believed in myself. You encouraged me to start my social media pages, and back then, you were the only person liking and commenting. Fast forward to now, you are still the first person to comment, but one of many. Thank you for loving me, and giving me a reason to love. My life is barely recognisable now, and that's because you've given me the space, grace and security I needed to grow. You are one in a million and I have no idea how I got so lucky.

First published in Great Britain in 2025 by Yellow Kite
An imprint of Hodder & Stoughton
An Hachette UK company

The authorised representative in the EEA is Hachette
Ireland, 8 Castlecourt Centre, Dublin 15, D15 XTP3, Ireland
(email: info@hbgi.ie)

4

A CIP catalogue record for this title is available from the
British Library

Hardback ISBN: 9781399736503
eBook ISBN: 9781399736510

Editorial Director: Nicky Ross
Senior Project Editor: Charlotte Macdonald
Designer: Claire Rochford
Photography: Lizzie Mayson
Food Stylist: Flossy McAslan and Rosie Reynolds
Props Stylist: Louie Waller
Senior Production Controller: Katy Aries

Colour origination by Alta Image London
Printed and bound in Italy by Lego Spa

Hodder & Stoughton policy is to use papers that are
natural, renewable and recyclable products and made
from wood grown in sustainable forests. The logging and
manufacturing processes are expected to conform to
the environmental regulations of the country of origin.

YELLOW KITE
Hodder & Stoughton Ltd
Carmelite House
50 Victoria Embankment
London
EC4Y 0DZ

www.yellowkitebooks.co.uk
www.hodder.co.uk

NOTES
The information and references contained herein are
for informational purposes only. They are designed to
support, not replace, any ongoing medical advice given by
a healthcare professional and should not be construed as
the giving of medical advice nor relied upon as a basis for
any decision or action. Readers should consult their doctor
before altering their diet, particularly if they are on a set
diet prescribed by their doctor or dietician.

The protein and fibre count for each recipe is an
estimate only and may vary depending on the brand
of ingredients used, and due to the natural biological
variations in the composition of foods such as meat, fish,
fruit and vegetables. It does not include the nutritional
content of garnishes or any optional accompaniments
recommended for taste/serving in the ingredients list.